19.99

M

This book is due for return on or before the last date shown below.

1 2 AUG 1999   16 Nov 2005

                  7 DEC 2005

4 SEP 1999   3 JAN 2006

                  24 JAN 2006

                  15 FEB 2006
2 2 NOV 2001

2 9 MAR 2002   - 2 JAN 2007

1 6 MAY 2002

- 8 AUG 2002

0 4 FEB 2004

Medic

- 8 JUN 2004

1 1 AUG 2005

0 7 OCT 2005
27 Oct 2005

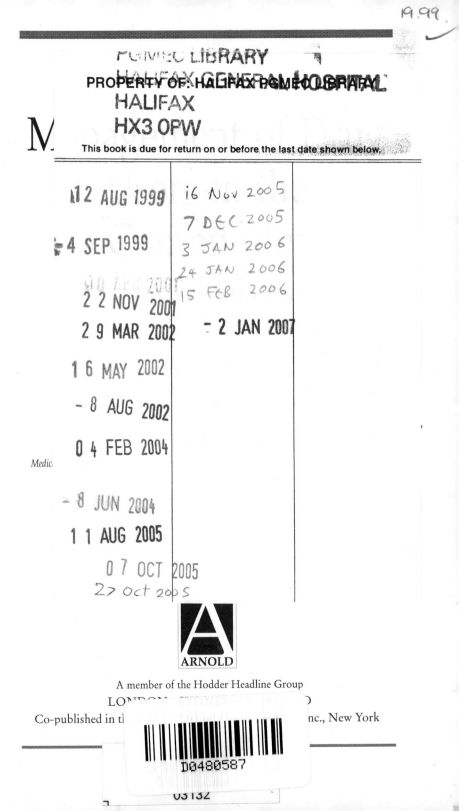

ARNOLD

A member of the Hodder Headline Group
LONDON

Co-published in t...   ...nc., New York

D0480587

03132

First published in Great Britain in 1998
Arnold, a member of the Hodder Headline group,
338 Euston Road, London NW1 3BH
http://www.arnoldpublishers.com

Co-published in the United States of America by
Oxford University Press, Inc.,
198 Madison Avenue, New York, NY10016
Oxford is a registered trademark of Oxford University Press

British Library Cataloging in Publication Data
A catalogue record for this book is available from the British Library

Library of Congress Cataloging-in-Publication Data
A catalog record for this book is available from the Library of Congress

Publisher: Georgina Bentliff
Project Editor: Catherine Barnes
Production Editor: James Rabson
Production Controller: Rose James
Cover designer: Mouse Mat Design

ISBN 0 340 70013 0

Typeset in $9\frac{1}{2}/11\frac{1}{2}$ pt Palatino by Photoprint, Torquay, Devon
Printed and bound in Great Britain by J.W. Arrowsmith Ltd, Bristol

Contents

Contributors

Carl Bickler
Medical Practitioner, Craigmillar Surgery, Edinburgh, Scotland

Judith Bury
Primary Care Facilitator (HIV/AIDS and Drugs), The Spittal Street Centre, Edinburgh, Scotland

Annette Dale-Perera
Head of Policy and Practice, Standing Conference on Drug Abuse (SCODA), Waterbridge House, London, UK

Don C. Des Jarlais
Director of Research, Beth Israel Medical Center, Chemical Dependency Institute, New York, USA

Michael Farrell
Consultant Psychiatrist, National Addiction Centre, London, UK

Claire Gerada
General Practitioner, Hurley Clinic, Ebenezer House, London, UK

Eilish Gilvarry
Consultant Psychiatrist, Northern Regional Drug and Alcohol Service, Carliol Place, Newcastle upon Tyne, UK

Marc N. Gourevitch
Director of HIV/AIDS, Montefiore Medical Group, Montefiore Medical Centre, Albert Einstein College of Medicine, Bronx, New York, USA

Fiona Hackland
Standing Conference on Drug Abuse (SCODA), Waterbridge House, London, UK

Frank D. Johnstone
Senior Lecturer, Centre for Reproductive Biology, Edinburgh, Scotland

John MacLeod
Clinical Research Fellow, The Medical School, The University of Birmingham, Birmingham, UK

Peter McDermott
is a freelance drug consultant working in Waterloo, Liverpool, UK

Patrick G. O'Connor
Director, Yale New Haven Hospital Primary Care Center, New Haven, Connecticut, USA

Fergus D. O'Kelly
General Medical Practitioner, Director of GP Training and Lecturer in the Department of General Practice, Trinity College, Dublin, Ireland

Marco Rizzi
Ospedali Riuniti di Bergamo, Divisione di Malattie Infettive, Largo Barozzi 1, Bergamo, Italy

Roy Robertson
Medical Practitioner at the Muirhouse Medical Group and part-time Senior Lecturer at the Department of General Practice, University of Edinburgh, Edinburgh, Scotland

Peter A. Selwyn
Associate Director, AIDS Program, Yale University School of Medicine, New Haven, Connecticut, USA

Richard Starmans
Director of Vocational Training in General Practice at the Department of General Practice, Erasmus University, Rotterdam and Medical Practitioner at the Nieuw Schilderswijk, The Hague, The Netherlands

Giel H.A. van Brussel
Head of Department, MHS Amsterdam, Nieuwe Achtergracht 100, Amsterdam, The Netherlands

Brian Wells
Consultant Psychiatrist, Riverside Mental Health, Substance Misuse Service, Central Assessment Unit, Earls Court, London, UK

Anne Whittaker
Project Manager, Community Care Resource Team (Drugs/HIV), Edinburgh, Scotland

Alex Wodak
Director, Alcohol and Drug Service, St Vincent's Hospital, Darlinghurst, Sydney, Australia

Foreword

For more than a decade, Roy Robertson has provided an inspiration through his compassionate committed attention to the healthcare problems and needs of drug takers in his care. His research studies and clinical examples have influenced a generation of practitioners and policy makers. With other colleagues working in the community (many of whom are contributors to this book), Dr Robertson has established the vital contribution of practitioners working in both the central and the various outer reaches of primary healthcare services. Without this care, there is many a drug user whose problems would be unnecessarily the greater, whose family and friends would be pointlessly exposed to exaggerated harm, and who would become a needlessly greater burden on the healthcare, social welfare and criminal justice systems.

Within this volume, the best of the field comes together, from diverse professional backgrounds, settings and countries, to chart the rationale underlying, and the methods of delivery of, the best of practice in their particular domains. As such, this collection of perspectives stands as an outstanding compilation of essays, many of which are leading texts in their own right and which, together, comprise an excellent primer for both clinicians working in the field and also for those responsible for the planning and purchase of services for this oft-overlooked group of people in need.

Professor John Strang
Director
National Addiction Centre
London

Preface

The preparation of this book is as a response to the growing complexity of illicit drug use in the community. Over many years, it has become increasingly clear that specialist hospital medical staff have less information and knowledge about illegal drug use than those working in the community and that there is a requirement for this information to be recorded and organized in some way. Several recent reports and government papers from a variety of countries have indicated the need for information and research and multinational organizations have been established in order to compare data and record trends on all aspects of drug use.

Inevitably, political and social pressures require law enforcement agencies to be heavily involved with all aspects of drug abuse and inevitably information and data arise out of law enforcement and legal involvement. Similarly, political requirements give rise to the need for numbers and trends but take little account of individuals or medical or social outcomes.

The text, therefore, is in recognition of the need to record the ongoing experience of clinical and social workers as well as those who have other firsthand experiences of drug use or working with drug users. The complex interactions of drugs with all aspects of society make television and newspapers intensely interested in drug use and drug users but, again, they tend to concentrate on short headlines indicating negative aspects of drug use or the impact of drugs on the lives of the famous or glamorous part of society.

The need for a text on treatment is brought about by the increase in contact between drug users and caring agents and the relatively small involvement of specialist and secondary care sectors of the health care and social care systems, making community care the repository of most care and information. Similarly, treatment is largely carried out outside specialist units and, for many reasons, not least economic ones, the trend is to encourage management and all aspects of treatment to be carried out as close as possible to home. Treatment is the theme of this text and is surprisingly complex. In Western countries, where alcohol misuse and abuse has been the source of such health care problems, it would seem that treatment for alcohol problems would be the logical prototype for managing illegal drug users. There are, however, many aspects to drug use, not least its illegality, which make individuals presenting with drug problems different and there are, of course, an increasing variety of drugs and social groups involved. The complex interaction therefore of ethical, legal medical and cultural problems has made national responses confused, conflicting and, at times, contradictory.

It is hoped that this book will offer a clear if not simple approach to a complex problem, concentrating on the consequences of all the problems and how a reasonable response might be made by a caring physician or health or social care worker. Without being unaware of the ethical and legal problems, it is possible to offer a humanitarian response to a debilitating constellation of symptoms. Hopefully, the carefully conceived contributions in the various chapters in this book will clarify our own involvement with drug users and help to discard some of the prejudice and fears of dealing with this group of individuals.

Roy Robertson
Edinburgh

Acknowledgements

The stimulus for organizing the production of this book has undoubtedly been brought about by contact with a large and varied number of drug users, many of whom have suffered severely from their dependence. Whilst they are portrayed as difficult individuals to work with, the reality is quite different. They are, in a way, a disenfranchised group of individuals leading impoverished lives and this is not often acknowledged by society.

The Partners of the Muirhouse Medical Group have been extremely patient and supportive throughout the project, as have the members of the Department of General Practice at Edinburgh University. The preparatory stages were supported by the Scottish Office and Lothian Health with a study leave grant.

The authors have responded enthusiastically and generously to our coaxing and Georgina Bentliff has been an inspirational editorial advisor. Lorraine Copeland has, throughout the project, organized all aspects of the preparation of the final drafts of each chapter and her attention to detail has been meticulous and allowed for progress which I would not have thought would have been possible. My wife Liz and family have been patient throughout. I am sure all the authors would share with me in hoping that the book does a lot of good in taking forward implementation of drug use treatment.

Introduction and background

Roy Robertson

Background

The massive pervasive presence of drugs on TV, on the radio, in newspapers and magazines, seems to increase year by year. Drugs appear to be present in schools, in sport, in the workplace, in prisons and in the entertainment industry. Those involved most commonly seem to be young people, those in public life, people living in poor communities and often the excessively well off. Information fatigue makes us less critical of press and media reports than we should be and too little informed of the superficiality of many of the sources of these reports. It does mean, however, that all of us are, at one level, better informed about drugs than we used to be but perhaps less aware of the complexity of the 'drugs issue'.

Although new information is useful and important, the concentration on escalating numbers, sudden deaths, emerging drugs and associated crime waves, does less to clarify the nature of drug problems than would longer term observations on what happens to drug users, why they have the problems which they have and a clearer analysis of whether the problem identified is caused by drugs, or just associated with drugs or whether it is merely just coexisting with drugs.

The purpose of this book is to look more clearly beneath the surface of the knowledge which everybody has today about drugs and to examine, particularly, approaches to treatment. Treatment has indeed been neglected by the communications industry in favour of the more easily portrayed problems of crime, prisons and drug associated scandal. For governments and the media the main issues in the drugs field are probably about control and prevention. This is understandable and leads to the major highlight being on drug trafficking and law enforcement nationally and internationally. Prisons and sentencing policies also loom large in the areas of public and political interest. The importance of prevention as the best form of treatment is widely accepted but the failure of this concept to translate into reality has, over the last 15 years, led to disappointment and disillusionment with successive policy approaches. A recognition of these failures has given rise to more support for treatment and the need to broaden attitudes to new forms of treatment. Treatment in its broadest sense encompasses prevention, minimization of harm, and management at the individual case level and these are the areas of interest in the following chapters. The important considerations of prevention and control are not the main interest of this text, but will be referred to where they are relevant to treatment or management of cases or populations.

As this book is principally aimed at healthcare workers and those interested in the management of drug users, treatment in its broadest context is their prime concern, as it is of course with those involved with taking drugs themselves. The nature of treatment, however, is equally complicated and this is perhaps the reason for its being low down in the media and political agenda. Drug use is common in young people, many of whom abstain after a short period. Addiction and dependence are difficult to define, and even in the committed drug user improvement occurs with age independently of other interventions. Treatment is expensive and difficult to evaluate and from decade to decade the focus of concern shifts to make treatment objectives less clear or convincing. To compound all these problems, society's view of drugs is constantly evolving and yesterday's drug problem is rapidly overtaken by something more sinister and corrupting.

Those involved with managing drug users, however, are pragmatic people not easily impressed with changing fashions and new reports. The issues for many healthcare workers are clear and uncomplicated. In a way that other afflictions can be separated out into those that require some support, help or attention, those that are long-term problems or only potential problems and those that are speculative, imaginary or ephemeral, drug issues can be addressed at many practical levels. Agencies, either statutory health or social services or non-statutory drug services, are often extremely focused on an area of drug treatment, examples of which occur throughout this book. They are increasingly required to work together and to provide flexible services which change along with an ever-changing drug scene.

In this text, the reader will be helped to identify the problems requiring the attention of health or social care workers and the wider issues that represent serious challenges to treatment agencies.

Definitions of drug dependency and terminology

Throughout the book the term 'drug dependency' will be used in preference to 'drug addiction' although the two may not be seen by all authorities as synonymous. Similarly 'drug user' will be preferred to 'drug addict' and 'injection drug user' to 'intravenous drug user'. These terms evolve from year to year and their meaning changes subtly, but consistency is required. Recreational drug use is a term in recent common usage and is taken in this text to be non-addictive or dependent use and can apply to the use of any drug. Two formal definitions of the 'dependence syndrome' are in common use. Firstly, that included in the International Statistical Classification of Diseases and Related Health Problems (WHO 1992) and, secondly, the American Psychiatric Association definition (American Psychiatric Association DSM–IV 1994).

The WHO definition includes the following description of the dependency syndrome:

'A cluster of behavioural, cognitive, and physiological phenomena that develop after repeated substance use and that typically include a strong desire to take the drug, difficulties in controlling its use, persisting in its use despite harmful consequences, a higher priority given to drug use than to other activity and obligations, increased tolerance, and sometimes a physical withdrawal state. The dependence syndrome may be present for a specific psychoactive substance (e.g. tobacco, alcohol or diazepam), for a class of substances (e.g. opioid drugs) or for a wider range of pharmacologically different psychoactive substances.' (ICD – 10 WHO Geneva 1992).

The diagnostic criteria for substances dependence published by the American Psychiatric Association requires three or more of the following seven criteria to be present in order to diagnose 'substance dependence'. They must have occurred within the same 12 month period.

1 Tolerance as defined by either of the following:
   - the need for markedly increased amounts of the substance to achieve intoxication or the desired effect
   - markedly diminished effect with continued use of the same amount of the substance

2 Withdrawal as manifested by either of the following:
   - the characteristic withdrawal syndrome for the substance
   - use of the same (or closely related) substance to relieve or avoid withdrawal symptoms

3 The substance often taken in larger amounts or over a longer period than was intended.

4 A persistent desire or unsuccessful efforts to cut or control substance use.

5 A great deal of time spent in activities necessary to obtain or use the substance to recover from its effects.

6 Important social, occupational or recreational activities, given up or reduced because of substance use.

7 Continued substance use despite knowledge of having had a persistent or recurrent physical or psychosocial problem that was likely to have been caused or exacerbated by the substance.

Both these standard definitions draw attention to the broad issues and illustrate that these are not necessarily drug specific. Many drug types are involved and overlap is present.

In the USA treatment is dependent very much on the presence of these diagnostic criteria, without which funding may not be available. In the UK and other countries attention to strict criteria are often not a requirement for entry into treatment.

Extent of treatment

In a complicated multidisciplinary problem such as drug misuse, treatment can be taken to mean intervention at any one of many levels. Treatment overlaps with prevention and even with law enforcement and working with drug users draws the healthcare worker into many unfamiliar areas. The text here is necessarily medical, but not to the exclusion of social care issues and is firmly committed to community care. This inevitably means addressing the effect of the environment and the economic environment on drug users when it affects treatment.

Treatment for drug dependency could, and does, fill many volumes. The variety of drugs and the great range of medical, social and legal problems that they cause is one of the reasons why confusion is present in the search for solutions or even for a sensible strategy. Many of the discussions about drugs are about different things and interest tends to focus on topics of importance but to draw on inappropriate data from unconnected sources. The debate about drugs and whether there is a best treatment or even a cure has to encompass the enormity of the problem and the absence of a single, or even a small cluster, of easily identified symptoms and complications. In this text therefore the reader has to be aware of the range of drug problems from experimental cannabis smoking, probably less dangerous than the longer term cigarette addiction it may lead to, to the seriously dependent and risky use of cocaine or heroin and all its consequences.

There is a, sometimes unwritten, assumption in most chapters that for seriously dependent persons there is no immediate cure. There is indeed ample evidence that for many individuals drug dependency is a problem lasting many years or decades. Treatment therefore is palliative and long-term and services designed for anything less are likely to be inadequate. Although most people are aware of the drug user who has been dramatically cured of the problem, the long-term nature of drug misuse and its resistance to treatment is a cornerstone concept in this text.

As much of the international experience in treating drug users has been in those using opiates or narcotics most of the treatment described and evaluated is for that problem. The main processes or modalities of treatment are:

- methadone maintenance
- in-patient drug free rehabilitation
- out-patient detoxification
- treatment of chemical dependency.

The broader concept of risk reduction or harm minimization can be applied in all areas of treatment as well as in prevention and in drugs policy.

Harm minimization

This is not a new concept, but since the anxiety about HIV during the 1980s it is an approach to treatment policy which has assumed a central role in thinking about therapy. Otherwise referred to as damage limitation or risk reduction the principal element is of palliative care for a group involved with potentially extremely dangerous and damaging behaviour. It involves accepting that a cure is not immediately available and that working closely with drug users is important. This gives rise to accusations of collusion with drug taking or, worse, giving in to an intolerable situation instead of looking for cures or eradication. It has however emerged from a time of anxiety about the failure of treatments in the 1960s and 1970s, and the recognition that for many individuals drug dependency is a long-term problem for them and their families.

Central to implementing harm reduction approaches for opiate injectors are such measures as provision of injecting equipment and provision of substitute drugs such as methadone. Equally important is the acceptance of ongoing treatment rather than short-term or abstinence-orientated approaches. There are, of course, many treatment approaches which are abstinence-directed, but harm reduction acknowledges abstinence to be best but sometimes not possible in the short-term or even elusive in many for the foreseeable future. Realistic aims which fall short of abstinence are manageable and have not inconsiderable rewards.

Adopted with some enthusiasm in Europe and Australia, harm minimization as a philosophy has had a more difficult time in North American centres where there is a long history of tightly controlled methadone provision and a large abstinence-orientated establishment. Whereas Italian drug users were able to purchase injecting equipment in the early 1980s in chemist shops and needle exchange was established in the UK and Amsterdam shortly afterwards, it was only in 1997 that Federal approval was given in the US (Kochems et al. 1996) and much anxiety still exists in many other countries.

The harm minimization approach has had a major impact on all treatment modalities and drug problems. Reducing the risk of injecting drugs leads on to reducing the risk of other ways of using drugs and limiting the damage done to the individual and society by lessening crime and illegal and antisocial behaviour. This provides a greater justification for other interventions such as substitute prescribing and a revived enthusiasm for prescribing other opiates and stimulants. The provision on prescription of alternatives or additional opiates include trials with heroin, dextromoramide and others as well as injectable heroin, methadone and amphetamine (Metrebian et al. 1996, Uchtenhagan et al. 1997, van Brussel et al. 1997). Harm minimization is therefore an approach to drug treatment compatible with other aims and inclusive of other therapeutic approaches. It does, however, represent a new approach to all types of care.

A variety of problems

Different drugs may have different patterns of use

For very good historical reasons opiates are at the present time the drugs of abuse about which we have most knowledge. This includes our understanding of the natural history of opiate dependence as well as the understanding of available treatment and responses. Much of what is written under the global heading of treatment for drug dependence is either specifically directed towards the management of opiate abuse or derived from an understanding of that problem. This creates difficulties if the assumption is made that drug dependants using other substances either pursue an exactly similar course or that they will respond identically given the same treatment. This is further complicated by the likelihood of multiple or polydrug use being present and the wide range of available substances which an individual may be using at any point in time.

Those responsible for funding, designing and delivering services are faced with a number of difficulties. Traditional treatment services for opiate users may be modified to include those using stimulants such as amphetamine or cocaine or to include the shorter, more volatile problems of recreational drug users using such substances as ecstasy or cannabis. Most likely, the service will be faced with a group of individuals with multiple drug use problems and therefore be required to provide a range of skills and approaches towards these problems. For practical reasons, as well as historical ones, divisions are often made upon arbitrary lines. Agencies geographically situated in a locality of high socioeconomic deprivation may find themselves providing services for a group of chronic polydrug users whereas a university campus facility may find the requirement for treatment is from younger, less experienced, non-injecting individuals who are using drugs such as amphetamine, cannabis or ecstasy. Most agencies, however, expand within the available resources to provide a range of services for drug users who can broadly be given one or more of the following headings:

- experimental drug users
- recreational drug users
- controlled drug users
- chaotic drug users
- polydrug users
- mature drug users.

These descriptive headings have all been used by drug workers to identify the present state of the drug user on the continuum of drug use which may last from adolescence to middle age. Similarly, most agencies see themselves as providing a variety of support services which may be summarized in the list of headings below:

- counselling
- psychological therapies
- psychiatric treatment
- prescribing of methadone

- harm minimization
- welfare rights
- medical referral
- legal and advocacy services.

Hidden epidemics of drug use

Drug use patterns or evolutions may become apparent for several reasons. A new drug may emerge and become a focus for media attention as ecstasy did in the early 1990s; a new complication may arise as HIV did in the 1980s; or a new treatment may become available drawing covert users into contact with treatment agencies. In the last decade a resurgence of interest in methadone treatment has expanded clinic contact with opiate users enormously. Conversely the absence of a specific therapy for cocaine or amphetamine use has allowed epidemic use to be comparatively less visible and the apparently benign nature of drug use such as cannabis keeps it less well-researched or quantified. Those less visible drugs do not necessarily have less in the way of side effects, but knowledge tends to be available on the basis of the ease with which it can be brought into contact with any agency capable of recording information. For example, the traditional methadone maintenance clinic is a huge source of information, not just about opiate use but its complications, including blood-borne viruses and many other drugs and drug effects. Onto therapy specific for opiate related problems can be built treatments for other drugs and management packages for psychiatric care, social problems and lifestyle and legal issues. These may or may not be directly connected to the presenting drug issue. Methadone in this instance is seen as an incentive into a variety of therapies and a 'glue' to keep drug users in contact with support agencies (Condelli 1993, Joe *et al.* 1991).

In the absence of such specific therapy the stimulants such as amphetamine, cocaine and methylenedioxymethamphetamine (MDMA: Ecstasy) enjoy a less well-researched position and share a smaller investment of medical and social care interest. Complications, however, can be equally serious. Injecting, particularly of cocaine but also of amphetamine, may be responsible for blood-borne virus spread and the short-acting nature of cocaine may account for epidemic spread in the USA and South America (Schoenbaum *et al.* 1989, Libonatti *et al.* 1993). Epidemic use of MDMA in the 1990s may give rise to serious problems in the longer term in the increased incidence of serious, and possibly treatment resistant, depression in later years (Seivewright and McMahon 1996, McCann *et al.* 1994, Steele *et al.* 1994).

For individual drugs, epidemic use depends on a variety of social and economic conditions and perhaps most importantly on availability. The emergence of complications similarly depends on rising levels of use, but also on the mode of administration. Examples of these phenomena are the rapid spread of HIV and other blood-borne viruses due to increased drug injecting in the 1980s (Burns *et al.* 1996, Des Jarlais *et al.* 1992). The increasing number of deaths observed in many centres in opiate users may be directly related to the increased availability of prescribed alternatives to illegal opiates. Perhaps the biggest epidemic among injecting drug users has been hepatitis C virus transmission. The many years during which this had been unrecognized have given rise to an emerging problem of staggering size. This is elaborated on in Chapter 6.

Epidemics and subcultural drug use are by their very nature covert, and this may sometimes be unimportant in medical terms. There is undoubtedly a hidden reservoir of untreated drug-related problems, most of which are important to the individual and many of which have implications for society.

Complications of different substances

Results of drug ingestion are notoriously unpredictable. Effects range from the expected and routine to the unanticipated and surprising. There are many variables which influence possible effects including idiosyncratic exposure to a single small dose of a drug, to overwhelming reaction to a dose higher in purity than usual or adulterated with an additional compound. Side effects depend upon previous experience of that substance, tolerance to a certain level of ingestion and even the physical environment of the drug taking (Zinberg 1984). Complications may be medical, social, psychological or economic and may vary in severity from trivial to catastrophic. The full extent of medical side effects are referred to in Chapter 6 and the specific problems associated with HIV in Chapter 7.

Many problems are related to the quantity of substance used, but side effects are also closely dependent on mode of administration. Those individuals injecting drugs are more at risk of a wider range of potential problems than individuals taking drugs by other routes.

Factors influencing complications:

- dose of drug
- mode of administration
- state of recipient (mental)
- state of recipient (tolerance)
- environment.

In the late 1980s and early 1990s, the need to engage drug users in methadone therapy in order to prevent HIV transmission became a major issue in Europe, North America and Australia (Yancowitz *et al.* 1991, Power *et al.* 1988, Wodak and Moss 1990). In many centres the HIV crisis in drug users was driven by epidemic use of heroin. In others, however, the injecting of cocaine and amphetamine was the main vector of HIV transmission making methadone substitution an inappropriate intervention (Libonatti *et al.* 1993, Friedman and Lipton 1991). A move towards engaging individuals at risk of HIV by any drug use began to include sexual risk groups, prostitutes, young sexually active people and women in general. Even among opiate users many do not enter treatment and others do not stay sufficiently long to receive the full benefits of treatment. Services need to expand to deal with increasingly complicated problems. Complications of drug taking are addressed at some length in various chapters following. These may be medical, psychiatric or social. Treating or managing the social consequences take up several other chapters.

Patients' needs and desires

Medical needs

Presentation of a drug problem to a medical agency is frequently recorded as the initial entry into treatment of any sort. This is increasingly a patient with a drug related problem presenting to a primary care doctor or nurse. In areas of high drug prevalence primary care organizations are often aware of drug problems in individual clients before the request for help is articulated and unlike secondary or tertiary care community care physicians are in a position to identify high risk behaviour before serious complications have occurred. In specialist clinics in North America the average age is often 25 to 35 years and in Australia two-thirds of entrants into methadone treatment are male with an average age of 28 years (Ward *et al.* 1992). The main period of drug use at entry into treatment may be seven years or more (Capelhorn and Bell 1991).

These characteristics seem to have changed over the last 20 years. Methadone patients in Europe, Australia and the US have become older; more women are applying for treatment and the patient's history of dependence is longer (Ward *et al.* 1992, van Ameijden *et al.* 1992). This is important at a time when drug use and presumably drug injecting is increasing in many continents. For many reasons therefore, the opportunity to engage a drug taker in therapy of some sort at the earliest opportunity, is available in community care and should be taken.

The possible medical complications of drug taking are endless and are developed in Chapters 6 and 7. Importantly the medical problem often identified by the drug user attending a clinic is the need for drugs, and in most countries the agency to supply legal addictive drugs is a medical one. The drug user may or may not be concerned about the medical problems, real or potential, which are present. Medical agencies therefore have a major opportunity to engage drug users early in supportive therapy, but have to strike a balance between the interventions seen by the doctor as important and those perceived by the drug user as required. In many established methadone maintenance clinics primary medical care is available (Selwyn *et al.* 1989) but evidence from New York is that these interventions are necessarily part of a long-term strategy if effective prevention of such complications as HIV infection is concerned. In 1988 while 50% of drug injectors were HIV antibody-positive, for those that had been in methadone maintenance therapy since 1978 the positive rate was almost zero (Hartel *et al.* 1988).

Table 1.1 shows an outline of the main interventions required. These are elaborated on in detail in subsequent chapters.

Table 1.1 Management and treatment opportunities for drug users

Intervention strategy	Comments
Contact with drug taker	May be educational input or attendance at a clinic or agency (the first major hurdle)
Assessment	May be first contact or one of many. Degree of problems needs careful consideration, including living situation, family issues and legal problems. Important to determine any need for urgent medical or social care.
Diagnosis	Co-existing pathology (social, psychiatric or physical needs to be evaluated). Referral to specialist worker in any or all of these areas may be necessary. Evaluation of presence and severity of opiate dependence and extent of other drug use.
Therapy	Various options depending on client choice, assessment and availability of individual therapies.
Follow-up and long-term support	Probably the most important, and neglected, area because of skills required, expense of worker time and frustration due to relapse and loss of contact.

Social needs

The other major entry of drug users into contact with a social care worker or healthcare worker is through an acute or chronic domestic problem. This may be a housing, lifestyle or legal issue and in many countries the agency contacted may deal with all these areas. Special groups may have particular problems, such as those affecting women, children of drug using parents, adolescents or the elderly. Sexual or ethnic minority groups may require workers with special experience (Baker *et al.* 1995) or language skills and those with co-morbidities might require close liaison between agencies. Confidentiality concerns among professional or employed drug users often give rise to late presentation of problems. All these areas require generic workers to be skilled in identifying problems and sympathetic to the situation. Specialist agencies find themselves requiring individual workers with special skills or increasingly developing a relationship with a wide range of agencies with complementary services (Table 1.2).

Table 1.2 Drug using groups requiring special skills

- Women
- Children of substance abusing parents
- Co-morbidity patients
- Co-dependent patients
- Adolescents
- Elderly
- Sexual groups
- Ethnic groups
- The homeless
- Health professionals
- The employed

Assessment of needs

Much of the text of subsequent chapters is about accurate assessment of the drug user's situation. Without this, opportunities are missed and interventions are inappropriate. A plan or strategy is as essential in drug use treatment as in other areas of therapy. Perhaps the most overlooked area of drug use treatment is the importance of the therapist and drug user understanding the problem they have, the likely developments and the aims and limitations of various treatment options. In recognition of rising treatment costs, largely due to increasing numbers requiring help, is the development of managed care. As a distinct entity this is an American development, and for many may be seen as an essential economic development. In many countries, the importance of funding a chronic relapsing disorder is only just being recognized (Armstrong 1997). Whilst the aims of treatment might be expressed simply as achieving abstinence, a range of further goals are best included in the assessment:

- therapy to achieve abstinence
- reduction in consumption
- reduction in risk-taking behaviour
- reducing street crime
- reducing foetal exposure to drugs
- improving general health
- improving psychological health
- restoring family functioning
- restoring employment.

Managed care in the US, as well as the process towards care in the community observed elsewhere, has three principal elements. First, increased access to primary healthcare is seen as an effective way of delivering healthcare, and also as a way of facilitating the second element of managed care, namely greater cost savings. The third element is improved quality of healthcare services. As a package this seems to fulfil anyone's needs, although seen as a way principally of saving money it may be a less than positive philosophy.

Natural history of drug dependence

Historical development of treatment

The clearest way to the provision of adequate treatment must surely depend upon the best understanding of the problem and this, to a certain extent, is one of the major difficulties in managing drug dependence. The concentration on the concept of drug takers as being slavishly addicted to an interminable life of drug use and drug withdrawal, obscured for many years the wider drug using issues. Subsequent broadening of interest in recreational drug use indulged in by the majority of young people in some localities led to confusion in the designing of appropriate services. The concept of a spectrum of disease similar to that observed in alcohol use and misuse may be helpful. A large part of the population indulges in some sort of drug taking, as they do with alcohol, the majority of the time coming to no apparent harm. A minority have a short exceptional crisis and a very small group fulfil the criteria of serious dependence or addiction and are likely to be in touch with drugs projects or using health services.

One further essential requirement in order to begin to understand drug use and drug dependence is the concept of the long-term nature of drug dependence. Behind the reports of sudden deaths, epidemic blood-borne virus spread and criminal involvement is a chronic remitting and relapsing disorder, for many people lasting years, if not decades. Approaching a disorder of this nature requires not only clear understanding of its natural history, but a separate range of services from those designed to treat acute emergencies. The Accident & Emergency Department of the local hospital is essential for managing the acute intoxication episode of an injecting drug user, but the same department has little or no involvement in long-term care, and assuming the individual survives the acute episode, little to do with the ultimate outcome. Although acute services are as much involved with drug users as long-term services, systematic approaches to treatment and agencies designed to provide therapy require understanding of the long view of drug dependence at the outset.

Faced with a patient with a problem of drug dependency, it is always of benefit if a clear view of the expected outcome or prognosis is available. The nature of drug dependency unfortunately rarely allows for a simple prediction of short-term, far less long-term outcome. There are, however, clear indicators which might influence the understanding of prognosis, the most obvious of which may be the drug being used. Additional features which at assessment may fairly confidently be used to predict outcome are factors such as age at onset, additional social or medical problems, the presence of multiple drug use and the previous history. Populations of opiate users have been studied over long periods (Marsh et al. 1990, Thorley 1981, Vaillant 1973, Tobutt et al. 1996 and Hser et al. 1993) and indicate a sizeable mortality per year associated with injecting drug use. These studies also refer to a recovery rate, although this may be in the absence of any details about lifestyles at follow-up. The concept of maturing out of drug dependency (Winick 1982) gives a further insight into drug taking as a phenomenon, and in the late 1970s and early 1980s allowed a shift from the concept that opiate addiction was inevitably destructive and a permanent state to the now, quite logical belief, that at least for some it is a reversible process and that the natural ageing and maturing process aids recovery.

The better understanding of the nature of opiate addiction has been refined by the research of Rounsaville et al. (1986) and Kosten (1991) as well as others who have looked more carefully at the inhibiting factors to change, and the indicators of who might relapse and who might continue with abstinence.

These ideas about what might happen to individual opiate users over a period of years or decades have been further developed by the observations of Newman (1983) and Daley and Marlatt (1997) who were able to develop the understanding of drug dependence as a remitting and relapsing disorder rather than a permanent or irreversible state. The importance for therapy of this line of thinking cannot be overstated as it allowed those involved a better understanding of the nature of treatment required rather than the pre-existing obsession with the failure and success of therapies. This approach was able to explain not only why the best efforts of the therapists seemed unsuccessful or ineffective, but to prevent the antagonism and loss of confidence which frequently arose for both therapist and patient in the event of relapse.

As well as the importance of the pharmacological properties of the drug being taken, the effect on an individual depends upon other factors. Zinberg's classic account of the effects of the personality in addition to the pharmacology of the drug and the social situation in which drug use occurs has been influential in understanding why different people behave differently when using drugs of addiction (Zinberg 1984). This built on the findings of Robins who had studied the drug use, or lack of use, of returning Vietnam troops (Robins *et al.* 1975). It is of some importance that these researches and other findings of 'controlled drug use' and long-term heroin 'chippers' (occasional users) (Powell 1973) have been unable to overcome the polarized arguments of the pro- and anti-drug lobbies. The presence of the other factors which so much affect recruitment and outcome is still largely neglected. Acceptance of social and educational inequalities as a significant factor in causing drug use is clearly difficult for societies. The division of drug use into the two alternatives of total abstinence or uncontrolled excess is perhaps a more comfortable philosophy.

Throughout the last 30 years, the therapeutic goals of treatment have constantly been challenged. The better understanding of the nature of dependency described above made many concerned about the use of large doses of heroin and cocaine (sometimes injectable) prescribed in the UK and methadone in the USA in the 1960s and 1970s. The awareness of other drugs such as barbiturates, amphetamines and vogues for methaqualone and more recently benzodiazepines and MDMA (Ecstasy), tested and continue to test the aims and goals set by those providing treatment facilities. The arrival of HIV infection provided something to treat at a time when the drugs issue was in danger of becoming too complicated for policy makers. Here was something tangible, and although controversial, important enough to use as a mechanism to sanction unpopular public health changes. One of these was spending scarce health resources on drug users.

More recently the importance of the type of drug related behaviour has concentrated on those characteristics of drug taking which cause the damage. It is therefore not necessarily the drug which causes the harm but the associated infection or side effect. Thus overdose, HIV or other virus transmission is associated with injecting. Whilst the concept of less damaging drug use is tenable, safe drug use is still an unacceptable public health policy in most countries. The transitions in type of drug taking are however extremely important (Strang *et al.* 1992, Gossop *et al.* 1992).

Development of treatment options

Three major 'modalities' of treatment dominate the provision for drug users. These are:

- out-patient methadone clinics
- residential detoxification (or therapeutic communities) and
- out-patients drug-free programmes.

Within these broad categories are a variety of therapies. Prochaska and DiClemente (1986) provided useful concepts and practical approaches to counselling and developing behaviour change. Marlatt (1985) introduced the concept of relapse prevention as a useful aide, not just to understanding the nature of the disorder but to preventing the basis of the problem, namely return to drug use, as opposed to treating the symptoms of the disorder, namely withdrawal symptoms. More recently, management of harm enshrined in the concept of harm minimization has arisen out of the concerns about blood-borne viruses. Whilst all these approaches to treatment are frequently promoted as individual circumscribed philosophies for managing the drug dependency problem, they are of course all interconnected, of use concurrently in any individual and useful when used appropriately rather than being panaceas.

Further research on the understanding of remission and relapse (Joe *et al.* 1991, Kauffman and Woody 1995) introduces the effects of factors which are positive and inhibiting factors to recovery. Factors such as criminal involvement, long history of drug dependency, coexisting psychiatric abnormality and coexisting physical disease are clearly negative influences on an individual's ability to respond to treatment, whereas young age, short length of dependency, higher educational attainment and preservation of family support and contacts are all positive indicators of a good prognosis. In a long-term follow-up study of Californian opiate users, the authors concluded that 'the eventual cessation of narcotic use is a very slow process, unlikely to occur for some addicts, especially if they have not ceased use by their late 30s' (Hser *et al.* 1993). Another US study concluded that 'getting high at a younger age and polydrug use correlated with more relapses and less overall control' (Marshall *et al.* 1994). Under-standing these positive and negative influences against the back-ground knowledge of the nature of the drug dependency syndrome and lifestyle allows the therapist to design treatment with more confidence and to select therapies which have a higher likelihood of success.

The availability of treatment

With a clear understanding of the range of individuals involved in drug use as well as the enormous array of possible outcomes, the provision of treatment services seems daunting. Two approaches are possible. The longitudinal nature of drug dependency and, in the majority, the expectation that it may pursue a relatively benign course for most of the time allows the possibility that drug users, like the rest of the population, might fit in to the available social and medical services. Their requirement for housing, primary medical care and even secondary medical care may be no different from the rest of the population and, even in the presence of a drug complication, generic services may be the most appropriate available agency. For example, a drug user who has a requirement for domiciliary care because of a drug-acquired illness may present no greater problem to social or medical services than an individual with the same medical problem acquired in a road traffic accident or as a result of a malignant disease. A drug user with an amputated limb or with a terminal liver or HIV related illness essentially requires the same services regardless of the underlying cause of the disorder. Alternatively special services, or those dedicated to the management exclusively of drug users, may be important. In areas unique to drug use and requiring the skills of a drug counsellor, therapist or case manager, specialist services are required. The provision of methadone, injecting equipment or de-toxification facilities may be pragmatically not possible from anything other than a specialist clinic or agency for operational and practical reasons. In practice both approaches are likely to be required. Services for drug users are unlikely to include the vast array of specialist medical and social provisions which may be needed. Referral to specialist services are therefore frequent and all specialists should have a basic knowledge of drug dependency problems.

Therapies are diverse and numerous and can be separated by subject matter whether it be medical, social, legal; or by function, namely domicilliary support, counselling, custodial, residential. They may, however, overlap and coexist so much that categorization is unrealistic and not necessary. The provision of psychological therapies to make available counselling, psychiatric treatment and methadone provision are as important as the harm minimization facility providing needles, syringes, sterilizing equipment and advice, as are the longer term supports, detoxification facilities and residential care programmes. The provision of all these in addition to welfare rights and legal representation in one agency or centre is unlikely. However, a move towards multimodal treatment agencies where a global view is taken of an individual's problem, and diversion into an appropriate selection of therapies is possible, is an attractive prospect.

For many agencies and clients, the selection of the most appropriate therapy depends on a range of choices and the availability of a variety of approaches to treatment. Unfortunately this variety of treatment choices is not always available and the patient may be slotted into the available treatment rather than the most appropriate therapy.

The relative expense of some management packages or treatment options is likely to be a further reason for lack of availability, although the lack of equal amount of evidence for the efficacy of different treatments is likely to preselect treatment opportunities for one in favour of another. Client acceptability is clearly an additional requirement for successful treatment and the nature of drug dependency and its satellite problems may be that treatment options such as methadone maintenance are more acceptable to a larger percentage of individuals than a more rigorous and demanding regime requiring psychological insights and aimed at abstinence. The wide variety of drug experiences and individuals involved require a full range of treatment services and opportunities. These will be discussed throughout the book, and recurring reference will be made to a variety of approaches in succeeding chapters.

Results of treatment

Studies of the results of treatment have identified associated problems, commonly referred to as comorbidities, as important in achieving and maintaining good results. Coexisting psychiatric problems (Rounsaville *et al.* 1986), previous criminal history (Simpson *et al.* 1982), associated benzodiazepine (Darke *et al.* 1993) and cocaine (Gottheil *et al.* 1993) use as well as alcohol use (Anglin and Hser 1990) are all associated with poorer outcome from treatment. Indications of more positive outcomes include older age, stable family and intact marriage and employment. Obviously longer term in treatment shows better outcome and much attention has been given to ways of getting drug users into treatment and the factors which prolong this treatment contact. The influences of social and sexual minority grouping are discussed in subsequent chapters as is, perhaps more fundamentally, the relationships between poverty, drug use, treatment access and prognosis. As a general rule, premorbid family or psycho-logical pathologies, early entry into drug use, multiple drugs of abuse (including alcohol) criminal involvement, past relapses and un-employment all indicate a poor prognosis and less successful out-come to subsequent therapy. As stated above, older age, stable background and intact marriage, higher social status and absence of other pathologies such as HIV, hepatitis B or C, depression and other psychiatric states, all correlate with better outcome and better response to treatment.

These observations and the more general appreciation of the variety of problems present in individuals presenting for treatment have stimulated the development of integrated programmes includ-ing modalities for addressing legal, social and multiple substance misuse problems (Avants et al. 1994).

For some time women have been known to pursue a different course in drug dependency. Positive features include better contact with health agencies, a positive relationship between childbirth and reducing drug use (Marsh and Simpson 1986, Finnegan 1991) and family responsibilities. Fewer women enter into drug use and fewer pursue a criminal career. Prostitution and the comparatively poor status of women are negative influences. There has been a relative lack of research in women compared with research on men and the association of HIV research with men. Despite this, the epidemic of HIV among drug users in the USA has had a greater relative impact on women. Over 50% of AIDS cases in women have been attributed to injecting drug use (Center for Disease Control 1991). Women may be more motivated to accept treatment (Anglin et al. 1987) and women-specific needs may be addressed in treatment programmes (Finnegan et al. 1993).

Evaluating success and outcome

As with other areas of drug research, most of the studies of outcome and evaluation of intervention with drug users have been carried out with groups of opiate users. Tools for measuring the extent of addiction present in an individual have been developed and include the Addiction Severity Index (McLellan et al. 1992) and the Opiate Treatment Index (Darke et al. 1992, Adelekan et al. 1996). These may be particularly useful as an initial assessment to direct the patient to the correct, or most likely to be useful, treatment option and have been used in short-term follow-up. They have however a lesser success rate as an ongoing monitoring tool in clinical practice (Macleod et al. 1996) and as a long-term way of evaluation of the success of a particular intervention, they have the same problems as other follow-up assessments. These problems include the enormous difficulties in tracing and contacting drug users over a period of years and the great difficulty of attributing outcome to any of the many interventions which may have had an influence on the behaviour of the individual. Many of these influences are caused by medical and social programmes, but other unconnected lifestyle changes may be equally if not more influential. The severity of dependence by whatever measure may for several reasons not correlate with outcome of treatment (Kosten *et al.* 1992a).

Issues for treatment of dependent users

Problems facing therapists

Many health and social care workers have low expectations of their success in treating drug users. This may arise from the lack of knowledge of the condition and the feeling that relapse of the client into further drug taking represents a failure of the therapy provided. This might be resolved by better education and support for doctors and healthcare workers. There are however other issues preventing many doctors and healthcare workers from involving themselves with such issues. These include lack of facilities or insurance cover, fear of malpractice suit, fear of loss of income due to reduced consultations from non-drug users, and fear of violence or other abuse. Inevitably a moral disapproval of addiction influences a large sector of the medical establishment against providing substance-dependency treatment. Finally, the cost of treatment may in some countries prohibit enrolment into even a baseline therapeutic relationship (Maddux *et al.* 1994).

In a recent treatment improvement protocol from the US Department of Health and Human Sciences the issues facing providers of treatment were summarized as a series of challenges (Kauffman and Woody 1995):

Challenge 1: The understanding that opiate addiction is a chronic, relapsing disorder.

Challenge 2: Providing comprehensive services to ensure successful opioid substitution therapy.

Challenge 3: Engaging and retraining the patient in treatment.

Challenge 4: Managing patient non-compliance in a positive manner.

Challenge 5: Expanding community awareness of the purpose and outcome of opioid substitution therapy.

The inclusion of these and other educational issues into undergraduate and postgraduate programmes is essential in the future provision of adequate therapy.

Violence and emergency treatment

The threat of violence and aggressive behaviour is a major source of anxiety for therapists and agencies providing care for drug users. Real incidents are not infrequent and are associated with the association of drug misuse and a disorganized lifestyle. Special training and experience of healthcare workers involved in such treatment settings are required in order to minimize stressful incidents. The need for a high staff-to-patient ratio leads to the requirement for disproportionately high funding in such clinics. Emergency room treatment of violent episodes are particularly associated with stimulant abuse and an estimated 142 000 incidents were reported in the USA in 1994. These incidents were highest for persons aged 26 to 34 years and the number of males was twice that for females.

Care in the community

Developing countries

Drug use is spreading rapidly in developing countries. Asia is of particular concern where traditional patterns of use of heroin are being replaced by injecting drug use. Discouraging injecting and changing behaviour of injectors are seen as vital (Stimson *et al.* 1997) and some successes have been reported in reducing risk activities by providing clean injecting equipment and education of those involved (Peak *et al.* 1995). Rapid spread of HIV and other blood-borne viruses have been identified however in Southern China, Myanmar, North East India and Malaysia (Wodak *et al.* 1993). Evidence of shifting patterns of drug use from cannabis and alcohol to cocaine and heroin cause concern in Africa (Obot 1990). Treatment efforts are aimed mainly at prevention by provision of educational activities, provision of condoms, and detoxification. Western-style clinics are less likely to be available, as is much needed information about medical complications. Bangkok continues to cause concern with 41% of injectors admitting to sharing syringes in the prior 6 months (Vanichseni *et al.* 1997) but the seroconversion rate for HIV is described as moderate (Des Jarlais *et al.* 1997) at 4.2% per year. Harm reduction policies have been implemented in New Delhi with syringe exchange and oral buprenorphine maintenance (Kanga 1997). In Brazil similar policies have been developed. The total number of countries where injecting drug use has been reported is now 121 (Stimson *et al.* 1997), an increase from 80 in 1992. HIV-1 among injecting drug users has now been reported in 81 countries, an increase from 52 in 1992. These countries depend increasingly on primary medical care to address their medical and public health problems. The models of care in subsequent chapters are relevant in all situations.

Prisons

Treatment of drug users in custody is a major problem for all countries. As with drug misuse outside prison, use by inmates has increased dramatically. For many their first drug use experience is when in jail (Gore *et al.* 1995a). The relationship between crime and going to prison is equally complicated but in one US study 50% of prisoners stated that they had taken drugs in the month prior to arrest (Mahon 1997). Epidemic spread of HIV in prison has demonstrated that the most severe problems are possible (Mutter *et al.* 1994, Yirrell *et al.* 1997). Custodial institutions have been shown to be a major focus of drug taking and actual and potential transmission of blood-borne viruses (Taylor *et al.* 1995). The failure of correctional facilities to correct behaviour, and the prospect of problems being made worse by custodial sentencing, is a social policy issue requiring considerable investment of resources. Reducing drug use in prison, harm reduction for those who do use drugs, methadone treatment for chronic opiate dependents in custody and rehabilitation of offenders are all areas of drug treatment with political constraints and practical difficulties. Strategies for prisons and real interventions are being discussed in most countries, often in an attempt to limit spread of HIV (Pont *et al.* 1994, Gore *et al.* 1995b, Jutta 1997, ACMD 1996). Peer education in prison, bleach distribution and heroin prescription/substitution programmes have been described in Zambia, Canada, and Switzerland respectively (Simooya and Sanjobo 1997, Nicol 1997, Beuchi *et al.* 1997). Few countries have been prepared to institute the provision of injecting equipment for prisoners using drugs. A recent report from Saxony indicates such an attempt (Jutta and Stover 1997).

Community versus specialists

In the UK the balance of contact between parts of the health service and newly presenting drug users has changed in recent years. From 1986 until 1990 general medical practitioners notified increasing numbers to the Addicts Index system. From 1990 until 1996 the largest percentage of notifications came from hospitals and treatment centres, probably reflecting the increase in numbers of community drug teams (which are classified as treatment centres). Interestingly, there was a large increase in notifications from prisons between 1994 and 1996, reflecting the increase in attention being given to drug dependents in custody (Figure 1.1). These changing patterns indicate

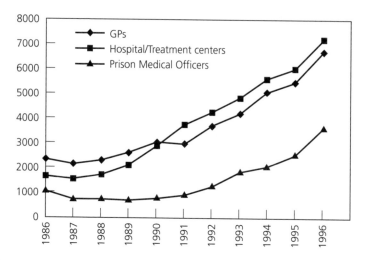

Figure 1.1 Source of notification of addicts in the UK 1986–1996 (Home Office Statistical Department)

the growth of new services and the new interest in drug users in traditional treatment agencies.

Treatment for drug users has historically been managed by specialists in hospital clinics in Europe and North America. Seen for many years as a psychiatric specialty, drug services, like alcohol services, have only recently emerged as a multidisciplinary problem. The development of hepatitis and HIV have encouraged this development and the move to primary and community based care has facilitated a generic rather than a hospital or specialist approach. The increasingly complicated nature of the problems experienced by drug users and the wide range of facilities required make a case management approach essential. The blurring of private and public funding in the US managed care system has further developed the need for better evaluated and shorter lasting treatment episodes. The recent enthusiasm of the general medical practitioner in the UK has provided for a model of management both cost effective and clinically robust (Greenwood 1992, Glanz 1994). Chapters 13 and 14 develop the concept and practical application of a more devolved structure for care of drug users, and include the role of social and community services in their treatment.

Integrated care

Similarly to the move to community care, the development of interrelating and complementary services are an evolution which makes some sense. The multidisciplinary nature of the providers of care for drug users can give rise to a disintegration and overlapping of services with loss of clinical and economic effectiveness. Often the responsibility for coordinating care has been with the physician responsible for prescribing, in the case of the methadone patient. The development of multimodal treatment clinics with an interest in a variety of substance-related problems, including cocaine and alcohol, gives the opportunity to provide a package tailored to the needs of the client (McLellan *et al.* 1983).

With the benefit of hindsight

Although there is an enormous and valuable literature associated with drug dependency treatments, there are large areas of information still required. Evaluation of treatment programmes was inadequate during the 1970s and 1980s, and the changing nature of the client population and the substances being used make the protocols and expectations of these services inadequate in today's environment. Systematic research is needed to evaluate treatment in community settings and this awaits completion. The expectations from treatment in the past mean that the full benefit was not given to clients and that outcomes previously considered to be a failure might be viewed differently today. Limited knowledge about cohorts of drug users from the 1960s onwards comes from limited investment in treatment and measurement of responses to treatment during these decades. A recent authoritative report from the Institute of Medicine suggested that 'although complete abstinence from illicit drugs is a desirable goal of treatment, the committee viewed the ability to function in society, to whatever degree possible, as an appropriate definition of recovery' (Gerstein and Lewin 1990). With the passage of time, the European HIV epidemic in injecting drug users has been largely attributed to the lack of knowledge among drug injectors of the dangers of needle sharing. The simple provision of sterile equipment and information is having a major impact (Goldberg *et al.* 1994). Whether this provision has had a similar impact on hepatitis C transmission is not yet proven. Learning from past inadequacies is an essential part of designing treatments for the future.

Political and legal considerations

International agreements

The two United Nations conventions which set about to control drug supply (Single Convention 1961 and Convention on Psychotropic

Substance 1971) have contrived to encourage member states to endorse policies on control of spread of drugs (United Nations 1990). These international agreements are about control and supply. Health agreements and resolutions including the World Health Organization Programme on Psychoactive Substance Abuse (WHO 1990) and the resolutions agreed at Alma Ata about the role of primary care in providing basic health (Chen and Cash 1988, Horder 1983) have firmly located health responses to drugs issues in primary care organizations. Other international organizations support sharing of medically useful information (European Monitoring Centre for Drugs and Drug Addiction, ECMDDA 1996).

It is left up to national organizations to consider the best response to managing their own drug problem. Treatment issues perhaps have less place in national strategy than control policy, as pressing concerns about the increase in drug use in young people, the potential spread of blood-borne diseases by needle sharing, and the changing perceptions of society to those drugs, such as cannabis, which seem less harmful, have given rise to government statements on these issues. The Australian ministerial endorsement of the 'harm minimization' strategy (MCDS 1996) and the establishment of task forces in the UK and Australia to look at these and other drug issues are indications of the pace of change (Department of Health 1996, National Drugs Strategy 1994). The appointment of drug supremos or 'czars' in the US and the UK indicates the recognition of the need for change (Strang et al. 1997) and legislative changes with profound effects on treatment services may be expected to follow (Smith 1995). Examples in Europe of evolving drug legislation within the constraints of international agreements are fascinating (Jepsen 1996, Alpheis 1996). These are exemplified by the experimentation in the Netherlands discussed in detail in Chapter 3.

Different countries, different opportunities

For several decades international comparisons have shown that the drug problems of different countries and their local health structure have determined different drug policies. The increase in communications, travel and availability have to some extent drawn common areas of consensus. Problems like the spread of HIV infection have concentrated minds on treatment interventions that will tackle the increase in numbers of this and other blood-borne virus disorders. Polarized attitudes towards abstinence only treatment or freely available drugs have perhaps been modified towards damage limitation strategies with some flexibility of approach. Legislation is some way behind rapidly changing clinical practice, but it is changing in an attempt to keep up with the reality. Better social integration of drug users is seen as a goal itself where as abstinence was previously the only meaningful objective (Nadelmann *et al.* 1997).

Research into drug treatment issues

Efficacy of treatment

The increase in drug use and the consequent escalating cost of treatment programmes have, understandably, stimulated a need for evaluation and cost-effectiveness. As most experience is with opiate users and these are the most widely injected drugs, research interest has been concentrated on treatment provision for this problem. There is, however, an absence of contemporary, appropriately designed outcome studies to assess change in drug taking or other measures. Table 1.3 indicates a possible list of aims for treatment and measures of change. Most research recognizes the importance of drug substitution therapy in reducing crime, deaths and increasing a broad range of indicators of social functioning (Treatment Works 1996). The longer term measures of substitution therapy demand clear study design.

Table 1.3 List of aims for treatment and outcome measures

Outcome domain	Measure
Drug use	<ul><li>Abstinence from drugs</li><li>Near abstinence from drugs</li><li>Reduction in quantity of drugs consumed</li><li>Abstinence from street drugs</li><li>Reduced use of street drugs</li><li>Change in drug taking behaviour from injecting to oral consumption</li><li>Reduction in the frequency of injecting</li></ul>
Physical and psychological health	<ul><li>Improvement in physical health</li><li>No deterioration in physical health</li><li>Improvement in psychological health</li><li>No deterioration in psychological health</li><li>Reduction in sharing injecting equipment</li><li>Reduction in sexual risk taking</li></ul>
Social functioning and life context	<ul><li>Reduction in criminal activity</li><li>Improvement in employment status</li><li>Fewer working/school days missed</li><li>Improved family relationships</li><li>Improved personal relationships</li><li>Domiciliary stability/improvement</li></ul>

Taken from *The Task Force to review services for drug misusers*. Department of Health 1995 London. Crown copyright is reproduced with the permission of the Controller of Her Majesty's Stationery Office.

Many studies have addressed different issues. Outcomes used have included deaths, abstinence, reduction in risk-taking, reduction in criminal activity, retention in treatment, recruitment into treatment, HIV and other viral seroconversion, other drugs used (including alcohol), family relationships, living arrangements, employment record and others.

Studies of optimal levels of methadone, best level of psychosocial services, use of take-home medicines, dual diagnosis treatments and managing behavioural problems in prescribing clinics are all examples of the research conducted into substitution programmes (Condelli 1993, Joe *et al.* 1991).

Previous research indicating the spontaneous recovery rate (Winick 1962) and optimism about recovery and the increasing numbers abstinent at follow-up are balanced by those studies which draw attention to the attrition rate due to overdose, suicide, HIV infection or violence (Stoneburner *et al.* 1988) and the persistence of narcotic addiction in a larger percentage (Skidmore *et al.* 1990, Hser *et al.* 1993). On balance research seems to indicate opiate dependence to be a chronic, often for decades, condition with an unpredictable spontaneous recovery rate but also a sizeable mortality (Shishodia *et al.* 1997) and a persistence into and beyond middle age in many (Gambert 1997).

Drug substitution as therapy

Having understood the complicated and long-term nature of drug dependence, the absence of an available and reliable short-term treatment and cure is self-evident. The concept of a long-term relapsing condition is not only important for therapists but for relatives and indeed for the drug dependent individual. It is often a turning point in the lives of individuals and their families when they begin to understand their problem at this level. The search for the elusive cure or even for the dramatic improvement recede and often a sense of control is experienced rather than hopelessness. Treatment modalities and treatment options are extensive and contemporary literature with an interest in drug treatment is currently interested in the long-term benefits of methadone prescribing for opiate addicts. The effects of such treatments on behaviour, both drug taking and criminal behaviour, the retention in treatment as a marker of some sort of success of methadone treatment as well as the frequency of relapse and psychosocial problems are all areas of attention for research. Research agendas include the study of individuals coming into treatment, their demographic profiles and how this may or may not be linked with outcome. The relative success of females over males in some studies (Kosten 1991), the difficulty of engaging young people and retaining them in treatment, and the inhibiting nature of those involved with crime, those socially isolated and lacking support (Gainey et al. 1993) all direct those providing the treatment towards the best possible selection and referral of patients. Different drugs clearly have different effects and are likely to require different approaches and the North American concern with cocaine addiction has directed research heavily toward the search for a pharmacological treatment for cocaine dependence similar to methadone in opiate users. Various contenders include Mazindol (Kosten et al. 1993), fluoxetine (Batki et al. 1993), buprenorphine (Gastfriend et al. 1993) and disulfiram in those also addicted to alcohol (Higgins et al. 1993). Similarly, for drugs other than heroin and cocaine, specific alternative pharmacological agents are rarely available although in many countries the legal status of drugs such as amphetamine, benzodiazepines and barbiturates allows for the same drug to be prescribed therapeutically. This clearly does not apply to cannabis which again in most countries is specifically not available from legal sources, and interestingly alcohol which is widely available at low cost and it is therefore not necessary to supply.

New developments

Changing legislation and regulations

Regulations and guidelines as well as legal superstructure are constantly changing and evolving in many countries. These changes often arise as the system becomes redundant due to new changes in drug usage or drug type. Guidelines for medical and other healthcare workers are required to regulate practice and to control poor practice. Examples of recent changes include UK recommendations to identify areas of expertise required to manage drug users with different severities of problems. This recommendation has the dual purpose of enforcing appropriate standards of education for doctors treating patients with drug dependency problems, and curtailing the use of more controversial treatment modalities such as prescription of injectable substitute drugs and the wider variety of oral substitute medications (Department of Health Guidelines for Good Clinical Practice, in press).

Decriminalization

As with treatment methods, availability of drugs is constantly changing and for the first time for many years a substantial degree of support is emerging for some form of decriminalization or even legalization. These arguments principally apply to the use of cannabis and arise out of the increasing belief that it is a non-toxic recreational drug. Some drug observers and experts advocate the decriminalization of all classes of drug and others still see the decriminalization debate as being not drug specific, but indicative of a pragmatic approach to a problem which not only has put the criminal justice system and healthcare systems in many countries under severe stress, but continues to cause political embarrassment. Whilst the range of options is constantly being examined and acceptable experiments are being viewed with great interest, it is likely that increased drug use and understanding of the effects of drugs will sooner or later lead to a normalization of some forms of drug taking throughout societies where previously it has been confined to minority groups. This may take many years.

Future research

The urgency to evaluate treatment to new standards and using other outcome measures relevant to present day worries about blood-borne viruses has given rise to national studies in several countries. In the UK, the outcome of treatment for four main interventions, methadone reduction programmes, methadone maintenance programmes, residential rehabilitation programmes and specialist in-patient drug dependence units are being evaluated using the outcome measures in Table 1.3 (Department of Health 1995). The Centres for Substance Abuse Treatment CSAT Study (NTIES 1996) has recently reported results on 5388 clients treated in public substance abuse treatment programmes. Among NTIES' findings were:

- clients served by CSAT-funded treatment programmes significantly reduces their alcohol and drug use
- treatment resulted in lasting benefits, with significant decreases in drug use and alcohol use one year after treatment
- clients also reported increases in employment, income and physical and mental health, and decreases in criminal activity, homelessness and risk behaviour for HIV/AIDS infection, one year after treatment.

Important areas identified by the British report as requiring further clarification are included in Table 1.4.

As already stated, the majority of research into treatment of dependency has been carried out with opiate or heroin dependent patients. Extrapolation to other substances may or may not be appropriate and specific initiatives to widen the base of research are needed. Serial reports and epidemiological studies provide information about current use and prevalence and major initiatives like the

Table 1.4 Key questions for future investigations

- Important to know the effects which particular interventions have on selected outcome measures
- The enduring effects once treatment has been completed
- The cost-effectiveness of different treatments
- The elements of treatment modules which are the effective ones
- The longer term effects of treatment, as distinct from the immediate impact
- The value of well-designed and the use of appropriate methodologies including randomized controlled trials
- The effectiveness of 'shared care' in primary care settings
- The impact of training on the behaviour of people working with drug users
- The comparative effectiveness of different types of counselling
- The feasibility of increased on site dispensing in drug services and supervised consumption of prescribed drugs
- Ways of enhancing the completion rates for detoxification, including the use of a range of drugs to assist in the process
- Whether drugs such as LAAM are appropriate alternatives to methadone
- The role and efficacy of injectable opioid prescribing
- The treatment of amphetamine dependence
- The treatment of cocaine dependence

Adapted from *The Task Force Report to review services for drug misusers.* Department of Health 1995 London. Crown copyright is reproduced with the permission of the Controller of Her Majesty's Stationery Office.

Drug Awareness Warning Network in the USA give a comparatively sensitive indicator of changing trends. National strategies such as the Australian Task Force have initiated strategic programmes to examine the under-researched area of drugs and have given over a short period of time some clearer insights into such previously neglected areas as the negative effects of cannabis abuse. The England and Wales Task Force Report 1996 stimulated a major study (NTORS 1996) on the efficacy of substitute prescribing for heroin users. The European Drug Dependency Monitoring Centre in Lisbon is likely to provide ongoing epidemiological basis for 13 member states of the European Union.

All these and other efforts provide new statistical information mainly concerning epidemiology and the introduction of new drugs of misuse. They give, however, comparatively little insight into issues germane to the design and provision of specific and appropriate treatment modules. As will be highlighted throughout this book, basic issues of understanding of the interaction between lifestyles and drug using, the precursors for change of drug taking and the inhibitors blocking recovery are required. Major issues such as the causes of mortality over a long period of time in populations of drug users remain cryptic and are difficult to research. Outcome studies of the wider range of newer drugs commonly in use will only be available with the passage of time. Similarly, the effect of treatment on drug users is poorly researched, largely because long-term evaluation is rarely built into treatment schedules. In a similar way to the evolution of drug use, the evolution of treatment means that current requirements of the results of treatment are different from those conceived of only a few years ago. There is, for example, a belief that counselling and support services with welfare rights and legal advice is likely to improve the outcome for most drug users experiencing difficulties in many areas of their lives. There is, however, very little chance of evaluating these items of input and measuring a successful or otherwise outcome. Even the evaluation of the efficacy of a specific treatment like methadone maintenance has proved extremely difficult over many years, especially in the absence of methodology to evaluate long-term survival and abstinence and attribute this to the treatment. Surrogate markers have been used to indicate the success of methadone treatment. These include reduction in criminality, retention in treatment, improvement of general health and, more recently, a reduced likelihood of continuing to inject and being HIV antibody positive. Common sense indicates that methadone is therefore an effective treatment, as does the belief that counselling and support with legal problems are likely to benefit the patient. Treatment is therefore often based less on good research and more on what society currently considers to be compassionate, affordable and pragmatic care.

References

ACMD. 1996: Advisory Council on the Misuse of Drugs. *Drug users and the criminal justice system. Part III, drug misusers and the prison system – an integrated approach*. HMSO, London.

Adelekan, M., Green, A., Dasgupta, N., Tallack, F., Stimson, G.V., Wells, B. 1996: Reliability and validity of the opiate treatment index among a sample of opioid users in the United Kingdom. *Drug and Alcohol Review* **15** (3), 261–70.

Alpheis, H. 1996: Hamburg: handling an open drug scene. In: Dorn, N., Jepsen, J., Savona, E. (eds). *European drug policies and enforcement*. MacMillan, London, pp. 55–73.

American Psychiatric Association DSM-IV. 1994: Diagnostic criteria for substance dependence. In: *Diagnostic and statistical manual*, 4th edn.

Anglin, M.D., Hser, Y.I. 1990: Treatment of drug abuse. In: Tonry, M. and Wilson, J.Q. (eds), *Drugs and crime*. University of Chicago Press, pp. 393–460.

Anglin, M.D., Hser, Y.I., Booth, M.W. 1987: Sex differences in addict careers. 4. Treatment. *American Journal of Drug and Alcohol Abuse* **13** (3), 253–80.

Armstrong, G. 1997: Managed care. In: Lowinson, J.H., Ruiz, P., Millman, R.B., Langrod, J.G. (eds). *Substance abuse. A comprehensive textbook*, 3rd edn. Williams & Wilkins, Baltimore, pp. 911–20.

Avants, S.K., Mangolni, A., Kosten, T.R. 1994: Cocaine abuse in methadone maintenance programmes: integrating pharmacotherapy with psychosocial interventions. *Journal of Psychoactive Drugs* **26** (2), 137–46.

Baker, A., Kochan, N., Dixon, J., Wodak, A., Heather, N. 1995: HIV risk taking behaviour among injecting drug users currently, previously and never enrolled in methadone treatment. *Addiction* **90** (4), 545–54.

Batki, S.L., Manfredi, L.B., Jacob, P., Jones, R.T. 1993: Fluoxetine for cocaine dependence in methadone maintenance: quantitative plasma and cocaine and benzodiazepine concentrations. *Journal of Clinical Psychopharmacology* **13** (4), 243–50.

Beuchi, M.L., Zeegers, P.D., Wasserfallen, F. 1997: *AIDS and drug prevention in Swiss prison system: a national overall strategy.* Vancouver XI Conference on AIDS. Abstract WED 353.

Burns, S.M., Brettle, R.P., Gore, S.M., Peutherer, J.F., Robertson, J.R. 1996: The epidemiology of HIV infection in Edinburgh related to the injecting of drugs: an historical perspective and new insight regarding the past incidence of HIV infection derived from retrospective HIV antibody testing of stored samples of serum. *Journal of Infection* **32**, 53–62.

Capelhorn, J.R, Bell, J. 1991: Methadone dosage and retention of patients in in maintenance treatment. *Medical Journal of Australia* **154** (3): 195–9.

Center for Disease Control 1991: *HIV/AIDS Surveillance Report, November 1–18*. Atlanta.

Chen, L.C., Cash, R.A. 1988: A decade after Alma Ata. Can primary care lead to health for all? *New England Journal of Medicine* **319** (14), 946–7.

Condelli, W.S. 1993: Strategies for increasing retention in methadone programmes. *Journal of Psychoactive Drugs* **25** (2), 143–7.

Daley, D.C., Marlatt, G.A. 1997: Relapse prevention. In: Lowinson, J.H., Ruiz, P., Millman, R.B., Langrod, J.G. *Substance abuse. A comprehensive textbook*, 3rd edn. Williams & Wilkins, Baltimore, pp. 458–67.

Darke, S., Hall, W., Heather, N., Wodak, A., Ward, J. 1992: Development and validation of a multi-dimensional instrument for assessing outcome of treatment among opiate users. The Opiate Treatment Index. *British Journal of Addiction* **87**, 733–42.

Darke, S., Swift, W., Hall, W., Ross, M. 1993: Drug use, HIV risk-taking and psychosocial correlates of benzodiazepine use among methadone maintenance clients. *Drug and Alcohol Dependency* **34** (1), 67–70.

Department of Health 1995. *The task force to review services for drug misusers*. London.

Department of Health Task Force 1996: *The task force to review services for drug misusers: report of an independent survey of drug treatment services in England*. Department of Health, London.

Des Jarlais, D.C., Friedman, S.R., Choopanya, K., Vanichseni, S., Ward, T.P 1992: International epidemiology of HIV and AIDS among injecting drug users. *AIDS* **6**, 1053–1068.

Des Jarlais, D.C., Friedman, S.R., Hagan, H., Paone, D., Vlahov, D. 1997: Drug use. Vancouver Conference Review. *AIDS Care* **9** (1), 53–7.

ECMDDA 1996: European Monitoring Centre for Drugs and Drug Addiction annual report on the state of the drug problem in the European Union. Lisbon.

Finnegan, L.P. 1991: Treatment issues for opiate dependent women during the perinatal period. *Journal of Psychoactive Drugs* **23** (2), 191–201.

Finnegan, L.P., Daveney, K., Hartel, D. 1993: Drug use in HIV-infected women. In Johnson, M.A., Johnstone, F.D. (eds). *HIV infection in women*. Churchill Livingstone, Edinburgh 133–57.

Friedman, S.R., Lipton, D.S. 1991: Cocaine, AIDS and intravenous drug use. *Journal of Addictive Disorders* **10** (4), 1–11.

Gainey, R.R., Wells, E, A., Hawkins, J.D., Catalano, R.F. 1993: Predicting treatment retention among cocaine users. *International Journal of Addiction* **28** (6), 487–505.

Gambert, S.R., 1997: The elderly. In: Lowinson, J.H., Ruiz, P., Millman, R.B., Langrod, J.G. (eds). *Substance abuse treatment. A comprehensive textbook*, 3rd edn. Williams & Wilkins, Baltimore.

Gastfriend, D.R., Mendelson, J.H., Mello, N.K., Teoh, S.K., Reif, S. 1993: Buprenorphine pharmacotherapy for concurrent heroin and cocaine dependence. *American Journal of Addiction* **2** (4), 269–78.

Gerstein, D.R., Lewin, L.S. 1990: Treating drug problems. Report from the National Academy of Sciences, Washington. *New England Journal of Medicine* **323**, 844–8.

Glanz, A., 1994: The fall and rise of the general practitioner. In: Strang, J., Gossop, M. (eds). *Heroin addiction and drug policy. The British system*. Oxford University Press, pp. 151–66.

Goldberg, D., Green, S., Taylor, A., Frisher, M. 1994: The heterogeneity of HIV prevalence among injecting drug users in Europe and the United Kingdom. *AIDS News Supplement*. Scottish Centre for Infection and Environmental Health 94/39.

Gore, S.M., Bird, A.G., Ross, A.J. 1995a: Prison rites: starting to inject inside. *British Medical Journal* **311**, 1135–6.

Gore, S.M., Bird, A.G., Burns, S.M., Goldberg, D.J., Ross, A.J., McGregor, J. 1995b: Drug injecting and HIV prevalance in inmates of Glenochle prison. *British Medical Journal* **310**: 292–6.

Gossop, M., Griffiths, P., Powis, B., Strang, J. 1992: Severity of dependence and route of administration of heroin, cocaine and amphetamines. *British Journal of Addiction* **87**, 1527–36.

Gottheil, E., Sterling, R.C., Weinstein, S.P. 1993: Diminished illicit drug use as a consequence of long term methadone maintenance. *Journal of Addictive Disorders* **12** (4), 45–57.

Greenwood, J. 1992: Services for problem drug users in Scotland. In: Plant, M., Ritson, B., Robertson, R. (eds). *Alcohol and drugs, the Scottish experience.* Edinburgh University Press, 138–44.

Hartel, D., Selwyn, P.A., Schoenbaum, E.E. 1988: *Methadone maintenance treatment and reduced risk of AIDS and AIDS–specific mortality in intravenous drug users.* 4th International Conference on AIDS, Stockholm.

Higgins, S.T., Budney, A.J., Bickel, W.K., Hughes, J.R., Foerg, F. 1993: Disulfiram therapy in patients abusing cocaine and alcohol. *American Journal of Psychiatry* **150** (4), 675–6.

Horder, J. 1983: General practice in 2000. Alma Ata declaration. *British Medical Journal* **286**, 191–4.

Hser, Y.I., Anglin, D., Powers, K. 1993: A 24–year follow-up of California narcotic addicts. *Archives of General Psychiatry* **50**, 577–84.

Jepsen, J. 1996: Copenhagen: A war on socially marginalized people. In: Dorn, N., Jepsen, J., Savona, E. (eds). *European drug policies and enforcement.* MacMillan, London, pp. 9–32.

Joe, G.W., Simpson, D.D., Hubbard, R.L. 1991: Treatment predictors of tenure in methadone maintenance. *Journal of Substance Abuse* **3** (1), 73–84.

Jutta, J., Stover, H. 1997: Shoot out in Germany prisons take charge. *Druglink* **12** (4), 9.

Kanga, K. 1996: *Drug intervention/awareness among IDVs in the slums.* XI International Conference on AIDS, Vancouver. Presentation Mo. D. 242.

Kauffman, J.F., Woody, G.E. 1995: In: *Matching treatment to patients needs in opioid substitution therapy.* Centre for Substance Abuse Treatment, Rockville, MD.

Kochems, L.M., Paone, D., Des Jarlais, D.C., Ness, I., Clark, J., Friedman, S.R. 1996: The transition from underground to legal syringe exchange: the New York City experience. *AIDS Education Preview* **83**, 471–89.

Kosten, T.A., Bianchi, M.S., Kosten, T.R. 1992a: The predictive validity of the dependence syndrome in opiate abusers. *American Journal of Drug and Alcohol Abuse* **18** (2), 145–56.

Kosten, T.R. 1991: Client issues in drug abuse treatment: addressing multiple drug abuse. In: Pickers, R.W., Leukfield, C.G., Schusfer, C.R. (eds). *Improving drug abuse treatment.* US Department of Health and Human Sciences. Research Monograph **106**, 136–51.

Kosten, T.R., Morgan, C.M., Falcione, H., Schottenfield, R.S. 1992b Pharmacotherapy for cocaine abusing methadone-maintained patients using amantadine or disipramine. *Archives of General Psychiatry* **49** (11), 894–8.

Kosten, T.R., Steinberg, M., Diakogiamnis, I.A. 1993: Crossover trial of mazindol for cocaine dependence. *American Journal of Addiction* **2** (2), 161–4.

Libonatti, O., Luria, E., Peruga, A., Gonzales, R., Zacarias, F., Weissenbacher, M. 1993: Role of drug injection in the spread of HIV in

Argentina and Brazil (editorial). *International Journal of STD and AIDS* **4** (3), 135–41.

Macleod, J., Scott, R., Elliot, L., Gruer, L., Cameron, J. 1996: The routine use of the Opiate Treatment Index in a clinical setting. *International Journal of Drug Policy* **7** (2), 130–32.

Maddux, J.F., Prihoda, T.J., Desmond, D.P. 1994: Treatment fees and retention on methadone maintenance. *Journal of Drug Issues* **24** (3), 429–43.

Mahon, N. 1997: Treatment in prisons and gaols. In: Lowinson, J.H., Ruiz, P., Millman, R.B., Langrod, J.G. (eds). *Substance abuse. A comprehensive textbook*, 3rd edn. Williams & Wilkins, Baltimore, pp. 455–8.

Marlatt, G.A. 1985: Relapse prevention: theoretical rationale and overview of the model. In: Marlatt, G.A., Gordon, J. (eds). *Relapse prevention: a self-control strategy in the maintenance of behaviour change.* Guildford, New York, pp. 3–70.

Marsh, K.J., Joe, G.W., Simpson, D.D., Lehman, W.E. 1990: Treatment history. In: Simpson, D.D., Sells, S.B., Malabar, F.L. (eds). *Opioid addiction and treatment: a 12 year follow-up.* Robert E. Krieger, New York, pp. 137–56.

Marsh, K.L., Simpson, D.D. 1986: Sex differences in opioid addiction careers. *American Journal of Drug and Alcohol Abuse* **12** (4), 309–29.

Marshall, M.J., Marshall, S., Heer, M.J. 1994: Characteristics of abstinent substance abusers who first sought treatment in adolescence. *Journal of Drug Education* **24** (2), 151–62.

MCDS 1996: *Statement on illicit drug harm minimization strategy.* Ministerial Council on Drug Strategy Communique. Australia's Commonwealth Department. Canberra AHMC 17/96.

McCann, U.D., Ridenour, A., Shaham, Y., Ricaurte, G.A. 1994: Serotonin neurotoxicity after 3,4-methylenedioxymethamphetamine (MDMA, 'Ecstasy'): a controlled study in humans. *Neuropsychopharmacology* **10** (2): 129–38.

McLellan, A.T., Kusnev, H., Metzzer, D., Peters, R., Smith, I., Grisson, G., Pettinali, H., Argeriou, M. 1992: In: The fifth edition of the Addiction Severity Index. *Journal of Substance Abuse Treatment* **9** (3), 199–213.

McLellan, A.T., Woody, G.E., Luborsky, L., O'Brien, C.P., Druley, K.A. 1983: Increased effectiveness of substance abuse treatment: a prospective study of patient treatment 'matching'. *Journal of Nervous Mental Diseases* **171**, 597–605.

Metrebian, N., Shanaham, W., Stimson, G.V. 1996: Heroin prescribing in the United Kingdom: an overview. *European Addiction Research* **2**, 194–200.

Mutter, R.C., Grimes, R.M., Labarthe, D. 1994: Evidence of intraprison spread of HIV infection. *Archives Internal Medicine* **4**, 793–5.

Nadelmann, E., McNeely, J., Drucker, E. 1997: International perspectives. In: Lowinson J.H., Ruiz, P., Millman, R.B., Langrod, J.G. (eds).

Substance abuse. A comprehensive textbook. 3rd edn. Williams & Wilkins, Baltimore, pp. 22–39.

National Drug Strategy 1994: *Legislative options for cannabis in Australia.* Monograph series No. 26. Australian Government Publishing Service, Canberra.

Newman, R.G. 1983: The need to redefine 'addiction'. *New England Journal of Medicine* **308** (18), 1096–8.

Nicol, T. 1997: *Bleach kit distribution pilot project in a Canadian federal institution.* Vancouver XI International Conference on AIDS Abstract WED 356.

NTIES 1996: The national treatment improvement evaluation study (NTIES) centre for substance abuse treatment, Rockville, MD.

NTORS 1996: *The National Treatment Outcomes Research Study.* National Addiction Centre, University of London.

Obot, I.S. 1990: Substance abuse, health and social welfare in Africa: an analysis of the Nigerian experience. *Social Science Medicine* **31** (6), 699–704.

Peak, A., Rana, S., Maharjan, S.H., Jolley, D., Crofts, N. 1995: Declining risk of HIV among injecting drug users in Kathmandu, Nepal: the impact of a harm-reduction programme. *Acquired Immune Deficiency Syndromes* **9**, 1067–70.

Pont, J., Strutz, H., Kahl, W., Salzner, G. 1994: HIV epidemiology and risk behaviour promoting HIV transmission in Austrian prisons. *European Journal of Epidemiology* **10** (3), 285–9.

Powell, D.H. 1973: A pilot study of occasional heroin users. *Archives of General Psychiatry* **32**, 955–61.

Power, R., Hartnoll, R., Daviaud, E. 1988: Drug injecting, AIDS. and risk behaviour: potential for change and intervention strategies. *British Journal of Addiction* **83**, 649–54.

Prochaska, J.O., DiClemente. C.C. 1986: Towards a comprehensive model of change. In: Miller, W.R., Heather, N. (eds). *Treating addictive behaviours: processes of change.* Plenum Press, NY pp. 3–27.

Robins, L.N., Helzer, J.E., Davis, D.H. 1975: Narcotic use in southeast Asia and afterward. *Archives of General Psychiatry* **32**, 955–61.

Rounsaville, B.J., Kosten, T.R., Weissman, M.M., Kleber, H.D. 1986: Prognostic significance of psychopathology in treated opiate addicts. A 25 year follow-up study. *Archives of General Psychiatry* **43** (8), 739–45.

Schoenbaum, E.E., Hartel, D., Selwyn, P.A., Klein, R.S., Davenny, K., Roges, M., Feiner, C., Friedland, G. 1989: Risk factors for human immunodeficiency virus in intravenous drug users. *New England Journal of Medicine* **321** (13), 874–9.

Seivewright, N., McMahon, C. 1996: Misuse of amphetamines and related drugs. *Advances in Psychiatric Treatment* **2**, 211–18.

Selwyn, P.A., Hartel, D., Wassermann, N., Drucker, E. 1989: Impact of the AIDS epidemic on the morbidity and mortality among intravenous drug users in New York City methadone maintenance programme. *American Journal of Public Health* **79**, 1358–63.

Shishodia, P., Robertson, J.R., Milne, A. 1998: Causes and frequencies of deaths in a cohort of drug users between 1981 and 1997 in a general Practice in Edinburgh. *Health Bulletin Scottish Office* **56** (2): 553–6.

Skidmore, C.A., Robertson, J.R., Robertson, A.A., Elton, R.A. 1990: After the epidemic: follow up study of HIV seroprevalence and changing patterns of drug use. *British Medical Journal* **300**, 219–23.

Simooya, O.O., Sanjobo, N. 1997: *'In but free' – an HIV/AIDS intervention in an African prison.* Vancouver XI International Conference on AIDS. Abstract WED 355.

Simpson, D.D., Joe, G.W., Bracy, S.A. 1982: Six year follow-up of opioid addicts after admission to treatment. *Archives of General Psychiatry* **39** (11), 1318–23.

Smith, R. 1995: The war on drugs. Prohibition isn't working - some legalization will help. *British Medical Journal* **311**, 1655–6.

Steele, T.D., McCann, U.D., Ricaurte, G.A. 1994: 3,4-methylenedioxymethamphetamine (MDMA, 'Ecstasy'): pharmacology and toxicology in animals and humans. *Addiction* **89** (5), 539–51.

Stimson, G.V. 1993: The global diffusion of injecting drug use: implications for human immunodeficiency virus infection. *Bulletin of Narcotics* **45** (1), 3–17.

Stimson, G.V., Hunter, G., Rhodes, T., Des Jarlais, D.C. 1997: *Continued global diffusion of injecting drug use has major implications for spread of HIV-1 infection.* Vancouver XI International Conference on AIDS. Abstract TH.C. 420.

Stoneburner, R.L., Des Jarlais, D.C., Benezra, D., Gorelkin, L., Sotheran, J.L., Friedman, S.R., Schultz, S., Marmor, M., Mildvan, D., Malansky, R. 1988: A larger spectrum of severe HIV-1 related disease in intravenous drug users in New York city. *Science* **24**, 916–18.

Strang, J., Clee, W.B., Gruer, L., Raistrick, D. 1997: Why Britain's drug czar mustn't wage war on drugs. *British Medical Journal* **315**, 325–6.

Strang, J., Des Jarlais, D.C., Griffiths, P., Gossop, M. 1992: The study of transitions in the route of drug use: The route from one route to the other. *British Journal of Addiction* **87**, 473–83.

Taylor, A., Goldberg, D., Emslie, J., Wrench, J., Gruer, L., Cameron, S., Black, J., Davis, B., McGregor, J., Follett, E., Harvey, J., Basson, J., McGavigan, J. 1995: Outbreak of HIV infection in a Scottish prison. *British Medical Journal* **310**, 289–92.

Thorley, A. 1981: Longitudinal studies of drug dependence. In: Edwards and Busch (eds). *Drug problems in Britain – a review of 10 years.* Academic Press, London, pp. 117–69.

Tobutt, C., Oppenheimer, E., Laranjeira, R. 1996: Health of a cohort of heroin addicts from London clinics: 22 years follow-up. *British Medical Journal* **312**, 1458.

Treatment Works 1996. Centre for substance abuse treatment. Department of Health and Human Services. Rockville, MD.

Uchtenhagen, A., Gutzwiller, F., Dobler-Mikola, A. (eds). 1997: *Summary of the synthesis programme for a medical prescription of narcotics*. Tages Anzeiger, 11th July.

United Nations 1990: A/Res/45/146. 69th Plenary Meeting, December 1990, New York.

Vaillant, G.E. 1973: A 20-year follow-up of New York narcotic addicts. *Archives of General Psychiatry* **29**, 237–41.

van Ameijden, E.J.C., van den Hoek, J.A.R., van Haastrecht, H.J.A., Couthino, R.A. 1992: The harm reduction approach and risk factors for human immunodeficiency virus (HIV) serconversion in injecting drug users, Amsterdam. *American Journal of Epidemiology* **136**, 236–43.

van Brussel, G.H.A., Buster, M.C.A., van der Woude, D.H. 1997: *Evaluation report. Palfium treatment for long-term heroin drug users*. Municipal Health Service, Amsterdam.

Vanichseni, S., Kitayaporn, D., Mastro, T.D., Kampanartsanyakorn, C., Raktham, S., Sujarita, S., Des Jarlais, D.C., Wasi, C., Esparza, J., Heyward, W.L. 1996: *HIV-1 incidence and follow-up in a prospective cohort of injecting drug users in Bankok*. XI International Conference on AIDS, Vancouver. Presentation Th. C 421.

Ward, J., Mattick, R., Hall, W. 1992: *Key issues in methadone maintenance treatment*. New South Wales University Press, pp. 272–4.

Winick, C. 1962: Maturing out of narcotic addiction. *Bulletin of Narcotics* **14**, 1–7.

Wodak, A., Crofts, N., Fisher, R. 1993: HIV infection among injecting drug users in Asia: an evolving public health crisis. *AIDS Care* 5 **(3)**, 313–20.

Wodak, A., Moss, A. 1990: HIV infection and injecting drug users: from epidemiology to public health. *AIDS* **4**, 105–109.

World Health Organization 1990: *Project on psychoactive substance use and primary health care/community involvement in health*. WHO resolution 33/1980, 42.20 of 1989 and 43.11 of 1990, Geneva.

World Health Organization 1992: *International statistical classification of diseases and related health problems*, 10th revision. WHO, Geneva.

Yancovitz, S.R., Des Jarlais, D.C., Peyser, N.P., Drew, E., Friedman, P., Trigg, H.L. Robinson, J.W. 1991: A randomized trial of an interim methadone maintenance clinic. *American Journal of Public Health* **81** (9), 1185–91.

Yirrell, D.L., Robertson, P., Goldberg, D.J., McMenamin, J., Cameron, S., Leigh-Brown, A.J. 1997: Molecular investigation into outbreak of HIV in a Scottish prison. *British Medical Journal* **314**, 1446–50.

Zinberg, N.E. 1984: *Drug, set and setting: the basis for controlled intoxicant use. Yale University*. Vail-Ballou Press, New York.

Systems issues

Don C Des Jarlais

Introduction

The use and misuse of illicit psychoactive drugs can be considered as a community, a national and increasingly as an international problem. Responses to the problem also need to occur at all of these levels. In this chapter, we will consider some of the international aspects of the problem of misuse of illicit drugs and some of the national responses to the problem. These international and national system issues form frameworks within which community-level management of illicit drug misuse can occur. The provision of drug abuse treatment and the prevention of HIV infection among injecting drug users (IDUs) will be used to illustrate possible responses to the problems of illicit drug use.

The international epidemic of injecting drug use

During the first half of the twentieth century, the injection of illicit drugs was sufficiently concentrated in one country that it was known as 'the American disease' (Musto 1973). (Non-injected use of psychoactive drugs, however, occurred throughout the world.) Over the last three decades, the practice of injecting illicit psychoactive drugs has spread rapidly. By 1989, drug injection had been reported in 80 different countries, with HIV infection among injecting drug users reported in 59 countries (Des Jarlais and Friedman 1989). Table 2.1 lists the 121 countries in which illicit drug injection has been reported

Table 2.1 Countries and territories with injecting drug use and HIV infection among IDUS, by December 1995

Americas	Europe	Africa	Asia	
Argentina*	Albania	Cote d'Ivoire	Azerbaijan	Kuwait
Bahamas*	Austria*	Egypt*	Bahrein*	Laos*
Bermuda	Belarus*	Gabon	Bangladesh	Macao*
Bolivia	Belgium*	Ghana	Brunei*	Malaysia*
Brazil*	Boznia-Herzegovina	Mauritius*	Cambodia*	Myanmar*
Canada*	Bulgaria*	Morocco*	China*	Nepal*
Chile*	Croatia*	Nigeria*	Georgia	Oman
Columbia*	Czech Republic*	Senegal	Hong Kong*	Pakistan*
Costa Rica*	Denmark*	South Africa	India*	Philippines*
Dominican Republic*	Estonia	Tanzania	Indonesia*	Saudi Arabia
Ecuador*	Finland*	Tunisia	Iran	Singapore*
El Salvador*	France*	Uganda	Iraq	Sri Lanka*
Guatemala	Germany*	Zambia	Israel*	Sudan
Haiti	Greece*		Japan*	Syria*
Honduras*	Hungary*		Jordan	Taiwan
Jamaica	Iceland*		Kazakhstan	Thailand*
Mexico*	Ireland*		Kirgystan	Turkmenistan
Nicaragua*	Italy*		Korea	Vietnam*
Panama*	Latvia*			
Paraguay*	Lituania			
Puerto Rico*	Luxembourg*			
Surinam	Macedonia			
Uruguay*	Malta*			
United States of America*	Moldova			
Venezuela*	Monaco*			
	Netherlands*			
Oceania	Norway*			
Australia*	Poland*			
Fiji*	Romania			
French Polynesia*	Russia			
Guam*	San Marino*			
New Caledonia*	Slovak Republic			
New Zealand*	Slovenia*			
	Spain*			
	Sweden*			
	Switzerland*			
	Turkey*			
	Ukraine*			
	United Kingdom*			
	Yugoslavia*			

*Countries reporting IDU with HIV infection.

through early 1996 (Des Jarlais *et al.* 1996) and the 80 countries in which HIV infection has been reported among drug injectors. There are now an estimated 5 million persons who inject illicit drugs throughout the world, and this number is probably growing rapidly (Mann and Tarantola 1996).

Understanding the rapid increase in both the number of countries with injection of illicit drugs and HIV infection among IDUs requires a context. Consider other aspects of communications, commerce and health in the late twentieth century:

- One cable television news network is available in hotels in over 200 countries
- There are outlets of a single fast-food restaurant chain in 101 countries.
- There are offices of a single advertising company in 91 countries.

It should also be noted that there have also been large increases in the use of 'legal' non-medical psychoactive drugs such as nicotine (Peto 1994, MacKay 1994) and alcohol (Barrow and Room 1991) and in the use of licit psychotropic medications (Trethowan 1975) over the last two decades.

The same factors underlying the globalization of international communications and trade also underlie the globalization of illicit drug injection. The improvements in communication and travel that facilitate trade in legal goods also facilitate trade in illicit goods.

The economies of scale in the production of illicit drugs also mean that substantial profits can be made selling drugs to 'poor' people. The very large profit margins from selling illicit drugs in industrialized nations can be used to underwrite the development of new markets in developing nations. Development of new markets is particularly likely along international drug distribution routes, as the marginal cost of putting additional supplies of drug into the distribution channels is relatively low, and the potential profits from developing new markets can be quite high.

Finally, it should be noted that injecting can be considered a 'technologically superior' method of administration of psychoactive drug. Injection produces a strong drug effect due to the rapid increase in the concentration of the drug in the brain. Injecting is also very cost-efficient in that almost all of the drug is actually delivered to the brain. Inexpensive technological advances tend to disperse widely, and are very difficult (though not necessarily impossible) to reverse (Rogers 1982).

While it is probably possible to improve current efforts to reduce the supplies of illicit psychoactive drugs, recent history suggests further growth in illicit drug markets rather than elimination of the illicit drug trade. To date, there have not been any societies that have been able to eliminate illicit drug injection after the practice had become established in the society. Public health officials should plan in terms of further world-wide increases in illicit psychoactive drug injection, with the potential for severe public health consequences, including transmission of blood-borne pathogens such as HIV. Clinicians involved in primary care, mental health, emergency care, and infectious diseases will need to become familiar with illicit drug injection and its health consequences.

National system responses to the problems of illicit drug use

The problem of illicit drug use is truly international, and there are international treaties, such as the Single Convention on Narcotic Drugs, and some international efforts, such as the United Nations International Drug Control Program, but the great majority of the activities to address problems related to illicit drug use are designed, funded and implemented as national programmes. This reflects the importance of the sovereign nation-state in world politics and the great difficulties in attempting to integrate drug policies among different countries. The next sections will therefore discuss societal/ national responses to the problem of illicit drug use. Three different types of responses will be examined.

Because of the illicit status of many psychoactive drugs, it is not possible to implement effective programmes to reduce problems associated with illicit drug use without utilizing a philosophic/ political framework that defines the 'nature of the problem' and what are and are not legitimate means for addressing the problems. Here we want to discuss briefly three different political perspectives on licit and illicit psychoactive drug use, and their implications for providing drug abuse treatment and for HIV prevention among drug users. These political perspectives are discussed as 'ideal types' and do not necessarily reflect the complexity of any specific country's policies towards psychoactive drug use. Nevertheless, these types provide an analytic framework for considering the possibilities of implementing effective drug abuse treatment and effective HIV prevention for drug users.

The traditional values immunity to drug use perspective

Many religious and cultural traditions ban or severely restrict the use of almost all psychoactive drugs. Followers of these traditions then tend to believe that their society will be immune to the 'modern decadence' of illicit drug use. One Islamic leader aptly summarized this position: 'Islam is preventative against alcohol, use of illegal drugs, and gambling. . . . because Islam rules against these behaviours' (Blans 1997). Similar prohibitions against many forms of psychoactive drug use can be found in almost all major religions, including Christianity, Buddhism, Hinduism, and Judaism. The 'traditional values' that are to protect against drug use need not be formulated in a religious framework. They may also be formulated as traditions of a specific country or ethnic group or of a political system with a strong ideology.

Within this traditional values perspective, the nature of the drug problem is thus that illicit drug use is both 'immoral' and 'foreign.'

There is little doubt that strong religious beliefs can have a protective effect against illicit drug use both at the individual and at the community level. At a policy level, there is a tendency for community leaders to assume that strong religious/traditional community beliefs will be sufficient protection against illicit drug use. The belief that traditional and religious values will provide a societal immunity against illicit drug use appears to be particularly common in developing nations (Stimson 1990). The data shown in Table 2.1, and in particular the 50% increase in the number of countries with illicit drug injection – from 80 countries in 1989 to 120 countries in 1996 – indicates that traditional/religious values will rarely be sufficient fully to protect a society against illicit drug use. To cite one particular example, production of opium for conversion to illicit heroin increased by 25% from 1995 to 1996 under the Taliban government in Afghanistan. The Taliban is one of the most fundamentalist of the Islamic governments and had officially banned production of opium. This ban was not enforced, however, for several reasons, including the lack of a suitable alternative cash crop for the farmers and a government need for tax revenues (Wren 1997).

Drug abuse treatment

The traditional values immunity perspective emphasizes the reasons why a particular nation will not develop drug use problems and usually provides little guidance for addressing such problems once they do develop. There are religious-based forms of drug treatment that are consonant with traditional values perspectives, e.g. the 12 step alcoholics anonymous programmes that have been extended to include illicit drugs and the Buddhism-based programmes in Thailand. Psychoactive medications may be used to alleviate acute withdrawal, but there is a strong sentiment against the use of any drugs to treat drug use. A primary treatment component of treatment is to re-inculcate the traditional values that would protect against future use of the drugs. While there is some evidence that these religious-based treatment programmes can reduce drug use, they are far from comprehensive approaches to either addressing drug addiction or to preventing HIV transmission among drug users.

HIV prevention

While many traditional values systems do emphasize providing care for the ill, the traditional values immunity perspective provides little positive guidance with respect to prevention of HIV among drug users. Because illicit drug use and having multiple sexual partners are usually viewed as foreign to the culture it is often difficult even to discuss HIV transmission publicly. The lack of public discussion itself can impede awareness of the threat of HIV/AIDS and reduce constructive coping with the threat. In the worst situation, AIDS may be seen as 'God's punishment' for the immoral behaviours, with a belief that no action to prevent HIV infection is needed.

The 'war on drugs' perspective

The 'war on drugs' or 'zero tolerance' perspective is probably the most common policy perspective among both industrialized and developing nations. There are both important similarities and differences between the 'traditional values immunity' perspective and the 'war on drugs' perspective. Both share a moral condemnation of illicit drug use as 'wrong'. The 'war on drugs' perspective, however, includes additional, more 'objective' reasons for opposing the use of illicit drugs. The drugs are seen as addicting, destroying the capacity for responsible behaviour of the individual. This view leads to a more complex view of the user. As in the traditional values perspective, the individual is still considered to be immoral for having used the drugs, but he or she is also a victim of the drugs themselves (and, of course, the persons who sell the drugs). Because the addicted user cannot control further drug use, he or she is also a victim of the drugs and is deserving of help to overcome his or her addiction. Thus the 'war on drugs' perspective does legitimize providing treatment to drug users, including treatment that utilizes psychoactive drugs.

Many community leaders who believe in the traditional values immunity perspective believe that their societies will not develop illicit drug use problems. Community leaders who subscribe to the 'war on drugs' perspective tend to see their societies as quite vulnerable to illicit drug use. Drug-free societies are seen as achievable goals within the 'war on drugs' perspective, but only with intense efforts.

Law enforcement at the international, national and local levels is the primary method for ridding society of the drug menace. Belief systems, such as religions, are not believed to be sufficiently powerful for eliminating illicit drug use. Criminal sanctions are needed to punish the individual users (criminalizing possession of the drugs even for personal use) and severe criminal sanctions are needed to punish distributors and sellers, including capital punishment in some countries.

Drug abuse treatment

Drug abuse treatment is also a potentially important method for reducing drug use within the 'war on drugs' perspective. As noted above, because the addicted user is seen as a victim of the drug, and addiction is – at least partially – seen as a disease, providing treatment is morally legitimated within the war on drugs perspective. There is also a strong pragmatic reason for providing drug abuse treatment. As long as there is a highly profitable demand to be met through marketing illicit drugs, law enforcement efforts to reduce the supply of drugs are likely to fail. This realization can lead to substantial funding for drug abuse treatment, but it does not overthrow the supremacy of law enforcement as the dominant method for reducing illicit drug use.

Treatment should include more than inculcating traditional values; it should also include use of the best scientific understanding of the mechanisms of drug addiction. A variety of different types of treatment programmes may be utilized, although there is usually an emphasis on abstinence-oriented forms of treatment. Psychoactive drugs may be utilized in drug abuse treatment, including maintenance treatment with psychoactive drugs. If psychoactive drugs are used in treatment, however, it is important to distinguish this type of drug medication from the drug abuse of using illicit drugs. Thus, an important aspect of methadone maintenance is that, with properly prescribed dosages, methadone does not produce the 'high' that heroin use does. If psychoactive drugs are used in the treatment of addiction, then it is likely that their use will be heavily regulated and restricted. Drug abuse treatment is often operated separately from 'regular' medical care, in some countries with a 'war on drugs' perspective, the drug abuse treatment programmes are operated by the police.

Abstinence from illegal drug use is the primary outcome for assessing treatment. Indeed, within the war on drugs perspective, the fact that methadone as a medication is specific to narcotic use, and does not biologically affect cocaine or alcohol use is seen as a failing for methadone maintenance treatment. When methadone maintenance treatment does not lead to cessation of cocaine use or of excessive alcohol use, the treatment modality is seen as failing.

HIV prevention

Since drug use is not only morally wrong, but also may lead to the disease of addiction, the preferred method for preventing HIV infection among drug users is treatment to eliminate the drug use. The threat of HIV infection is seen as one more reason why drug users should stop using drugs.

While drug abuse treatment is the preferred method for preventing HIV infection within the 'war on drugs' perspective, other prevention activities are also used. Outreach programmes, to provide information/education about HIV and AIDS, and HIV counselling and testing have been utilized in many countries with 'war on drugs' perspectives. Bleach distribution to disinfect used syringes has also been used, though syringe exchange and decriminalizing the possession of syringes as 'narcotics paraphernalia' are usually seen as antithetical to a 'war on drugs.' Here it is interesting to note that the conflict is not over the actual effects of syringe exchanges – they do not lead to increased use of illicit drugs (Normand et al. 1995) – but over the symbolic quality of government funded workers providing drug users with the actual means (needles and syringes) for using illicit drugs. The concern is that officially-approved syringe exchanges appear to 'condone' illicit drug use and 'send the wrong message' about illicit drug use. The need for consistent symbolism of government actions as 'tough on drugs' may thus substantially limit implementation of HIV prevention activities.

Full strength household bleach is a relatively strong disinfectant and can inactivate HIV. Bleach is, of course, relatively inexpensive. Household bleach has been distributed to drug injectors as an anti-HIV disinfectant in many cities in the United States, and many IDUs in the country have adopted bleach disinfection (Normand et al. 1995).

There are, however, important limitations on the use of bleach for disinfecting drug injection equipment. Bleach is not currently available in all areas where drugs are currently injected. Bleach is chemically unstable in heat and in sunlight. Perhaps most importantly, while bleach is a powerful disinfectant, it may be difficult for IDUs to disinfect needles and syringes successfully under field conditions. There have been three studies that examined the effectiveness of (self-reported) bleach use with new HIV infections as the outcome measure. In two of these studies, there was no protective effect of self-reported bleach use against HIV infection (Titus *et al.* 1994, Vlahov *et al.* 1991) while one study did find a protective effect against new HIV infection (McCoy *et al.* 1994). Current laboratory results suggest that HIV can remain active within a needle and syringe for two weeks or more (R. Heimer, personal communication) and that at least 30 seconds of contact time is needed for bleach to deactivate HIV. In order to increase the likelihood of successful disinfection, current recommendations for bleach use include rinsing the needle and syringe prior to using bleach, using bleach for 30 seconds or longer, and then rinsing the needle and syringes again. Clean water is preferred for the rinses, or, at the very least, water that has not been used to rinse others' drug injection equipment.

The 'war on drugs' perspective can in some situations actively impede HIV risk reduction among drug injectors. Prescriptions may be required for the purchase of sterile injection equipment, possession of injection equipment by itself (without possession of drugs) may be made a criminal offence, and/or police may harass drug users for carrying drug injection equipment. All of these can serve to limit the effective availability of sterile injection equipment, and thus lead to an increased likelihood that drug injectors will share injection equipment, and transmit HIV and other blood-borne pathogens.

The United States is often identified with the 'war on drugs' perspective. Historically, this perspective with its emphasis on law enforcement developed in the United States and was then exported to other countries, both industrialized and developing (Musto 1973). While there are not yet good comparative studies of drug abuse and HIV prevention policies, based on our experience, the 'war on drugs' perspective is the dominant perspective on drug abuse problems in the majority of developing countries.

Harm reduction

The world-wide epidemic of HIV infection among injecting drug users has led to important conceptual developments on injecting drug use as a health problem. HIV and AIDS have dramatically increased the adverse health consequences of injecting drug use, and thus have led to seeing psychoactive drug use as more of a health problem and not just a criminal justice problem. At the same time, HIV infection can be prevented without requiring the cessation of injecting drug use. This potential separation of a severe adverse consequence of drug use from the drug use itself has encouraged analysis of other areas in which adverse consequences of drug use might be reduced without requiring cessation of drug use. The ability of many injecting drug users to modify their behaviour to reduce the chances of HIV infection has also led to consideration of drug addicts as both concerned about their health and as capable of acting on that concern (without denying the compulsive nature of drug dependence).

These ideas have formed much of the basis for what has been termed the 'harm reduction' perspective on psychoactive drug use (Brettle 1991, Des Jarlais *et al.* 1993, Heather *et al.* 1993). This perspective emphasizes the pragmatic need to reduce harmful consequences of psychoactive drug use while acknowledging that eliminating psychoactive drug use and misuse is not likely to be feasible in the foreseeable future. Thus, community and public health officials need to implement programmes based on the assumptions that psychoactive drug use will continue and that it is possible to reduce drug-related harm without necessarily reducing drug use itself.

The harm reduction perspective was first developed in industrialized countries, with important developmental work originating in the Netherlands, the UK and Australia. Harm reduction concepts and programs are, however, spreading to many developing countries. Syringe exchange programmes have been implemented in Nepal, Thailand and India. There is an Asian Harm Reduction Network for persons interested in implementing harm reduction efforts throughout Asia.

Harm reduction should not be confused with 'legalization' of currently illicit drugs. Unrestrained commercial exploitation of psychoactive drug – as occurs with currently legal non-medical psychoactive drugs – can be expected to lead to great amounts of drug-related harm. The case of nicotine in cigarettes illustrates this very well. Rather than legalization, harm reduction requires a balance of criminal law, civil law, education, prevention, treatment and other health programmes to address the many problems associated with psychoactive drug use.

Harm reduction is essentially pragmatic. Programmes that work to reduce drug-related harms are preferred to programmes whose value is symbolic, i.e. they send a message that society is against drugs without necessarily having any demonstrable positive effect on drug use or drug-related harm. Because of its essential pragmatism, harm reduction programmes will often not appear to be symbolically consistent with either a libertarian (adults should be free to take whatever drugs they want to take) or a temperance (no-one to use mood altering substances) perspective.

Harm reduction thus does not offer a solution to all psychoactive drug problems. Indeed, the harm reduction perspective presumes that psychoactive drug use will continue and that problems associated with psychoactive drug use will also continue.

Drug abuse treatment

A wide variety of drug abuse treatment programmes have been implemented under harm reduction perspectives. These include abstinence-oriented therapies with long-term resocialization of drug users and 'substitution' therapies which use medications such as methadone for maintenance treatment of narcotic addition. Harm reduction-oriented drug abuse treatment also includes 'low threshold' drug treatment programmes, in which the clients are encouraged to abstain from illicit drugs, but are permitted to remain in treatment even if they continue to use illicit drugs.

Harm reduction treatment has also included experimental treatment with injectable morphine, and more recently with heroin as substitutes for illicitly obtained heroin (Lewis *et al.* 1995, Wren 1997). These experiments have been conducted with 'multiproblem' heroin addicts who have not responded positively to conventional forms of drug addiction treatment. These experiments have included comparisons of the functioning of the 'multiproblem' addicts while on morphine or heroin to their functioning while in conventional treatment and to their functioning when not in treatment (and using drugs obtained from illicit sources). The experiments have been confined to addicts who have repeatedly failed to respond positively to conventional forms of drug addiction treatment, and in the absence of new forms of treatment, would be expected to continue using illegally obtained drugs. There are, of course, good reasons to believe that these multiproblem addicts may function better with legally obtained drugs rather than having to obtain drugs on the illegal market, and that there may also be societal benefits from removing these addicts from the illicit drug market. These experiments thus illustrate the willingness of officials with a harm reduction orientation to explore pragmatically a wide range of possible means to reducing drug-related harms, even if these means may appear to 'condone' rather than 'condemn' the use of illegal drugs. This illustrates a basic principal of harm reduction that drug-related harms may be the result not only of the use of specific drugs, but also of the circumstances under which the drugs are used.

While is important to note that the harm reduction perspective does include experimentation with unconventional forms of drug abuse treatment, it is also important to state that these are unusual. The bigger difference between drug abuse treatment as provided under a 'war on drugs' perspective and under a 'harm reduction' perspective is in the availability of treatment for drug addiction.

Under a 'war on drugs' perspective, treatment for addiction is typically provided only to a modest fraction of addicts, while under a 'harm reduction' perspective, attempts are made to provide treatment to all persons who request such treatment.

Drug addiction treatment is also more likely to be integrated with mainstream medical care under a harm reduction perspective. Rather than addiction treatment being provided only in specialty clinics, as often occurs under a 'war on drugs' perspective, addiction treatment under a 'harm reduction' perspective may be provided by either specialists with the 'regular' healthcare system, or by primary care physicians (with appropriate training and with back-up specialist services).

HIV prevention

While interesting developments in providing drug abuse treatment have occurred under the 'harm reduction' perspective, it is the harm reduction approach to preventing HIV infection among drug users that has undoubtedly led to the greatest elaboration of the principles of harm reduction. The harm reduction approach to preventing HIV infection among drug users is best expressed in terms of a hierarchy of recommended actions. First, the drug user is encouraged to cease using psychoactive drugs. If this is not practical, the drug user is encouraged to cease injecting psychoactive drugs. If this is not practical, the drug user is encouraged not to share drug injection equipment with others. Finally, if this is not practical, the drug user is encouraged to disinfect drug injection equipment before it is re-used. This hierarchical set of recommendations illustrates the priority of abstaining from psychoactive drug use as the preferred method for reducing drug-related harms and the willingness of harm reduction advocates to utilize other means for reducing harm when abstinence is not likely to occur. A wide variety of methods for reducing HIV transmission have been implemented under harm reduction, including expansion of drug abuse treatment, community outreach, pharmacy sale of injection equipment, and disinfection of used injection equipment. The harm reduction perspective is, however, most closely identified with syringe exchange as a method of preventing HIV infection among injecting drug users syringe exchanges not only provide injecting drug users with a source of sterile injection equipment, they also provide a means for safe disposal of potentially HIV-contaminated injection equipment and continuing contact between health workers and injecting drug users. This continuing contact can then serve as a basis for providing other services, including condom distribution (to reduce sexual transmission of HIV and other sexually transmitted diseases), entry into drug abuse treatment, social services, primary healthcare, HIV counselling and testing, and tuberculosis screening and treatment. These additional services may be provided either on site or through referral.

Summary

Over the last several decades, the use of illicit psychoactive drugs has spread rapidly to many countries throughout the world. This diffusion has occurred in parallel with the increased use of illicit psychoactive drugs, improvements in communication and transportation and the 'globalization' of the world economy. While there are probably many things that could be done to reduce the distribution of illicit drugs, it would be unreasonable to expect a reversal of the world-wide distribution of illicit drugs without a similar reversal in the world-wide distribution of legal trade. Thus, public health authorities need to develop policies to address the continuing use of illicit psychoactive drugs.

Injection may be considered a 'technologically superior' method of psychoactive drug administration, in that it produces a very strong drug effect because of the rapidity with which the drug reaches the brain and because a very large percentage of the drug can be delivered to the brain. Inexpensive technological innovations tend to diffuse widely, particularly innovations that are highly cost-effective, and once such innovations have been adopted, it is usually very difficult to return to previous practices (Rogers 1982). Unfortunately, the injection of illicit drugs is also highly likely to transmit HIV and other blood-borne viruses. The illicit nature of the drug use tends to lead drug users to cooperate in obtaining drugs and then to inject together. If injection equipment is scarce at the time of drug use, then the drug users are very likely to share the equipment, and possibly transmit HIV and other blood-borne pathogens.

While the problems of illicit drug injection and the spread of blood-borne pathogens are truly international in scope, responses to these problems vary greatly among different countries. Three different types of national responses were discussed: the traditional values immunity perspective, the 'war on drugs' perspective and the harm reduction perspective. The traditional values perspective primarily utilizes the inculcation of social/religious values to prevent use of drugs, and the war on drugs perspective primarily utilizes law enforcement efforts to reduce the supply of drugs. The harm reduction perspective utilizes law enforcement, but also emphasizes providing a wide variety of types of drug abuse treatment and specific programmes to reduce problems such as the threat of HIV infection.

All actual societies are likely to utilize a mixture of these three perspectives in addressing the problems of illicit drug use. There are, however, many points on which the perspectives are not compatible. Which perspective is primarily utilized within a country will determine to a great extent what resources will be available for community-level management of illicit drug use.

References

Barrow, S., Room, R. (eds). 1991: *Drinking behaviour and belief in modern history.* University of California Press, Berkeley, CA.

Blans, J. 1997: Pills solve problem Islam. *Jellinek Quarterly* 4 (1/2), 9.

Brettle, R.P. 1991: HIV and harm reduction for injection drug users. *AIDS* 5, 125–36.

Des Jarlais, D.C., Stimson, G.V., Hagan, H. 1996: Emerging infectious diseases and the injection of illicit psychoactive drugs. *Current Issues in Public Health* 2, 102–37.

Des Jarlais, D.C., Friedman, S.R. 1989: AIDS and IV drug use. *Science* 245, 578–9.

Des Jarlais, D.C., Friedman, S.R., Ward, T.P. 1993: Harm reduction: a public health response to the AIDS epidemic among injecting drug users. *Annual Review of Public Health* 4, 413–50.

Heather, N., Wodak, A., Nadelmann, E., O'Hare, P. (eds). 1993: *Psychoactive drugs and harm reduction: from faith to science.* Whurr, London.

Lewis, D., Gear, C., Rihs-Middel, M. 1995: *The medical prescription of narcotics.* Huber Verlag, Fribourg, Switzerland.

Mackay, J.L. 1994: The fight against tobacco in developing countries. *Tubercle and Lung Disease* 75, 8–24.

Mann, J.M., Tarantola, D.J.M. (eds). 1996: *AIDS in the world II.* Oxford University Press, New York and Oxford.

McCoy, C.B., Rivers, J.E., McCoy, H.V., Shapshak, P., Weatherby, N.L., Chitwood, D.D., Page, J.B., Inciardi, J.A., McBride, D.C. 1994: Compliance to bleach disinfection protocols among injection drug users in Miami. *Journal of the Acquired Immune Deficiency Syndrome* 7, 773.

Musto, D. 1973: *The American disease: origins of narcotic control.* Yale University Press, New Haven, CT.

Normand, J., Vlahov, D., Moses, L.E. (eds). 1995: Preventing HIV transmission: the role of sterile needles and bleach. National Academics Press/National Research Council/ Institute of Medicine, Washington, DC.

Peto, R. 1994: Smoking and death: the past 40 years and the next 40. *British Medical Journal* 309, 937–9.

Rogers, E. 1982: Diffusion of innovations, vol. 3. The Free Press, New York.

Stimson, G.V. 1990: The prevention of HIV infection in injecting drug users: Recent advances and remaining obstacles. 6th International Conference on AIDS. San Francisco, CA.

Titus, S., Marmor, M., Des Jarlais, D.C., Kim, M., Wolfe, H., Beatrice, S. 1994: Bleach use and HIV seroconversion among New York City injection drug users. *Journal of Acquired Immune Deficiency Syndrome* **7**, 700–704.

Trethowan, W. 1975: Pills for personal problems. *British Medical Journal* **3**, 749–51.

Vlahov, D., Celentano, D.D., Mufloz, A., Cohn, S., Anthony, J.C., Nelson, K.E. 1991: *Bleach disinfection of needles by intravenous drug users: association with HIV seroconversion.* Seventh International Conference on AIDS, Florence, Italy.

Wren, C. 1997: Despite Taliban vow, Afghan opium production is up, UN says. *New York Times* September 11, p. Al 3.

3 Services – the Amsterdam model

Giel H A van Brussel

Introduction

The development of drug treatment services depends upon the nature of the problem, the speed with which it emerges, the size of the problem (number of new and chronic drug users) and the available infrastructure of services and systems. The rapid emergence of an overlapping series of problems in Amsterdam between 1974 and 1984 and the subsequent response by medical and public health authorities demonstrate such a response. Similar responses to their own type and size of problems were happening elsewhere in Europe and the USA round about the same time. However, it is possible by observing the Amsterdam authorities' actions and their effects as a case study, to understand certain critically important things about drug use problems, the response of drug users to appropriate services, and the outcome after a period of time. Some of the responses and resulting services are unique to the Amsterdam situation because of the political structure and organization of the health and social services. Many parts of the service have been adopted elsewhere or modified for other situations.

Other cities with acute drug problems acknowledge interest in the Amsterdam attempts to provide flexible responsive care as problems evolve. Examples are reported from Hamburg, Zurich and Copenhagen (Alpheis 1996, Fahrenkrug 1996, Laursen 1996) of similar problems and attempts to respond. National governments watch cannabis control experiments with interest (Horstink-von Meyenfeldt 1996).

Social and medical services for the management of drug users vary internationally according to social, economic and medical perspectives and traditions. The context of the drug problem in any centre depends upon the values and attitudes of that society. Several issues influence policy. Does drug addiction as a health problem belong primarily in the realm of psychiatric or of public health and primary care? What has failed in the approaches until now and is this failing recognized by the public and the politicians and care providers? Often this policy-context is linked to the length in years in which the problem has existed. Drug problems are a treacherous subject for political debate. It takes some time, if ever, for the public and politicians to see through rhetoric and recognize effects of interventions for what they are. As well as the basic approach to drug misuse, the prevalent pattern of use has a major influence on treatment policy. The dominant use of opiates requires a different response to that of cocaine or amphetamine and intravenous use requires a distinct approach.

These points indicate that the approach to the drug problem must, of necessity, differ between countries; there is no 'universal good answer'. They indicate the need to develop an effective local policy. Such a policy must take a broad view as to what works elsewhere, what does not and why, and then adapt it for local use.

Considering the development of a drugs policy it is essential to observe the basic similarities and differences between the country and the policy studied. In Amsterdam harm reduction emerged as the main focus of the multilevel drug treatment approach as early as 1981. During that year absolute drug abstinence was abandoned as the primary goal of all treatment efforts. Instead the policy was defined as 'in the absence of a curative treatment for the majority of drug users, the next best aim is to try to limit harm, e.g. overdose death, infections and social degradation as the foremost goal of intervention'. This led to the formation of low threshold methadone programmes (1981), needle exchange (1984) and a close cooperation with classic abstinence-oriented treatment approaches such as high threshold American styled methadone programmes and therapeutic communities. Also it was the base on which the city General Practitioners declared themselves willing to act as a middle level methadone facility for those drug users, who while often still engaged in low level drug abuse were socially regulated in housing, income and orderly behaviour. To explain the working of the Amsterdam system some background information is necessary about historical developments and the differences between drug users in an exploding drug epidemic (1977) and one that is in regression (1997).

In an exploding drug epidemic, deviant drug experimenting behaviour is adopted by normal, young people of all social classes as well as by the extremely marginalized underprivileged social classes. In the regression phase one has to deal with those who have not been able to mature out of addiction, especially clients with social and psychiatric stigmata. This latter problem profile also extends to new entrants coming into drug use in the regression phase.

In this chapter on services using the Dutch perspective, the following subjects will be outlined:

- The historical development of the drug problem in Amsterdam
- Drug use client characteristics, mortality and morbidity patterns to date
- The policy of harm minimization; a developmental overview
- The low, medium and high threshold service system
- Medical health service in general and drug use associated pathology, specific shared care demands in view of HIV, hepatitis C, chronic psychosis
- Expected future trends, problems and solutions.

The historical development of the Amsterdam drug problem

Amsterdam is the capital of the Netherlands. It is a fairly small, compact city of 700 000 inhabitants in a small, densely populated (15 million), affluent country. Though small, the city has always had a cosmopolitan nature, characterized by being the haven for religious refugees (Jews and French Protestants) as early as 1700 AD. The social climate is traditionally tolerant. Dramatic change occurred in the population during the 1970s due to the influx of migrant Mediterranean labourers and the migration of a large part of the Surinamese population after the declaration of independence of that country in 1974.

In keeping with the traditional tolerant nature of the Dutch, Amsterdam was a core city of the hippie subculture at the end of the 1960s. In this subculture new ways of dressing, long hair, music and illegal drugs such as cannabis and LSD were introduced. Heroin was not available. Half-refined opium used by the traditionally numerous, in large part illegal, Chinese community was also used, but it then emerged as a drug used intravenously in artist circles (jazz musicians, poets, painters). Injecting amphetamine users ('speedfreaks'), whose problems included chronic paranoid delusions and sometimes true chronic psychoses due to amphetamine, began to use opium. For the first group, opium was a creativity enhancing substance, for the latter group it was self-medication for anxiety and distress, caused by psychosis. The anxiolytic, sedative effect of opiates reduces these troublesome complaints. The total number of Dutch opium users at that time, 1972, was estimated to be 150 persons. Soon it became apparent that dressing differently and smoking pot as a relaxed manner of changing the world and its moral standards was a passing phenomenon. The world remained as it was; most hippies became regular citizens. Cannabis use integrated into normal society as a passing adolescent experimenting behaviour; LSD became less fashionable. As a result, use of illegal drugs of all types was seen by many as innocent, passing and self-limiting experimental behaviour.

This setting therefore was of a great demographic population change, combined with a decreasing economic growth in the mid-1970s (first oil crisis), and an innocent naive view of illegal drugs. This combined to create a situation of extreme vulnerability to dependent heroin use. Cheap heroin in large quantities was introduced in the summer of 1972 in the wake of American Vietnam deserters. At the same time, coincidentally, the foreign police cracked down on the illegal Chinese community due to some brutal public Triad murders in the city. As a result the opium disappeared overnight and heroin was available. This created 150 heroin users who displayed, soon after prices went up, traditional criminal 'junkie behaviour'. This was especially problematic among the former amphetamine users.

Young male Surinamese immigrants, massively migrated in 1974 from a friendly Caribbean culture and climate, to Holland with its totally different climate and living conditions, including a shortage of housing. Many ended up in improvized night shelters and spent most of the time on the street, be it with a Dutch passport, a social security check and an application for the housing waiting list. The number of people involved was staggering. In the course of approximately 2 years, 150 000 Surinamese citizens migrated to Holland, with more than one-third of those ending up in Amsterdam. As the women, children and old people spent most of their time in crowded boarding houses the young males and adolescents took to the streets as they were used to in their native Caribbean country. These young male Surinamese adolescents and adults appeared to be extremely vulnerable to dependent heroin use. Remarkable was the technique of 'chasing the dragon' which they introduced, inhaling heated (not smoked, and thus burned) heroin vapours from tin foil. This became known as 'chinesing'. The heroin abuse was not so much of a problem as a solution for this group. Feeling warm in a cold land and maintaining the traditional streetlife meant that they encountered each other continuously in specific parts of the 'Red Light' zone of the city.

Heroin was an alternative currency and a job on the street, especially so when in 1975/77 the heroin problem reached a third phase, with the introduction of a great number of white Amsterdam adolescents to heroin addiction. In contrast to the first two waves, many female users (30%) made their introduction to the drug scene, often forced into prostitution to finance their habit. The drug users belonging to this third wave adopted, in 50% of cases, the Surinamese way of oral use; the others used drugs intravenously. In the following years the drug epidemic grew, particularly because of a massive influx of foreign drug users, especially from Germany. It reached a peak in 1984 when the drug using population was estimated to be about 10 000. In the ensuing period, cocaine has become a major substance of abuse, though for most heroin is still the dominant drug. Due to the swamping of all Western Europe by heroin and cocaine, the image of Amsterdam as a drug users 'Mecca' has diminished, resulting in far fewer foreign users. Good quality, inexpensive heroin has been found everywhere in Europe since 1989.

The original introduction of individuals to drug use is an important indicator of the way the problem presents itself in the various subpopulations. It is very clear that the problem profiles for all these patients differ individually, although similar problems remain.

* For Surinamese drug users drug use has a strong social function; traditionally they avoid physical damage caused by intravenous-drug use. In the majority, the dependence is limited to heroin and cocaine. Alcohol and prescribed drugs such as benzodiazepines are avoided. These clients have the longest dependency career and life expectancy. They stayed true to their original pattern of dependence to illegal drugs.
* Drug users originating from Holland often exhibit a combination of drug dependency with underlying or coexistent psychopathology, especially in combination with injecting drug use, and if present a polydrug use pattern with alcohol and benzodiazepines that causes extreme social degradation.
* Despite the diminishing reputation of Amsterdam as 'dope-city' specific problems are still associated with foreign drug users. Many have become settled in the city. For those with no criminal background, it was possible to register officially and obtain the

rights and privileges associated with Dutch citizen status in respect of housing, social security and health insurance. For illegal foreign drug users, life has become extra hard.

The drug problem today

Quantitative data and methods

The picture in 1997 is one of a stable drug culture. Two groups seem to exist. First, the classic chronically dependent opiate user who is mainly dependent for his/her day to day functioning on heroin and or methadone, used on a daily basis. Often opiate dependence is combined with cocaine use varying from extensive use a few days a month to extremely intensive use among the drug prostitutes.

The second group consists of those involved with recreational abuse of MDMA (ecstasy) and its analogous substances, and cocaine abuse not combined with opiates. This tends to be a self-limiting and passing behaviour pattern. The main burden in the sense of morbidity and mortality, as well as the intensive chronic dependency on drug treatment as a way of surviving is limited to the opiate dependent individuals. This also goes for hospitalization and drug-related crime. In the public eye and thus the eye of the politician, this differentiation between true chronic dependency (opiates) and experimenting self-limiting behaviour often is not clearly understood. This is an important distinction for healthcare workers who need to understand treatment approaches.

The epidemiological data on the course of the opiate use-dominated population are generated by the Municipal Health Service. The MHS is a large public health organization responsible for preventive youth healthcare, for infants but also primary school students, control of infectious diseases such as tuberculosis (TB), sexually transmitted diseases (STD), AIDS and public psychiatric care. In the division of public psychiatric care, the drug department is responsible for low threshold methadone programmes including a central registration for all methadone dispensed in the city by General Practitioners, as well as by low threshold programmes. Case management projects are available for AIDS/drugs patients and for dependent parents. The department has outreach activities in which all arrested drug users are treated for withdrawal symptoms in the city police stations. Also all drug-dependent patients who are hospitalized in general hospitals for a variety of morbidities are regulated by means of a case management contact in the hospital. All activities have been recorded in detail over many years. This practice of registration was greatly enhanced on the one hand by the fact that

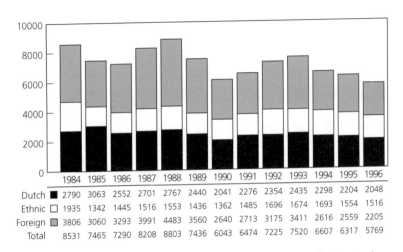

		1984	1985	1986	1987	1988	1989	1990	1991	1992	1993	1994	1995	1996
Dutch	■	2790	3063	2552	2701	2767	2440	2041	2276	2354	2435	2298	2204	2048
Ethnic	□	1935	1342	1445	1516	1553	1436	1362	1485	1696	1674	1693	1554	1516
Foreign	▨	3806	3060	3293	3991	4483	3560	2640	2713	3175	3411	2616	2559	2205
Total		8531	7465	7290	8208	8803	7436	6043	6474	7225	7520	6607	6317	5769

Figure 3.1 Estimated total numbers of opiate drug users in Amsterdam between 1985–1996. (Capture/recapture estimates)

methadone is an opiate and as such there is a need for registration of all prescriptions, dosages, dates and patient data, and on the other hand by the public health-derived need to have a high quality surveillance of data such as TB, AIDS, overdosage, death etc.

Estimates of the total number of drug users in the city are made using a capture/recapture technique based on the assumption that the same population is registered in the low threshold methadone programmes as well as in the police registrations. With both fractions known, as well as the overlap, the total number can be computed. This technique is not completely reliable. This applies especially to non-resident populations, such as the subsegment of foreign drug users. Repetition over the years with the same procedures gives some insight into the development of trends, especially if the data are in conjunction with other observations.

The mean age of the drug users in methadone programmes has been rising through the years. The mean age in 1996 for drug users born in Holland was 37 years. For those born in Suriname it was 41 years; for the foreign opiate users 38 years.

Shift from injecting to oral use

There has been a steady decline in the number of drug users using intravenously. This is due to three factors:

- a yearly surplus in mortality among injecting users compared with non-injecting users (see section on mortality below)

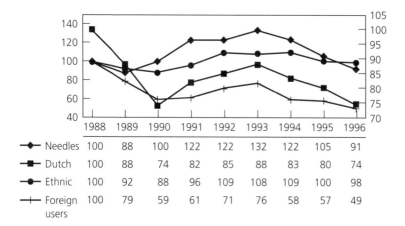

	1988	1989	1990	1991	1992	1993	1994	1995	1996
Needles	100	88	100	122	122	132	122	105	91
Dutch	100	88	74	82	85	88	83	80	74
Ethnic	100	92	88	96	109	108	109	100	98
Foreign users	100	79	59	61	71	76	58	57	49

Figure 3.2   Needle exchange in Amsterdam, 1988–1996. Index: 1988 = 100

- a shift from injecting use to oral use because of health concerns, but also because the Amsterdam opiate users are dependent for many years and have great difficulty with finding veins in which they can inject
- a decreasing number of foreign opiate users.

Morbidity

Drug-related morbidity centres in the injecting part of the drug population. Despite the greater proportion of drug users coming from ethnic minorities, especially the Surinamese, there are relatively far less intravenously transmitted viral diseases among this subpopulation because they do not inject. This is the background to their expected long survival of drug use.

HIV

For a correct interpretation of the numbers of HIV-infected drug users, one must realize that the harm reduction low threshold methadone programmes came in to existence in 1981. This was a period during which AIDS was regarded as a new American disease that did not create a risk for injecting drug users in the Netherlands. The needle exchange was started in 1984 because of a hepatitis B epidemic among injecting drug users. This resulted from the cessation of the sale of syringes by a pharmacist in the centre of the city which had

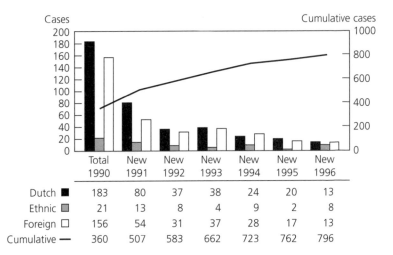

Cases   Cumulative cases

	Total 1990	New 1991	New 1992	New 1993	New 1994	New 1995	New 1996
Dutch ■	183	80	37	38	24	20	13
Ethnic ▨	21	13	8	4	9	2	8
Foreign □	156	54	31	37	28	17	13
Cumulative —	360	507	583	662	723	762	796

Figure 3.3 New cases of symptomatic HIV-infection among injecting drug users in Amsterdam

catered for the greater part of the inner-city injecting drug users. In 1985 the HIV antibody test became available. In a cohort of Amsterdam injecting drug prostitutes the prevalence of HIV was 29% (van der Hoek *et al.* 1988). When that public health calamity became known, the needle exchange was vigorously expanded, in conjunction with many HIV preventive measures which since that time have been more or less effective (van Ameijden 1994). In retrospect, because of the internationally-oriented drug use as well as the international gay community in Amsterdam, HIV infection was introduced very early into the drug scene in the city. For this reason Amsterdam was too late in avoiding a considerable HIV problem among drug injectors. In the rest of Holland the preventive measures launched in 1986 were taken in time. Epidemiological research data (Wiessing *et al.* 1996) shows the following HIV prevalence among injecting drug users. Rotterdam: 12% (1994); Maastricht: 10% (1994); Arnhem: 2% (1995); Deventer: 0% (1991); Utrecht: 5% (1996).

Observing the mode of presentation of symptomatic HIV, the incubation period passed and the declining numbers of cases, it seems correct to assume that the majority of infections can be dated back to the early/middle 1980s. It is also clear that the estimated number of 398 HIV/drug patients alive in January 1997 has put a great burden on the medical care in Amsterdam, especially since the treatment of HIV has been improved with the introduction of new effective antiviral drugs. This necessitates a further enhancement of the shared care principle between the hospital specialist, GPs and public health drug services.

Hepatitis C

A reliable antibody test for diagnosing hepatitis C infection has been available since 1992. There are indications that a great majority of injecting drug users are suffering from this chronic infection (van de Poel *et al.* 1994) as they are in other centres where drug injecting is common (Burns *et al.* 1996). A parallel exists with the problem of HIV infection. In the fated years 1982–83 the many jaundiced injecting drug users were probably not only contaminated with hepatitis B and HIV, but also with hepatitis C virus (HCV). In view of the serious consequences of chronic HCV hepatitis, such as liver cirrhosis and hepatoma after a span of 20–30 years in a substantial proportion of infected cases, depending on the type of virus, individual susceptibility and especially concomitant alcohol abuse, many HCV-infected drug users are likely to come into treatment. Recently it appears that improvement in therapy is pending. Trials under way with interferon and ribavirine point to approximately 50% of treated cases resulting in viral clearance (Bisceglie *et al.* 1995). It is clear that this expensive treatment will only work in a compliant drug user, and should be applied with reason. It is also essential that the treated HCV carriers do not resume infective injecting drug abuse after clearance of the virus.

Tuberculosis (TB)

There is a clear correlation between the incidence of tuberculosis, drug abuse, homelessness and HIV infection. Pulmonary tuberculosis is a risk, not only for drug users, but also for society in general. In the MHS low threshold programmes, half-yearly TB screening is obligatory, not only for the benefit of the TB-infected patients that can thus be treated as early as possible, but also for society in general. The still uninfected HIV positive drug user is also a very vulnerable patient.

Good results in compliance are possible when tuberculostatic agents are used along with methadone treatment. Because of liver enzyme induction by rifampicin, very high dosages of methadone are necessary. In cases where compliance is a problem, Direct Observed Therapy (DOT) is offered.

The need to be on the alert for the spread of TB among drug users in New York has been clearly demonstrated (Selwyn *et al.* 1989). It is also found in Amsterdam. In MHS methadone programmes, the yearly incidence of TB among drug users in the period 1989–93 was 386 per 100 000. This is 38 times higher than the TB incidence in the

Table 3.1 TB cases among drug users in Amsterdam 1992–1996

	1992	1993	1994	1995	1996
Male	17	21	23	21	20
Female	2	3	6	7	5
HIV-pos.	11	16	15	17	14
Dutch	6	12	12	11	11
Ethnic minorities	9	4	5	6	6
Foreigners	4	8	12	11	8
Total	19	24	29	28	25

same period observed in the general population in Holland (van Brussel *et al.* 1995).

Mortality

Mortality among drug users is strongly associated with injecting drug use. The toll of fatal overdose in Amsterdam is low, especially among those drug users using the low threshold methadone programmes. Illegal and passing foreign drug users are excluded because of city regulations. In conjunction with other indices such as capture/recapture estimates, the decreasing numbers of needles exchanged (foreign drug users practically all use intravenously), the decrease in the number of foreign overdose cases confirms the overall trend, indicated above. The studies of Grönbladh *et al.* in Sweden (1990) clearly demonstrated that in a waiting list group of drug users, the relative risk for lethal overdose was as high as 5% per year, compared with the clients who were admitted to the methadone programme before the intake to this programme was blocked for political reasons. Recent preliminary evidence in Amsterdam suggests a relation with the dose of methadone, meaning clients in dosage schemes of 60 mg or more had a lower chance of death by overdose compared with the ones with a lower dosage or only incidentally using the programme. However, care should be taken to induce clients to methadone gradually and under close observation, with gradually increasing dosages, otherwise there is a real danger of methadone overdose.

The rate of indirect mortality depends on the effect of infections caused by injecting drug abuse. The only way to prevent this would be a total change to oral use or complete asepsis when injecting. Endocarditis and abscesses are bacterial consequences of such poor

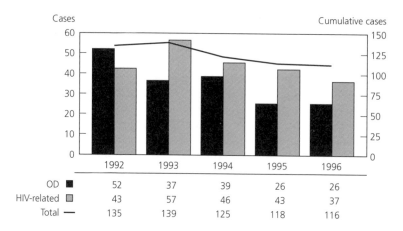

	1992	1993	1994	1995	1996
OD ■	52	37	39	26	26
HIV-related ▨	43	57	46	43	37
Total —	135	139	125	118	116

Figure 3.4 Mortality among opiate drug users in Amsterdam: direct overdose and indirect drug-related causes 1992–1996

hygiene problems. The prevention of HIV and HCV is of course of paramount importance.

Because of the time sequence of HIV infection in relation to the incubation period before immune problems emerge, HIV-related mortality is expected to decrease gradually in the coming years. The tragedy is that despite more or less effective prevention methods, the majority of HIV-negative injecting users are HCV infected. This is also the case in a great number of persons who have had drug dependency problems in the distant past, and see themselves as no longer drug users.

The development of harm reduction, a general overview

Harm reduction in Amsterdam came into being as a direct result of the enormous drug use explosion in the 1970s. Treatment facilities were literally swamped. Large amounts of public funds were invested in all sorts of approaches varying from the very strictest of the therapeutic communities to the religious movements in the form of Hare Krihsna or Christian groups, to subsidized private foundations that exploited centres where heroin dependents could inject. It was a period of political strife and dissension fuelled by public (and political) fear that asked the question: 'where will this end?' Also influential were money-hungry aid institutions. It became very clear in 1981 that truly nothing had worked. The keen disappointment was also occasioned by the false promises that many of these aid institutions had made in the recent past with an eye on that year's budget. Local political upheaval resulted in the resignation of the alderman responsible for public health.

The 'grand' scheme of methadone dispensing as it exists now came into being in 1981 (van Brussel 1996). The core of the system consisted of methadone prescription and dispensing, not only by the MHS, but also by the Amsterdam GP community, the pharmacists and various treatment centres. A specific role for these institutions had to be carved out by concensus according to needs, capabilities, and strong and weak points. An essential part consisted of the creation of a central methadone registration (CMR 1979) to avoid the double prescription of methadone resulting in overdosage, and the resale of methadone on the 'black market'.

It also meant the creation of a consultative support system for the General Practitioners, because they were not trained to treat drug patients, and in the rest of Holland were not supposed to treat drug users, especially not by prescribing methadone. Methadone prescription by the Amsterdam GP community was limited to drug patients belonging to their practices who had a satisfactory social regulation status. To integrate the Amsterdam GPs in the municipal network for the treatment of drug users, a specific primary care support project was financed. Two part-time doctors, experts in drug treatment, were made available by the MHS to support individual GPs. This included visiting individual practices and joint consultations with problematic patients.

An important feature of this development had to be the integration of the existing conventional abstinence-oriented drug-free treatment into this new system. These partners in the multilevel treatment system were afraid that if it was so easy to obtain methadone, particularly for those patients unable to quit their use of illegal drugs, nobody would want to use their facilities any more. However, intake into drug-free treatment soared. These new clients were in a better state of mind, and motivated not by the misery of the gutter, but because they truly wanted to kick the habit. This encouraging fact created a total consensus in the first part of the 1980s among almost all professionals engaged in the various parts of the multilevel Amsterdam treatment system.

This state of consensus on the need to maintain the multilevel treatment system still exists. Less is expected of abstinence-oriented treatment. It is now recognized that the methadone system may be capable of delaying morbidity and mortality, but not totally preventing it. Concern about this apparent inadequacy gave rise to new institutions of 'coerced treatment' or alternatively, to plans for heroin distribution.

The participants

The Amsterdam drug treatment consists of three levels depending on the demands that are made of patients. The better they are structured/motivated, the higher the level. Patients circulate between levels depending on their status with regard to the addiction severity index profile and to their ability and willingness to establish and to maintain a relationship with the professional and the treatment services.

Low threshold and specific programmes

These are offered by the Municipal Health Service, outreach field-work organizations and the institutions for the homeless. Basically no demands are made for abstinence as a performance criterion. The demands made consist of essential behaviour, such as no aggression or intimidation. Compliance with simple house rules such as no drug use on the premises is essential.

Public health

The MHS methadone programmes are highly structured. Strict obligatory diagnostic procedures are followed with every client, including: TB check every 6 months, 3-monthly general check-up using an adapted ASI (Addiction Severity Index) schedule in which all relevant facets are examined.

In principle, all drug users are admitted to the MHS programmes provided that they are Amsterdam registered citizens. Specific crisis intervention aimed at repatriation is available for those drug users from other parts of the country or who are of foreign origin.

The following issues are addressed in this 3-monthly examination:

- addiction severity status (amount and nature of substances used, frequency of use per day/days per month, mode of use, place of use, hygienic measures etc.) broad spectrum urine analysis
- HIV test counselling, safe use/safe sex practices
- medical status at the time of examination, including the use of medical services such as General Practitioner, dentist, hospital specialist, appointment with these providers in time, that may need to be monitored on fulfilment
- medication monitoring
- psychiatric complaints
- social status; is everything all right in regard to insurance, social security, housing, relationship with family and friends etc.

This periodic general examination provides clues/points of focus for intervention, communication with other providers, referral if necessary/possible with regard to patient compliance and past experiences, to General Practitioners or other therapeutic facilities.

The effectiveness of the programmes is determined in large part by:

- the reach and 'holding capacity' of the methadone programme
- the measure in which a structured way of providing can be applied, without being too demanding and developing into a 'high threshold' attitude, leading to exclusion of the more difficult patients
- the cooperation interrelationship with other providers, social security management and especially the city General Practitioners. An important medium of stimulation is information, preferably in the form of a detailed individual letter of a quality comparable with 'good' hospital discharge letters to the GP over his/her patient that is treated by the MHS.

Specific programmes exist for:

Drug dependent prostitutes

Because of their specific health problems, a separate methadone programme is available for these multiproblem patients, often with a background of sexual abuse as a child. Prostitution is a health-hazardous way of obtaining money for drugs. HIV counselling and anticonception prescription, control of sexually transmitted diseases (STD) and integrated outreach are important ingredients, as well as the normal structured diagnostic procedures.

Crisis intervention for illegal foreign drug users

Crisis intervention aimed at repatriation is offered to these clients. The care is combined with the care for drug dependent prostitutes. The clinic can provide long-term methadone and somatic care for those illegal foreign drug users who refuse to go back to their country of origin if they have serious health problems such as AIDS, recurrent STD episodes or other serious illnesses. To a great extent, these foreign drug users, most of them German, have lived in Amsterdam for many years and have taken on a Dutch identity. Important factors in their not having gone back to Germany are often problems with the police in their country of origin. Prostitution is an important source of money for these damaged people.

Drug dependent parents

At the beginning of the drug epidemic at the end of the 1970s and 1980s, many female drug users became pregnant, often caused by a mistaken belief that secondary amenorrhoea caused by heroin resulted in infertility. This was an important reason for stressing the need for effective contraception in combination with methadone treatment. A specific city-wide case management project was set up to ensure the safety of any children. This was to encourage the drug-using parents to provide essential family conditions including food, housing of a minimum standard of quality, and care for their child(ren). Within this project approximately half of the families are able to provide for their child. The other half of the children are under judicial monitoring or placed in another family or a foster home.

Case management for hospitalized drug patients

Often it is necessary to hospitalize, mostly acute, drug patients. AIDS-related infections were the cause in approximately half the 510 drug patient hospitalizations in Amsterdam during 1996. Drug patients have a right to quality medical treatment, during and after hospitalization. This is especially important in the case of ambulatory poli-clinical AIDS care. This means that these patients have to be compliant with the treatment, but also have to behave themselves in the hospital in an orderly, regulated fashion. Outreach case management techniques are used in which the case manager is the intermediary agent between the drug patient and nursing staff. This prevents a lot of problems, and escalations over minor issues. The goal is reached in the great majority of sick drug patients. Like other patients, drug users are very hopeful of living a normal life expectancy.

Medical care for arrested drug users

The city police arrest yearly a large number of drug users charged with drug-related crimes. The MHS traditionally provides medical support for the police such as forensic and coronertasks, but also in safeguarding the medical condition of the prisoners in the police stations. During the imprisonment of drug users, the first days are critical due to the acuteness of the onset of opiate withdrawal. Making daily medical visits to these drug users to provide medication for withdrawal and ensuring that there are no other serious medical conditions provides a good opportunity to motivate drug users to use the MHS methadone programmes when they are released. Approximately 8000 visits are made to the estimated 1800 drug users who are in custody per year.

Social support

Having an extensive network of social benefit providers is essential to the integrated working of a harm reduction system. Our society has quite a number of specific social services for the Amsterdam citizens in general. Drug users tend to be excluded because of inability to maintain appointments and disorderly behaviour in general. These characteristics applied especially during the early phase of the epidemic. Specific social services aimed at being an intermediary between client and city institutions were therefore created. These services are provided by specific institutions, often with a religious background.

One of the specific and important social services is outreach. Great importance has always been placed on specialized social workers going out into the city to look for drug users in the drug scene. These approaches are based on a confidential relationship with the drug users in an attempt to motivate them into the low threshold methadone providing programmes. This function was very important in the early stages of the epidemic when the users were young, relatively inexperienced and ignorant of the various treatment facilities. At the present time it is still important especially for the drug-using prostitutes and those drug users who are unwilling to re-enter the methadone programme. A lot of drug users with a Surinamese background choose to stay away from methadone programmes, because they prefer the continued heavy oral use of heroin and cocaine. Their main fear is fostering an extra dependency on methadone. When they develop illnesses, caused especially by cocaine base smoking (pneumonia), they come for treatment to the MHS, often motivated by the street corner outreach workers. Similar approaches are used in large US centres with ethnic minority groups (Friedman *et al.* 1987, 1992).

Social security management

A large number of drug users including non-dependent chronic psychiatric patients, have found recourse to the social security management service operated, among others, by the outreach fieldwork organizations for drug users. This service handles all administrative demands and details needed to implement the individual right to social security checks. As part of the most intensive management offered, the clients obtain their social security money twice a week, after necessary costs for paying off old debts to various state and city organizations (rent and energy debts). This service is very valuable, because it gives the opportunity to start a new social life, especially in housing. The city house cooperatives demand some guarantee of payment and of other behaviour, before they are willing to provide a new home. It is clear that with regard to the high mean age of the Surinamese drug users (over 40 years) they need to have reasonable housing. Traditionally it is possible to provide 'accompanied living' in the form of an apartment that is let on probation for a period of 3 or more months. If the drug user is able to live there without disturbing the peace, the rent contract can become indefinite.

Housing

Providing some sort of housing for the homeless drug-dependant is a core facility. In the early phase of the epidemic, housing problems existed because of the general shortage in the city of cheap housing at that time. At that time deviant behaviour associated with drug use was a complication that occasioned many involuntary removals from the house.

At the present stage of the epidemic, the main reason for not having a house is associated with dual diagnosis morbidity. Often psychiatric problems have arisen during the dependency, or have been aggravated by the chronic dependency if pre-existent before it started. This means that the qualitative nature of the homeless problem has changed from direct drug-related causes (debts, drug dealing in the house, disorder by drug use and quarrels with other users and neighbours) to psychopathology-based disturbance. The majority of the current homeless drug users cannot live independently. This has led to the plan to create 'social medical pensions', a form of halfway houses with a tolerant view of ongoing illegal drug use if at least a minimum of socially acceptable behaviour can be enforced. In the case of these social pensions, which are at the moment in the planning stage, a mixture of persons with problems will be housed. Homeless drug users will be limited to one-third of the population, the rest being chronic psychiatric patients that do not fit into regular psychiatric care. The third part will consist of homeless alcoholics and others. The institutions will be operated by existing care providers for the homeless, such as the Salvation Army and other charities.

Because it is expected that order problems will be generated by the drug users, special measures are taken to ensure a good and safe behaviour. These measures consist of the 'carrot and stick' approach, the carrot being the housing service in itself in combination with good food, a private room, linen, bed etc. These clients will also have recourse to 'heroin equivalent' euphoriating opiates, prescribed by the MHS. These opiates consist of Palfium (dextromoramide), an oral short-acting strong lipofile opiate that is popular among the older Surinamese drug users, injectable methadone and injectable morphine. The stick part of the contract includes expulsion to the street again and a less benevolent approach by the police towards public drug use, loitering and other behaviour.

Middle level programmes

In these General Practitioners programmes, clients participate with an ongoing history of active illegal drug use, without serious impairment of social life (van Brussel 1996). This means that there is not too much money spent on 'dope', no disruptive behaviour and also an acceptable presentation in the public. The crime rate among these clients is low and their medical condition is such that they do not need the frequent observation, if need be daily, that is available in the MHS programmes. With regard to methadone they must be able to self-control with a weekly or bi-weekly prescription. Clients tend to change levels periodically. Occasionally, however, after a good period, a time of disarray may follow caused by some life crisis such as the selling of prescribed methadone on the black market, unkempt looks and disruptive behaviour in the GP practice. A referral back to the MHS is the usual response. Vice versa, an MHS client can have a good period, be trained (under observation) in the way that he or she manages on a two-weekly or weekly dosage scheme with the MHS, and if successful be referred to his or her GP, who is yearly informed of her or his status. This way of operating ensures a high degree of GP willingness to take on such a client when contacted by the MHS with this request.

General Practitioners

In the Netherlands, as in some other European countries such as the UK and Germany, the General Practitioner is the gate keeper to specialized medical care. This implies that he/she sees all citizens with a medical complaint. If needed by the patient, the GP makes the referral to specific medical specialist care. All Dutch citizens have a health insurance, in the great majority 'ziekenfonds', a collective public insurance. Only in Amsterdam do GPs participate in the methadone prescription to regulated opiate drug users. This arose after a dispute in 1981 in which the local GP community refused to let itself be prohibited by the State Inspection from prescribing methadone. This stand was facilitated by the City Government and supported in practice by the MHS. Today approximately 70% of all 400 GPs in Amsterdam treat opiate drug users in their practices. They use guidelines developed by the City Professional Association, in accordance with the City Association of Pharmacists, the MHS and City Hall. These guidelines consist of the following: GP methadone clients should be:

- registered with the practice, they should be a 'known' client
- socially regulated, meaning insured, stable, with source of income, housing
- no extreme drug use
- the patient must be able to behave his/herself correctly, e.g. keeping appointments, satisfactory self-care etc.
- the patient must be able to handle a weekly prescription of methadone
- the GP is not obliged to take on the drug user. When he/she wants to stop the treatment the MHS must take the patient back immediately
- not more than ten drug patients per practice
- consultation possibilities with specialized service
- an efficient medically operated Central Methadone Register, to preclude the possibility of double prescription

In 1996, 1160 different opiate drug users were prescribed methadone by 259 different GPs. For these General Practice services, no extra income was provided.

A focus for attention in the future will be assisting the GP and evaluating the ongoing dependency history of his/her dependent patients on a specialist level. Before patients are referred to the GP, they are examined very thoroughly over a prolonged period of time. Of necessity, when treated by a GP who has no specialist training in public health addiction care, not too much attention is paid to TB screening, HIV counselling, or hepatitis C monitoring. One could choose to make arrangements directing and encouraging GPs themselves to undertake these essential heroin addiction treatment features, but it is highly unlikely that this would work. As General Practitioners are reluctant to take on large amounts of drug-related work, it has not been possible to extend their responsibilities this far.

In a recent survey among GPs they were asked about satisfaction concerning prevalent practices, information and care decisions. The resulting response of 70% of the total GP community of 400 physicians was extremely high. The greater part of respondents were satisfied. Typically they referred the complex aspects of care to specialized agencies while they embraced as their own the tasks they normally do already such as contraception, sexually transmitted disease control, diagnosis and care of physical and psychiatric problems.

Social care

There are no specific middle level institutions that provide social care to drug users. The clients of General Practitioners use, if needed because they are 'socially regulated' to begin with, the existing social facilities for normal non-dependent people.

High level programmes

These centre around the notion of the patient or client shortly reaching or actually having reached drug abstinence. These programmes consist mainly of the long-term therapeutic admissions of 6 to 8 months. The term 'high level' applies originally to traditional methadone programmes in which all medication is 'dope' and therefore tapered off. Patients should see the world with clear eyes and thus overcome their 'junky-existence' and become normal people who participate in society like everyone else.

This is politically a very attractive message because it appeals to the notion of 'healing', a cure to a 'status before' addiction, 'a drug-free nation', 'just say no' etc. One can ask the question if this pre-drug status was so satisfactory for most patients, why have they become dependent on drugs in the first place? The answer to that is that after having reached abstinence, one works into the therapy the principle of further developing one's identity, and of learning new ways to cope with the frustrations and living modalities that have led to the original drug dependence.

This concept is applied in therapeutic communities, but also in out-patient care, for instance in the form of naltrexone-assisted abstinence, reached in a few days in ambulatory form or acutely under narcosis (Legarda and Gossop 1994). Group and individual therapy are elements in an abstinence-oriented treatment. This approach is integrated in a small, structured methadone programme in the city. Of all drug treatment facilities, the high threshold programmes are by far the most attractive to the general public and politicians because they are aimed at a 'cure'. Low threshold programs tend to be seen as 'defeatist' and soft, continuing and maintaining the addiction.

In Amsterdam a great deal of money, yearly approximately £4 million (2.8 million Dutch guilders), is invested in these therapeutic high level programmes. Data on the number of intakes, dropout rates and number of patients having finished the programme are not available.

Follow-up data on continuance of abstinence after discharge are also not available.

In practice, high level programmes are a worthwhile adjunct, to keep hope alive especially in the family. The patients most benefiting from them are those who are shortly addicted, not too heavily involved in the drug scene, and not too seriously disturbed with disorders such as psychosis, borderline personality disorder, or serious depression. The indication criteria used in acute high-dosage naltrexone-induced, anaesthesia-supported ultra rapid detox, are: having a caring non-drug using involved partner or family, with substantial means to finance this expensive treatment and the guarantee of daily observed naltrexone intake over one year.

Coercive treatment

In Dutch law it is prohibited to treat a patient against his or her will. This also applies to psychiatric patients. A clear distinction is made between the right of the community to hospitalize, when necessary involuntarily, a psychiatric patient in the case of (acute) danger to the patient or the community. This might be caused by, for instance, imperative hallucinations and psychotic delusions.

The notion of coercive treatment for drug users arises in political debate from time to time, as does the debate for drug legalization. It is based on collective fear in society, and is also a measure of the discontent with interventions such as methadone treatment and therapeutic communities.

The message of drug dependence being a chronic illness for which there is no effective cure is not a popular one.

In Amsterdam, the debate on coercive treatment, led in 1987 to the 'Street-junky' project. In this activity, criminal drug users expecting a sentence of some months in jail were forced to choose between jail and a therapeutic intramural programme. As a result a large number of criminal street-junkies were hospitalized with the more or less expected result of practically immediate 'dropout', often as early as a few hours after admission in the great majority of clients. This resulted in the rules concerning the receiving of a therapeutic facility being changed and methadone maintenance being offered. However, the drug users finishing the programme mostly reverted to street drug use a few months after discharge. No hard, scientific, data are available. Expectations from residential programmes have become limited in Amsterdam as they have elsewhere (Gerstein and Lewin 1990).

Notwithstanding (or because of) this state of affairs, plans are being made to create a prison-based educational programme in some new jail complexes. The legal aspects of this new proposal which are possibly against the constitution because of human rights deprivation, are not yet consented to by the Dutch parliament. If this scheme goes through, the results may well be disappointing, for the same reasons as other coercive schemes have been unsuccessful.

Medical attitudes to drug dependent patients, shared care options

Relations between drug dependent patients and the medical profession are often strained. This is due to a reciprocal misunderstanding between patient and doctor. Typically drug patients have learned that 'dope works against anything' and it does. Opiates mask serious debilitating symptoms that would put a non-opiate user in a bed immediately. He or she tends to see doctors as people who can prescribe 'dope' or dope-like medication, but who often nag about this or that behaviour. Typically these stressful relationships develop in the work situation of physicians who have to deal with drug patients on a daily basis. The consequent loss of good relations can cause serious problems if the need arises to hospitalize a drug patient with, for instance, pneumonia, endocarditis or a soft tissue infection. Patients may not let themselves be hospitalized or leave the hospital prematurely. There may also be situations when hospitalization of drug users occurs for no obvious medical reasons.

In this situation it helps when drug dependent patients are seen in a structured situation such as a GP practice for a periodic methadone prescription. The interaction between hospital practice and general practice allows for the sharing of experience and information. The fact that so many Amsterdam physicians have some experience in methadone treatment for drug patients helps to destigmatize the drug patients in the general health systems as such. Fear of disruptive behaviour is thus lessened. There is a case management support team from the MHS that works in hospitals. These factors result in a satisfactory open climate in hospitals for drug patients. It is also possible to avoid hospitalization of all drug dependent patients in one hospital unit, which can create stigmatization and accumulation of problems in these wards and clinics.

In 1996, 510 drug dependent patients were hospitalized in Amsterdam hospitals. Fifty percent of all admissions were with an HIV-related health condition. Quality of treatment for HIV positive drug clients is associated with the degree to which they are able to participate in extramural polyclinic care after discharge. This means keeping appointments, complying with diagnostic and treatment arrangements, not being unkempt in appearance, not constantly asking for prescriptions of benzodiazepines and other drugs. Up until now, there has been a high level of success in enabling HIV positive drug clients to participate with new pharmacological therapies. In future hepatitis C will also be a major focus of attention.

Future trends

Of necessity, remarks on future trends have a speculative nature. Trends in drug use and problems associated with drug use are dominated by the question: is experimenting drug use behaviour (excluding heroin abuse), for instance with ecstasy, a passing phenomenon? Will there be no consequential pathology for the greater part of experimenters such as is the case over many years for cannabis users? Or is experimental use of ecstasy an indicator of vulnerability for other drugs such as heroin? In Amsterdam and elsewhere, an exploding heroin epidemic came out of the blue in the 1970s. It is also a fact, however, that the cocaine crack epidemic that engulfed the USA in the 1980s has not expanded to Europe, despite warnings by American experts and politicians.

It is very clear from more than a decade of experience that heroin in Amsterdam has lost its allure for young people. It is a drug for 'losers' not 'winners' and everybody, especially the young, want to be winners. This epidemiological fact means that the remaining hard-core heroin dependent patients will more and more be seen by the public for what they are: patients with a truly chronic heroin dependence with a lot of concomitant problems, who will probably be dependent on heroin and other less dominant substances for the rest of their lives.

Heroin prescription

Because of this growing recognition in the medical community of the chronic nature of the heroin dependence problem, the logical measure is to implement heroin prescription in our existing multilevel treatment system. With an eye on the Swiss (Broers 1997, Farrell and Hall 1998) but also the UK (Metrebian et al. 1996) experiences, this could mean a major step forward. Up until now heroin is not registered as a medicament that can be prescribed in Dutch pharmacopaea. The Amsterdam MHS has experimented because of the unavailability of medical heroin with the dispensing of morphine and methadone in injectable ampoules and also with Palfium (dextromoramide) in oral form. The results have been positive in 40% (morphine/methadone ampoules) to 60% (Palfium tablets) of patients. Very clearly the drug users prefer the original substance. Still the 'treatment working relationship' has bettered significantly. However especially in the case of Palfium, a euphoriating lipofile opiate that has an even shorter effect than heroin, a very intensely controlled dispensing situation is necessary to avoid overconsumption. A daily dispensing system has been essential in order to avoid excessive use resulting from powerful withdrawal effects.

Heroin is easier to handle than Palfium. Still the results generated by following 53 patients during a 1.5 year treatment programme (van Brussel *et al.* 1997) have been very satisfying. One element in the success of this project is clearly the way in which the dispensing is implemented. Daily dispensing is required and an individual treatment contract with the patient in which specific goals are enumerated, e.g. reparation of family ties, social security arrangements, medical specialist care for somatic pathology and other basic provisions.

An important new development is also the growing cooperation between MHS, police and charity organizations that exploit halfway houses for chronic psychiatric patients who were living in the streets, but possibly also for older street drug users who are offered a substitution therapy with palfium besides methadone maintenance. This is a supervised contract format including the agreement that the drug patients use their rooms in the halfway facility in an ordered, supervised fashion.

'New drugs'

Slightly alarming is the massive drug use experimenting behaviour of young people. Although we have been used to transient experimenting behaviour among youngsters with cannabis for many years, this has changed with the advent of MDMA (ecstasy) and its analogues. These are clearly 'hard drugs', not in the sense of dependency, but in the sense of danger of physical side effects, caused by toxicity or by individual susceptibility. These include hyperthermia, dehydration, hepatic failure and sudden death. Equally alarming is the neurotoxicity in simians of the substance MDMA in dosages very close to those used in recreational settings such as the rave scenes. There is also an increase in the use of 'ecodrugs' such as psylocibine containing mushrooms and South American products as guarana. The danger of these drugs is not so much dependency, but the possibility of side effects comparable to MDMA. Luckily, up until now these have been practically non-existent.

Another pattern of drug use causing some concern is the growing tendency to use anything to feel good. Luckily heroin is not yet among the substances 'en vogue', although reports from the American Drug Awareness Warning Network (DAWN) indicates an increase in heroin use among middle class citizens.

Conclusions

Drug use subcultures can emerge as a result of international changes and political decisions. In the case of Amsterdam, an immigrant population after the independence of a South American colony and the migration of young people within Europe had an influential effect on drug taking. Equally changes elsewhere can reduce or improve drug taking. In Amsterdam the widespread availability of heroin throughout Europe in the early 1980s meant less of a drug problem in that city. As many of these events are essentially outside the control of local or even national governments, flexibility over a period is required and with it the ability to respond to existing and emerging problems.

The Amsterdam system is effective in preventing part of drug use-associated morbidity and mortality. Especially overdose mortality can be practically eliminated. With HIV prevention, moderate success can be achieved, although prevention was instituted too late for a large number of chronic drug users who became infected in the early 1980s. The current harm minimization approach has prevented further spread by needle and syringe sharing. This preventative measure seems less effective for hepatitis C which seems to be more infectious, and serious thought needs to be given to this issue.

Because of the engagement of the GP community and specific support measures, drug users can and do have the same qualities of medical care as other non-drug using patients. This makes good economic as well as ethical sense.

It is possible to regulate to a high degree many of our drug users to a more or less satisfying life provided with basic necessities.

It is impossible to eliminate all drug-associated problems. Heroin prescription is a necessary step forward, but a substantial proportion of drug users will not be reached and regulated, even when medically prescribed heroin is available.

References

Alpheis, H. 1996: Hamburg: Handling an open drug scene 1996. In: Dorn, N., Jepsen., Savona, E. (eds). *European drug policies and enforcement.* Macmillan, London, pp. 55–74.

Bisceglie, A.M.D., Conjeevaran, H.S., Fried, M.W., Sallie, R., Park, Y., Yurdaydin, C., Swain, M., Kleiner, D.E., Mahaney, K., Hoofnagle, J.H. 1995: Ribavorin as therapy for chronic hepatitis C. A randomized, double blind, placebo controlled trial. *Annals of Internal Medicine* **123** (12), 897–903.

Broers, B. 1997: *Success in heroin prescribing program in Switzerland* – personal communication.

Burns, S.M., Brettle, R.P., Gore, S., Peutherer, J.F., Robertson, J.R. 1996: The epidemiology of HIV infection in Edinburgh related to the injection of drugs: an historic perspective and new insights regarding the past incidences of HIV infection derived from retrospective HIV antibody testing of stored samples of serum. *Journal of Infection* **32**, 53–62.

Fahrenkrug, H. 1996: Drug control in a federal system: Zurich, Switzerland. In: Dorn, N., Jepsen, J., Savona, E. (eds). *European drug policies and enforcement*. Macmillan, London, pp. 171–95.

Farrell, M., Hall, W. 1998: The Swiss heroin trials: testing alternative approaches. *British Medical Journal* **316**, 639.

Friedman, S.R., Des Jarlais, D.C., Sotheran, J.L., Garber, J., Cohen, H., Smith, D. 1987: AIDS and self-organization among intravenous drug users. *International Journal of Addiction* **22**, 201–19.

Friedman, S.R., Neaigus, Des Jarlais, D.C., Sotheran, J.L., Woods, J., Sufian, M., Stephenson, B., Sterk, C. 1992: Social intervention against AIDS among injecting drug users. *British Journal of Addiction* **87**, 393–404.

Gerstein, D.R., Lewin, L.S. 1990: Treating drug problems. *New England Journal of Medicine* **323**, 844–8.

Horstink-von Mayenfeldt, L. 1996: The Netherlands: tightening up of the café's policy. In: Dorn, N., Jepsen, J., Savona, E. (eds). *European drug policies and enforcement*. Macmillan, London, pp. 97–106.

Grönbladh, L., Öhlund, L.S. and Gunne, L.M. 1990: Mortality in heroin addiction; impact of methadone treatment. *Acta Psychiatrica Scandinavica* **82**, 223–7.

Laursen, L. 1996: Denmark and the Nordic union: regional pressures in policy development. In: Dorn, N., Jepsen, J., Savona, E. (eds). *European drug policies and enforcement*. Macmillan, London, pp. 151–3.

Legarda, J.L., Gossop, M. 1994: A 24 hour inpatient detoxification treatment for heroin drug users: a preliminary investigation. *Drug and Alcohol Dependence* **35**, 91–3.

Metrebian, N., Shanahan, W., Stimson, G.V. 1996: Heroin prescribing in the United Kingdom: an overview. *European Addiction Research* **2**, 194–200.

Selwyn, P.A., Hartel D., Lewis, V.A., Schoenbaum, E.E., Vermund, S.H., Klein, R.S., Walker, A.T., Friedland, G.H. 1989: A prospective study of the risk of TB among IV-drug users with HIV-infection. *New England Journal of Medicine* **320**, 545–50.

van Ameijden, E. 1994: *Evaluation of AIDS prevention measures among drug users, the Amsterdam Experience*. Dissertation, University of Amsterdam.

van Brussel, G.H.A. Buster, M.C.A., Kambiz Nasseri, van Limbeek, J., van Deutekom, H., van den Brink, W. 1995: Incidence of tuberculosis among drug users in Amsterdam methadone programs. *European Journal of Public Health* **5** (4), 253–9.

van Brussel, G.H.A. 1996: Methadone treatment in Amsterdam: the critical role of General Practitioners. *Addiction Research* **3** (4), 363–8.

van Brussel, G.H.A., Buster, M.C.A., van der Woude, D. 1997: *Evaluation report. Palfium treatment for long-term heroin drug users.* Municipal Health Service, Amsterdam.

van den Hoek, J.A.R., van Haastrecht, H.J.A., van Zadelhoff, A.W., Goudsmit, J., Coutinho, R.A. 1988: Prevalence and risk factors of HIV-infections among drug users and drug using prostitutes in Amsterdam. *AIDS* **2**, 55–60.

van der Poel, C.L., Cuijpers, H.T., Reesink, H.W. 1994: Hepatitis C virus, six years on. *Lancet* **344**, 1475–9.

Wiessing, L.G., Houweling, H., Spruit, I.P., Korf D.J., van Duynhoven, Y.T., Fennema, J.S., Borgdorff, M.W. 1996: HIV among drug users in regional towns near the initial focus of the Dutch epidemic. *AIDS* **10**, 1448–9.

4 Contemporary drug taking problems

Peter McDermott

Introduction

If one were to rely solely on the mass media for information about drugs and drug use, it might seem very difficult to comprehend why there is such a growing drug problem. Popular representations of illicit drugs and drug users all too often casts the issue in terms of a limited number of binary oppositions: sin and morality, health and sickness, criminals and victims.

Of course, reporters are not alone in falling foul of this sort of oversimplification. For far too long, expert discussion on the issue followed much the same lines. There has been a symbiotic relationship between the discourse of the popular media and that of those who worked in drug treatment, and this tendency has played an important role in directing past enquiry into drug use and drug problems. As a consequence, drug treatment and research into drug-related problems have remained in what the philosophy of science calls a 'pre-paradigmatic state'.

According to Kuhn (1970), a discipline only reaches maturity when a majority of those who work in that field have reached a broad consensus about the nature of the problem, the basic assumptions that underlie our thinking on the issue, and the tools that we use to enquire into it. While these features do not remain fixed, progress in a field will often come through the process of a 'scientific revolution', when aspects of the paradigm, or even the whole paradigm itself, are called into question and ultimately replaced; nevertheless there is sufficient agreement amongst those working in the field on a wide range of basic assumptions and beliefs.

It would be very hard to argue that drug treatment and scholarship has yet reached that stage. This is not to say that outstanding scholarship and treatment models do not exist – although both are far rarer than one would wish – but it remains extremely difficult to find any basic assumption about what it is that actually constitutes a drug problem that can secure a consensus who will support it.

In light of this, those charged with the responsibility of responding to drug problems have tended to be unduly influenced by intellectual fashions of one sort or another. Wherever you have a vacuum it becomes all too easy for poor quality ideas and theories to sweep in and take hold, and the drug treatment field has been only too susceptible to this tendency since it first began to emerge at the end of the last century. Sadly, it has not been unusual for some of the remedies that have been advocated actually to do more harm than the original problem would ever have done. Examples such as the use of heroin as a cure for cocaine addiction, or leucotomy as a treatment for heroin dependency both spring to mind.

What do we mean when we talk about 'drug problems'? It is vital to consider such definitions before approaches to treatment can be addressed. It might be helpful, therefore, before we proceed any further, to try to define exactly what it is we mean when we talk about 'drug problems'. All too often, the term evades and conceals as much as it illuminates.

Confusingly, the term is used to refer to phenomena at two levels. We talk about society having a 'drug problem', an expression that is often used to say that some proportion of our society is using drugs of one sort or another. On the other hand, we talk about an individual having a 'drug problem', and just as when talking about society, for many people this may mean little more than the fact that the said individual is using some sort of drug, more often than not, a drug that we don't approve of.

Before we proceed then, perhaps we should try and unpack these common sense definitions a little further. What exactly does it mean when we talk about the existence of a 'drug problem' at the societal level? Or rather, now that we have been forced to recognize that unlimited resources will no longer be available to tackle any problem, perhaps it may be more profitable to pose the question of what problems we face as a society as a consequence of drug use, recreational and more seriously dependent.

The notion that the existence of illegal drug use in and of itself is society's drug problem is flawed in a number of ways – most obviously because it completely obscures the problems that result from the use of alcohol and tobacco. Conspiracy theorists might even argue that it was framed in that way for precisely that reason. This definition highlights the historically and culturally determined nature of the problem. Such a definition came into being at a time when the recreational use of these substances was a new and alien phenomenon. It wasn't that we believed that recreational drug use *per se* was immoral, but rather that these particular substances were a new and undetermined risk. Racism and minority group involvement and prejudice also played its part in shaping our view as substances such as cocaine, the opiates and cannabis were associated with races and groups with marginal status. Recreational drug use had long been seen as a threat to the social order, in the form of time and work discipline, which was why legislation had been introduced governing the opening times of pubs in the UK. The link between work discipline, morality and alcohol use had also been forged in various branches of protestantism and the temperance movement. In light of this, it would seem fairly logical that the recreational use of such substances would be prohibited, and that moral disapproval would accrue to their use. The rationale behind prohibition is almost always presented in terms of health risks, but as there is now an abundance of evidence demonstrating that alcohol and tobacco are at least as harmful as many illegal drugs, and in some cases much more so, this is less of an argument. (Szasz 1987, Smith 1995).

Increasing numbers of people now reject the argument that it is inherently immoral to use one particular substance for the purposes of intoxication, while no moral connotations accrue to the use of another. Because of the relative health risks, the law is growingly seen as arbitrary and unjust, and this may be why increasing numbers of people are choosing to disregard it. The point is often made that one of the most common harms that stem from the use of illegal drugs are solely caused by their legal status.

Regardless of how one feels about the issue of prohibition or legalization then, it has become extremely difficult to sustain the claim that simple drug use is the major drug problem that we face as societies. As Nadelmann and others illustrate, the problem is not whether or not to legalize drugs, but how best to regulate the production, distribution and consumption of a large number of psychoactive substances already in use (Nadelmann 1993, Zimring and Hawkins 1992).

Changing conceptions of the nature of the problem

Let us take what is perhaps the most archetypal manifestation of problem drug use – that of heroin dependency. Looked at through one lens, it appears that what we are seeing is a problem that is pharmacologically determined. A person tries the drug, likes the way that it makes them feel, and then uses the drug repeatedly until they become physically dependent. While they have adequate supplies, they might display no obvious signs of dependence. However, when these supplies run out, the withdrawal syndrome becomes apparent. The drug user becomes physically sick, and experiences an overwhelming desire for the drug. In some people, the discomfort is so extreme that people who had previously been completely honest will now lie, cheat or steal to secure the drug.

Looked at in this way, it seems obvious that heroin addiction is solely a consequence of using heroin, a pharmacologically determined problem. For many years, this was precisely how international addiction medicine tended to regard the problem. This was not an unreasonable assumption as alcoholism seemed to model the problem fairly closely. Cast in this light, it seems obvious that prohibition is the best way to deal with it. If heroin is not available, nobody will become dependent and the problem is solved. And while such an approach may seem naive today, we should remember that it was much more enlightened than the approach that dominated in the USA, where heroin addiction was regarded solely as a criminal act. An approach which gave birth to the British System of heroin maintenance, the Americans increased control in prescribing programmes and increased custodial sentences for drug-related offences (Strang and Gossop 1994).

The pharmacological determinist model of drug dependency may have been as successful as it was because it had an obvious appeal for doctors, focusing as it did on the body and the effects of chemicals on the metabolism. However, as they gained an increasing familiarity with the subject throughout the 1960s, it became apparent that there were a number of contradictions that caused problems for this view of addiction. How could it be that some people were exposed to heroin managed to become dependent, while others, who had had a similar number of exposures, managed to avoid it? Some users seemed to be able to manage to avoid developing a dependence by spacing out their use, whereas others seemed to get addicted from the very first shot.

Given these variations, it became apparent that there was more at work than the effects of just chemicals on the human metabolism. Psychology obviously played some role in all this, but the precise role that it played remained unclear. A great deal of time and effort was expended on the search for the 'addictive personality'. Perhaps people were addicts because they had a personality of emotional problem. They looked, and sure enough, they found some people with a personality or emotional problem. But they found more people who didn't. Perhaps addicts had sociopathic tendencies? Research seemed to indicate that this was true, but back in the 1950s, a very high proportion of addicts were doctors and nurses. Could sociopathic tendencies really be that heavily over-represented in the medical profession?

As more and more psychological research was conducted, it became fairly apparent that addicts didn't suffer from a disproportionate number of psychological defects. Nor did they seem to suffer from much higher levels of mental illness. In fact, the psychological profile of the drug dependent population didn't look that different from the population in general. (Although recent research from the USA suggests that this may no longer be the case as growing numbers of 'dual diagnoses' patients – people who suffer from both drug dependency and from mental illness – are coming to light. However, it seems likely that such cases have more to do with the growing use of addictive substances in such marginal populations rather than being an inherent feature of the phenomenon of addiction.)

And so once again, just as we thought we were starting to get a handle on the issue, the complex and contradictory nature of the problem resisted all attempts to come up with any simple statements about exactly what the problem of dependency was, and how it arose.

The Vietnam war was to provide another insight that was to destroy the myth once and for all that addiction was a problem whose roots lay in individual pathology. There were a number of factors that led large numbers of US soldiers to experiment with heroin during the Vietnam war. The cultural climate of the period, political objections to the war, anger at having been conscripted, the emotional stress of being in a combat zone and the extremely low price of heroin in a producing nation all combined. The result was that an inordinately high proportion of GIs used heroin in Vietnam, with many becoming physically dependent (Robins et al. 1974, 1975).

What was surprising though, was that when these GIs returned to the USA, the vast majority of them gave up heroin without any problem at all. While this had previously been seen with people who received the drug for therapeutic purposes, the fact that such a large number of addicts who had started using heroin for recreational purposes were able to stop using without any apparent effort completely undermined all of our previous ideas about drug dependency. Subsequent studies of the men who needed heroin in Vietnam showed that about half of them used heroin on returning to the US, but only 12% became re-addicted (Robins *et al.* 1979).

One conclusion that was eventually drawn from these findings was that we could no longer continue to regard drug dependency as a phenomenon that was located solely within a pathological individual. Addiction, indeed, the effects of any psychoactive drug, was more than a simple interaction between a chemical and the human metabolism, or the chemical and its effects on the human psyche. The social and cultural context in which the drug was used was at least as important, perhaps even more important, than these other factors and any explanation or discussion of the impact of drug use on either individuals or society that didn't integrate all of these dimensions would almost certainly be lacking in explanatory power.

Drug, set and setting

Although there had been other attempts to explain and discuss drug use in sociological terms, these were almost invariably framed in terms of the discourse of the sociology of deviance, and as a consequence could only provide a partial explanation for the negative aspects of illicit drug use. Such explanations saw drug use as a response to alienation, or cultural anomie, or presented drug users as the passive victims of labelling theory. Once again, they were partial accounts of the phenomenon, predicated primarily on pathology, albeit a social pathology, rather than a more limited individual pathology. As with the pharmacological and psychological models, they concealed as much as they explained, offering no rational explanation as to why the number of illegal drug users was continuing to grow steadily despite all the death, doom and destruction that framed all of our public discourse on drugs.

The most elegant system then, for thinking about the effects of any psychoactive drug, has to take into account three specific processes, all of which interact and over-determine each other in shaping the outcome. These processes are usually referred to as 'drug, set and setting' (Zinberg 1984).

The word 'drug', as one might expect, refers to the actions of the particular pharmacological agent involved. 'Set' is shorthand for the mind-set of the user, his or her expectations, values, etc. The final variable, 'setting', refers to the physical location in which the drug is being taken. This formulation was originally devised by Timothy Leary who originally conceived of it with regard to the effects of LSD. Due to the somewhat volatile nature of an acid trip, Leary, at the time a Harvard professor of psychology, was seeking ways of attempting to make the experience more predictably positive, and so he would recommend ways to try and encourage a positive mind-set and a conducive setting in an attempt to avoid bad trips. However, it wasn't long before the wider ramifications of the equation became apparent, and the notion of 'setting' was taken to refer to the whole cultural and social context in which the drug was used, as well as the narrower micro-context of the setting in which any particular act of drug taking occurred.

Despite seeming so apparently obvious to us now, it is hard to convey the extent to which this single small insight has revolution-ized the study of drug problems, and the various strategies for dealing with them. For the first time, a coherent model was available to explain effects of drugs and drug use that could account for both positive and negative experiences of illicit psychoactive drug use, and a model that provided a meaningful way of framing and responding to drug-related problems.

Drugs and drug subcultures: a historical survey

As has been explained, attempts to get to grips with either the effects of drugs or drug problems without a good grasp of the context in which that use occurs is largely pointless, and responses that are not grounded in such an understanding are almost certain to be doomed to failure. Consequently, it is important to have some understanding of the subcultures in which use occurs, and as with any such phenomenon, the historical trends will invariably offer more in-sights than a static snapshot of this dynamic and ever-changing phenomenon.

Some of the most illuminating insights into the social and cultur-ally determined nature of drug problems can be discovered by looking at the changing face of drug use and drug users. In the 19th century, drugs like cannabis, opium and cocaine were freely available, and opium use in particular was extremely common. It could be bought in a variety of forms, from the raw tar, to soothing syrups for children that were intended to help the baby sleep, and while overdose was not unknown, it was also not particularly common. At this time, the unsanctioned use of refined drugs like heroin, morphine and cocaine were largely limited to the middle classes due to the much greater cost of such preparations. However, notions such as 'abuse' or 'problem drug use' were meaningless at the time. Such drugs were simply part of the normal repertoire, or equipment for living, and the distinction between medical use and recreational use was an arbitrary one.

It was only as the century drew on that the first signs of concern about these issues became apparent. An important part of the process of creating professional status is the process by which access to the tools of those professions is restricted to its members in a process that is referred to as 'closure'. So, for example, in the law, only barristers have the right to argue before the courts. Berridge (1984) has drawn our attention to the conflict between doctors and pharmacists in the last half of the 19th century, as each struggled for the exclusive rights to supply certain services to the public. As the most common remedy for a variety of ailments was opium, it's not surprising that much of this struggle was focused upon the unrestricted trade in the drug.

And so for the first time, in the last quarter of the 20th century, the discussion about opium use became shaped in moral terms as doctors and pharmacists began to object to the fact that a certain section of the population were using the drug for the purposes of intoxication.

In the UK, however, the pressure was primarily aimed at securing professional privilege. Concern was also growing about a similar situation in the USA. However, in the USA, the primary difference is that the moral entrepreneurs who were forming the arguments were politicians, and their arguments took on a far less benevolent tone. This was due to the fact that the USA was and is a much more diverse population comprised, in the 19th century, largely of immigrants. The discussion over drug control became phrased primarily in terms of race. As usual, the real concerns were economic, most notably the desire to break Britain's monopoly of trade with China that was founded on opium, but the politicians played to public anxieties by making racist claims, suggesting that drugs like cannabis, opium and cocaine incited black men to rape white women, endowed them with superhuman strength, and white women were being enslaved in opium dens by wily Orientals who then sold them into slavery. Eventually, the USA introduced domestic prohibition, and then went on to become the driving force behind a number of international treaties that led to drug prohibition world-wide. The most important international agreements relating to drugs control are the United Nations (1961) resolution known as the Single Convention and the (1971) Convention on Psychotropic Substances (United Nations 1990).

These measures played a crucial role in changing the shape of drug use, and also in changing the shape of the population of drug users, and the differing cultural contexts in which those changes occur can be clearly seen in the differences between the drug using populations of the two countries.

The first drug prohibition laws were originally pushed through the US congress as revenue measures, e.g. 'United States 63rd Congress. Public Law No. 233 – *to provide for the registration of, with collectors of internal revenue, and to impose a special tax on all persons who produce, import, manufacture, compound, deal in, dispense, sell, distribute or give away opium or coca leaves, their salts, derivatives or preparations'* (approved 17 December 1914). Thereafter a law enforcement bureaucracy sprang up that was determined to treat the issue as a criminal justice problem. Although some doctors attempted to provide maintenance prescriptions to their addict patients, the already existing Harrison Act (1914) was strengthened to prevent professionals from dispensing narcotics to persons whose only problem was addiction itself (Musto 1997). Hundreds of doctors were prosecuted and many were imprisoned for their humanitarian stance towards addicts and addiction. The result was that the addict population shifted dramatically. 'Respectable' people either quit, shifted their drug of addiction or were rapidly marginalized, and drug use became associated exclusively with more marginal groups.

Britain, in contrast, established a policy in the 1920s of maintaining addicts on their drug of choice, effectively operating a 'quarantine' system that was intended to allow addicts to live as normal a life as possible, while preventing other people from taking up the habit. This led to a dramatic contrast between the addict population in the two countries, and by the late 1950s drug use and addiction was limited to the criminal classes in the USA, and predominantly to therapeutic addicts in the UK, some of whom were those who worked in the medical professions and other employment.

Both systems enjoyed a measure of success in curtailing the drug problem for some 30 years or so, but in the 1950s, things began to change (Spear 1994). Drug use had always been a feature of the jazz scene, coming as it did, out of America's black urban culture. However, it might well have remained limited to that milieux had it not been for the 'beats', an American literary movement centred around figures like Jack Kerouac, Allen Ginsberg and William S. Burroughs (Kerouac 1997). These writers were influenced by both jazz music and the French Romantic poets, and so it was hardly surprising that they would go on to experiment with drugs themselves. Though controversial, they had an enormous influence with young people, both in Europe in the USA, and one of the ways in which that influence was manifested was by growing numbers of people emulating their drug use.

As a consequence, towards the end of the 1950s the trend of ever decreasing numbers of drug addicts known to the Home Office turned upwards for the first time, as the UK witnessed the birth of its first indigenous recreational drug-using subculture. While there had been small pockets of recreational use prior to this date, they tended to be associated with either immigrants or haute bourgeois bohemian types. The distinctive feature of these new drug users was their youth and their association with newly emerging pop culture. This phenomenon first came to public attention in 1950, when a raid on the 'Scott Club' in Soho netted several young people, including musician and club owner Ronnie Scott (Cohn 1987).

The growing increase in the number of addicts known to the Home Office over the next few years became a matter of increasing public concern. Whereas in the past, most notified addicts had been either medical professionals or therapeutic addicts – patients who had become addicted throughout the course of medical treatment – these new drug users were seen as delinquents rather than people suffering from a medical problem, and the old policy of quarantining addicts through maintenance prescribing started to come under question as the practice began to spread rapidly to other young people. This concern resulted in the start of a questioning of the utility of the old British System, and over the next decade, the UK was to follow increasingly the lead of the USA in the shape of its policy responses to the problems of drug use and addiction.

Drugs and British youth subculture

In his ethnographic studies of the hippy and biker subcultures, sociologist Paul Willis utilizes the concept of 'homology' to describe the symbolic fit between the lifestyles and the values of such groups, in an attempt to demonstrate a coherence between their subjective experiences of its members and the cultural artefacts that they use to express a sense of identity (Willis 1976, 1978). While use of the concept has since been largely limited to discussions of clothes, musical forms, design, etc., Willis's original study made much of the role that drugs played in this homology, arguing that it was the homology between the alternative value system (i.e., 'turn on, tune in, drop out'), hallucinogenic drugs, and the acid rock music of the era that was to make hippy culture cohese as a 'whole way of life' for the individual members.

This phenomenon of a homology between the preferred intoxicant of a youth subculture, and its attitudes, values and cultural artefacts seems to run throughout the whole history of British youth sub-cultures, and has probably played an increasingly important role in shaping them since the issue first emerged at the end of the 1950s.

After their appearance in the jazz clubs of Soho, the next context that illegal drug use surfaced into the public arena was in the growing 'mod' subculture of the early 1960s, and once again, we can see the fit between the sharp, fashion conscious style of the mods, their concerns with status and superiority and their preference for various forms of dance music and 'all nighters' with their drug of choice – amphetamines. Indeed, so close is the fit between the pharmacological effects of speed and the various values and symbolic practices of the mod subculture, that it begins to become apparent that the relationship between culture and drug use may well be a dialectic – with the pharmacology of various drugs shaping aspects of our social and cultural life, which then go on to determine the boundaries of how we experience the effects of those drugs.

Drug subcultures today

The role that drug use has played in shaping youth subcultures is far from being limited to the 1960s, and its effects can be traced through later subcultures such as Punk. However, the influence was probably never greater or more profound than it has been in the last 10 years.

As yet, we are still too close fully to comprehend the full impact that MDMA (ecstasy) has had on British society, but there can be little question about the profound and dramatic impact that it has had on young people's lives. As with earlier youth subcultures, we can see a very close fit between the effects of the drug, its most valued primary effect being the capacity to induce intense feelings of empathy between those who use it, and the club culture that developed as its use spread. From the end of the 1980s onwards, Britain's nightclubs were increasingly becoming locations designed for the optimum enjoyment of the drug experience, as MDMA's effects began to shape not only the psyche of the user, but ultimately, large sections of the British leisure industry as well.

Not only was it the music, the lighting, and the effects in clubs that were influenced by the drug, but fashion came under its influence as clubgoers eschewed designer clothes and 'dressed to sweat'. The geography of the clubs was altered as well, with many initiating 'chill out' spaces, where music was slower and people could relax after a period of compulsively repetitive dancing. As ecstasy displaced the use of alcohol, clubs began to stock ever increasing varieties of soft drinks (often charging similar prices to those charged for alcohol), and the alcohol industry faced a minor crisis over their loss of the use market. They responded to this challenge with the introduction of 'alco-pops', a move that cynics may see as aimed at capturing an even younger market.

However, MDMA was not the only drug in the clubgoer's pharmacopea, and since the initial boom of the late 1980s and early 1990s, British club culture has fragmented once more, with each fraction having their own distinctive music, dress style and preferred drug. The 'techno' scene is fuelled by acid and amphetamine; the 'hip-hop' scene by cannabis; 'jungle clubs' are associated with crack and cocaine; 'speed-garage' with champagne; while 'handbag house' clubgoers stick with the now conservative favourite, MDMA. As ever, the music played is made by the clubgoers themselves and so is directly influenced by the effects of the drugs that they use on the dance floor.

The failure of drugs prevention

There have been two primary strategies that governments have used to deal with the 'drug problem' at the macro level, interdiction and demand reduction. Neither has had any apparent impact, beyond the continued appeasement of the USA, for whom the 'war on drugs' has replaced the Cold War as their prime foreign policy objective.

Arising from the Maastricht treaty, the establishment of Europol in 1993 has strengthened pre-existing attempts to reduce supply and trafficking of drugs into and within Europe. The consequent national implementations of drug prevention initiatives were conceived as a strategy to reduce demand as the second line of prevention – in the expectation that reduction in supply to anything less than current levels is likely to be an unobtainable goal. Different European countries showed a wide diversity of policies on drug users. These ranged from a relaxation of police activity against cannabis use and possession, to decriminalization of possession of any drug in Italy and Spain, to increasing social reaction against drug users in France, and targeting of users of 'crack' cocaine by police in the UK (Dorn et al. 1996).

Until very recently, all drug prevention was primary prevention that was grounded in the premise that the problem was drug use itself, rather than the problems associated with use. As a result, drug prevention initiatives did little more than confirm the beliefs of those people who were never at risk of using in the first place, while having little or no impact whatsoever on those people who were going to use drugs.

Of course, the reason such initiatives have little visible impact on drug taking is because illegal drugs have now become an integral part of British youth culture. While illicit drug use was still limited to a deviant minority, it remained possible to disseminate the sort of information that is characteristic of such campaigns. However, once drugs had reached the sort of levels that they have in the last 10 years, campaigns based on scaremongering portrayals of the negative effects of such drugs, and exhortations to young people to 'just say no' had lost any possibility of having any significant impact. There are two central problems that are inherent prevention campaigns of this nature: firstly, the information presented is contradicted by most young people's experience of drugs and drug users, and secondly, illegal drug use is extremely fashionable among young people. It has been for the last 40 years now, and as yet this trend shows no signs of abating.

Consequently, it has become less and less convincing to regard drug use as a deviant activity that is the prerogative of delinquent youths; in fact it is becoming increasingly likely that soon it will be those young people who do *not* use illegal drugs who are regarded as deviant. Illegal drug use has become an integral part of the lifestyle of a major section of our community, and in light of these changes, our definition of what we mean when we talk about a 'drug problem' have also had to change.

In the early 1970s, there was often a surplus of resources aimed at tackling drug problems. So much so that it wasn't that unusual to find people who were doing hospital in-patient detoxification, and even longer spells in a therapeutic community for nothing more than a parent's concern about their smoking cannabis. Today, in contrast, the numbers of people seeking in-patient treatment for heroin or cocaine addiction far outnumber the available places – even if the local authority has the funds to pay for such a treatment.

Therefore it has become essential that those who are charged with dealing with drug users learn to prioritize, and come up with innovative strategies that enable us to tackle these problems with the efficiency that characterizes our responses to other medico-social problems.

Of course, such things are far easier said than done, but in order to move forward in tackling these issues, a break with the paradigms of the past is necessary. One such issue is the tendency to focus on pharmacology in isolation from culture – both of which collaboratively interact to shape the psychology of the problem drug user. For example, one area that seems to be vitally important in our understanding of drug problems and how we can best address them is the role that drugs play in shaping the user's sense of identity. Anyone who has much experience of talking to drug users outside the constraints imposed by the unequal power dynamic of the criminal justice system or some of the more coercive treatment facilities, is well aware of how old-fashioned concepts such as the role of 'peer pressure' are inadequate when it comes to describing the positive ways in which many users actively embrace the opportunity to try illegal drugs for the first time.

This issue also plays an extremely important role in determining the likelihood of relapse. Many addicts acknowledge that the physical withdrawal is the least of their worries. While there has been a significant amount of work done on the subject of craving, the focus may be too narrow, focusing mainly on responses to cues. In fact, the decision to use again is often made long before people are exposed to any cues. When they try to leave behind their drug use, they are leaving behind a central part of their sense of identity, their community, their status. Not just the things that they feel bad about, but also everything that ever made them feel good about themselves. In order to help people to reconstruct these identities in a more positive and less damaging ways, some insight into the internal logic of these identities is required.

One mistake that many people who work with drug users make is to regard the drug subculture as a single, monolithic culture and this tendency to lump all drug users together can often be extremely damaging to any attempt to form a therapeutic alliance with the client/patient. Most drug users prefer professionals who will acknowledge their lack of experience of their culture, but show a preparedness to be non-judgmental and a willingness to learn about it, to the sort of 'know-it-all' types who smoked pot once in the 1960s and profess insight that they are all too obviously lacking.

Rather than present the usual taxonomical list of the various illegal drugs and their associated problems then, it may be far more helpful to attempt to try to view the problems created for individuals by the drugs they use rather than concern ourselves with the individual drugs. The view of the severity of drug use is often wrongly based on an incomplete understanding of a drug type or worse still upon its legal status. Looking at the problems encountered by drug use is a more pragmatic way of designing helpful intervention and a successful way of engaging drug users who may not share the drugs workers' concerns about drug use. This idea of identifying the problems rather than the drug has been the basis of the intensely practical approach taken by the Manchester 'Life-line' Project.

Division of drug users into groups depending upon their likely problems and needs makes a practical structure for designing appropriate interventions. It effectively seeks to divide the population of drug users into two halves – Group A refers to those whose use is occasional, recreational and relatively unproblematic, while Group B refers to those people whose drug use is more chaotic, dependent or risky. As with any model, this greatly oversimplifies the true range of patterns in the ecology of drug use, and conceals the great extent to which there is overlap between these ecologies. The distinction was, however, responsible for some important advances in the way that services began to think about targeting client groups and producing new strategies for secondary drug prevention campaigns. Rather than continuing to pursue the impossible goal of attempting to prevent drug use altogether, such campaigns focused on seeking to delay or prevent that transition between Group A and Group B – often involving members of those groups themselves in the production of the materials, in an attempt to guarantee the insight into the culture that is believed to be necessary if the material was to speak to those groups with a credible voice.

While Lifeline's use of this typology of Group A and Group B is a sophisticated one based primarily on the differing cultures of the two groups, it is also possible to allocate drug users to one group or other in a much cruder fashion – simply by determining their drug or drugs of choice. The main drugs favoured by Group A include cannabis, LSD, amphetamine, MDMA and possibly cocaine if used intranasally (snorted). Those users allocated to Group B tend to use heroin and other opiates, benzodiazapines, and cocaine either smoked in the form of crack (cocaine freebase) or injected intravenously. Again, it is important to stress that the boundaries between such groups are not hard and fast, and it would be a mistake to see these cultures as being totally pharmacologically determined.

Nevertheless, both pharmacology and, almost just as important, the method by which the drug is administered, play an important role in determining which group to which a user belongs. Someone who injects amphetamine regularly will almost certainly share more characteristics with Group B, despite the fact that amphetamine is usually seen as a Group A drug. Likewise, someone who has only ever snorted coke has very little in common with the chaotic cocaine injectors and crack users that inhabit Group B.

Group A users are much more likely to be employed, much less likely to have a criminal record, tend to have better relations with family and friends, and a much better support system to deal with problems. All of these factors make members of Group A much less likely to experience drug-related problems, and much better equipped to deal with them should they arise. This is not to say that professional help is not sometimes necessary for members of this group, but simply that it is the members of Group B who suffer the more intractable problems and consequently make the greatest demands on services.

Commonly used drugs and their effects

Despite having spent so much of this chapter discussing the importance of culture in the production of the subjective experience of drugs, drug use and thus upon drug-related problems, it is important to remember that these things are not solely culturally determined and that pharmacology still plays an important corresponding role in these processes. It remains essential then, for those with the responsibility of working with these problems, to have a good understanding of these substances, how they are used, their subjective effects and any problems associated with their use. While much fuller accounts of these issues can be found elsewhere (Andrew Tyler's book, 'Street Drugs' being one particularly comprehensive and accessible guide to this subject), what follows is a brief look at some of the key issues that each of these substances raises.

Cannabis

Cannabis is the meat and potatoes of illegal drug use in the UK, and is used by literally millions of people. The drug comes in a number of forms:

Marijuana is comprised of the top leaves and flowers of the cannabis plant, and is referred to as grass, weed, ganga, sensimillia or sensi, etc. In recent years, there has been an increasing tendency towards high potency strains of marijuana bred in Amsterdam and grown indoors under lights. Although there is a wide range of varietal names given to these strains by the seed breeders such as Northern Lights, Haze, Big Bud, etc. this type of marijuana seems to be most commonly referred to by the name of the most popular strain – Skunk. Although there has been a fair amount of scaremongering about these particular high potency strains in the media, there is no evidence to suggest that they are any more harmful than any other strain of cannabis.

Hashish is another cannabis product, made from the compressed resin of the marijuana plant. Known as dope, puff, rocky, slate, draw and a host of other names, it looks completely unlike marijuana, which appears as a green dried herbal product. Hashish appears in block form, in colours that vary from pale blonde to dark black, and consistencies ranging from soft and pliable like modelling clay, to hard and unyielding, almost like a stone. This is the form most commonly available in Europe. The third and least common form of cannabis product is hash oil. Sometimes misleadingly referred to as THC, the major psychoactive ingredient of cannabis, this product is made by dissolving the resins from the plant into a solvent, which is then evaporated off leaving a brown, viscous substance that is usually smeared onto cigarette papers which are then rolled around the tobacco from a cigarette.

The most common method of using cannabis is by smoking, although it can also be eaten as well. There is often some ambiguity when trying to classify cannabis by its effects, because so many of its qualities are unique to the drug and often dependent upon the individual user. In small doses, it makes one relaxed and happy. In larger doses, particularly when eaten, the effects are similar to psychedelic drugs like LSD and can cause severe anxiety and paranoia. However, all effects wear off in a couple of hours.

Cannabis is probably the safest of all of the illegal drugs. It is not physically addictive, but like most pleasurable activities, it can be extremely habit forming and many cannabis smokers become mildly agitated when supplies run low. Some experts have argued that this is evidence that cannabis is, in fact, addictive, but among other experts this view is not commonly shared. Although there is no conclusive evidence that the active ingredients in cannabis can do any harm and there have been no deaths attributed to cannabis overdose, this does not make it totally harmless. Any substance that is smoked is bound to have a detrimental impact on the respiratory tract, but perhaps the most obvious harm that derives from smoking cannabis are the legal consequences. Around 40 000 people are prosecuted for cannabis offences every year in the UK and such a prosecution can put an end to any possibility of a career in many occupations. Summary data suggest cannabis is increasing in Europe, Australia and New Zealand and has been extremely high for some years in the USA (Hall *et al.* 1994).

Psychedelics

Lysergic acid diethylamide (LSD)

LSD (Also known as acid, trips, cardboard and microdots) is the archetypal psychedelic drug. The term psychedelic comes from researcher Humphrey Osmond, who was irritated by the way that psychedelics were then seen as psychotomimetics (drugs that induce a psychosis-like state). Osmond also argued that the term hallucinogens was regarded as a misnomer, because LSD produces pseudo-hallucinations as the user knows that the visions are produced by the drug, in contrast with the hallucinations produced by amphetamine or cocaine psychosis. These are 'true' hallucinations as the user believes that those dwarfs that he sees following him out of the corner of his eye are really there (Osmond 1973).

LSD initially became popular in the 1960s when a number of influential people decided that the drug was capable of astonishing effects (Leary and Burroughs 1989). Not only did it produce profoundly mystical experiences, it cured various mental illnesses, most notably alcoholism and could enhance one's creativity. Unfortunately, it also inspired huge amounts of pretentious and trivial nonsense that some people deluded themselves into believing to be profound in some way. LSD had the strange quality of imbuing almost everything with some sense of deep meaning.

LSD today is usually sold in much lower doses than it did in the 1960s and 1970s. The average tablet or microdot then was around 200 microgrammes, whereas today's 'blotting paper' is more likely to be around 50. However, popular rumours about acid being adulterated with amphetamine or strychnine are as untrue now as they ever were. Differences in effect are due to the differences in dosage, or just the fact that the subjective experience of the drug is inherently diverse.

Like cannabis, LSD is not physically addictive and has no adverse physical side effects. There are many people who after taking the drug had some difficulty returning from the states that they achieved. It may well be that these people were already predisposed to psychological problems or mental illness before they ever took acid, and anyone who is a high potential risk for such problems should be advised to avoid taking the drug.

Most bad experiences are simply panic or anxiety reactions and are temporary. In such circumstances, the best treatment is often a change of environment to a place where the user can feel more secure, and a sympathetic friend who can offer reassurance and talk the user down. If this proves ineffective and more drastic measures are required, a sedative will end the trip by putting the user to sleep.

Phenylethylamines – the psychedelic amphetamines

MDMA, MDA and MDEA are the most common substances that are sold as ecstasy. All members of the phenylethylamine family, these are structurally related to both speed and also to mescaline (an LSD-like psychedelic that is rarely seen in the UK).

Although MDA has been available on the American black market since the 1960s, it never really made a significant appearance in the UK until after the demand for MDMA among British clubgoers started dramatically to outstrip supplies at the end of the 1980s.

MDMA (methylenedioxymethamphetamine, ecstasy)

MDMA, or 3,4 methylenedioxymethamphetamine, had an extraordinary impact on the British drug scene. A totally new category of drug, unlike all previous substances, ecstasy seemed to be an extremely safe, extremely manageable substance when it first appeared on the market. A well-kept secret for most of the 1970s and early 1980s, MDMA was increasingly being used in the USA by therapists, who valued the chemical for its remarkable ability to create a sense of empathy and facilitate communication. Clients seemed able to talk about very traumatic incidents without experiencing any pain, and it invariably left users feeling that their lives had changed in some subtle but positive way. Eventually, the drug slowly made the transition from the therapist's office onto the street.

MDMA acts primarily on the emotions and feelings by creating a sense of empathy. It is short-acting, a dose lasting around 3–4 hours, compared with LSD's 8 hours and more. Initially, users noticed that it didn't have the uncomfortable side effects associated with amphetamine. People weren't kept awake all night, grinding their teeth. For a brief period, it seemed to be the perfect recreational drug. Then, gradually, people started to notice that perhaps it wasn't quite as benign as it had originally appeared. Inexplicable collapses, many of which resulted in death, began to be reported. At the same time, the enormous growth in demand led to a massive growth in counterfeit MDMA. Much of this was actually MDA, a stronger, longer acting and more psychedelic substance which may be more toxic than MDMA. Other tablets proved to be MDEA, a similar substance but lacking MDMA's capacity to produce the strong feelings of empathy that the drug was valued for. Other tablets sold as ecstasy included ketamine, a dissociative anaesthetic related to PCP, and many others which contained no active drug whatsoever – dog worming tablets, oxygenating tablets for fish tanks, paracetamol. You name it, somebody, somewhere was passing it off as an 'E'.

However, it wasn't the counterfeit tablets that caused these deaths; they were all caused by real MDMA, in many cases, as little as a single dose. At present, the exact mechanism of this collapse is not known. Some researchers have speculated that these incidents may be related to heat-stroke, but at present the reasons behind them are unclear.

These accidental deaths are not the only problem associated with ecstasy. Research with primates conclusively shows that drug damage to the neurotransmitter nerve terminals of the brain, and while this has yet to be found in humans, there are strong reasons to suppose that it is a possibility. The drug has also been implicated in an increase in various psychiatric problems, most notably depression, which is probably caused by depletion in the neurotransmitter serotonin.

Stimulants

Amphetamines

During the 1960s and early 1970s, almost all the amphetamines consumed came as legitimately produced pharmaceuticals that were diverted from medical supplies. Originally prescribed for people dieting, by the 1970s the medical profession recognized that the risks far outweighed the benefits, and now they are only prescribed for conditions such as narcolepsy. Today, virtually all of the amphetamine sold on the black market is illicitly produced. The usual form is a white powder, although haphazard production methods mean that the colour can vary widely. According to police analysis, the average amphetamine content in a wrap of speed tends to be about 4%.

Referred to on the street as speed, whizz, billy, go-faster, amphetamine is taken intranasally, swallowed in a drink or injected, and though not physically addictive, excessive use can lead to psychological dependence. Many amphetamine users engage in long periods of use, during which they go without sleep. This can result in depression or amphetamine psychosis, a form of temporary psychosis that appears similar to schizophrenia. The user sees things that aren't there, often little men in the periphery of his or her vision, or bugs crawling on or beneath the skin, and may also suffer from intense paranoia or hear voices. Usually, these symptoms will pass after a period of abstention and sleep. However, as with LSD, in those subjects with a predisposition towards mental disorders, amphetamine use can be the catalyst for a chronic mental illness.

Cocaine

During the 1970s and early 1980s, cocaine had a reputation for being the rich man's drug of choice. Its high price and short duration put it beyond the reach of most drug users on anything other than special occasions. By the middle of the 1980s, however, the price of cocaine was steadily dropping, and as American markets became saturated, South American drug cartels began to expand into the European market. In 1977, the average price of a gram of cocaine in the UK was around £80. Today, 20 years later, the same gram can be bought for £50 or even less.

Sold either as cocaine hydrochloride (coke, charlie, white) for snorting or injecting, or in its freebase form (crack, rock, stones, wash, base) for smoking, cocaine is prized for its intense but very short acting rush. The peak effect of a snort of coke lasts maybe 30 minutes, whereas the peak effect from a hit of crack lasts maybe three minutes. The intense, exciting high, is followed by an equally intense crushing depression that users feel can only be relieved with another hit, and compulsive users may go through as much as a quarter ounce a day, often more, just smoking and smoking until they go crazy or the money or the drugs run out. Some people spend everything that they have in the attempt to avoid the crash and just keep on basing. (For diagnostic criteria of dependency, see Table 4.1.) Like amphetamines, cocaine was long regarded as a drug that wasn't physically addictive. However, as the price has dropped, and the use of freebase has become more common, we began to see patterns of use that were actually more compulsive and more self-destructive than that of heroin and it rapidly became apparent that the issue of physical addiction was moot. The depression that followed a period of cocaine use was just as much of a prompt for the user to go out and use again, regardless of the negative consequences, as physical withdrawal was

Table 4.1 Diagnostic criteria for cocaine dependency

Loss of control:
- Inability to stop using or refuse cocaine
- Failure to self-limit use
- Predictable or regular use
- Binges for 24 hours or longer
- Urges and cravings for cocaine

Exaggerated involvement
- Self-proclaimed need for cocaine
- Fear of distress without cocaine
- Feelings of dependency on cocaine
- Feelings of guilt about using cocaine and fear of being discovered
- Preference of cocaine over family, friends and recreational activities

Continued use despite adverse effects:
- Medical problems (e.g. fatigue, insomnia, headaches, nasal problems, bronchitis)
- Psychological problems (e.g. irritability, depression, loss of sex drive, lack of motivation, memory impairment)
- Social/interpersonal problems (e.g. loss of friends or spouse, job difficulties, social withdrawal, involvement in road traffic accidents, excuse-making behaviour)

Washton AM, Gold MS, Pottash AC, Opiate and cocaine dependencies: techniques to help counter the rising tide. *Postgrad Med* 1985; **77**: 293–300.

for any heroin addict. What's more, there is no 'magic bullet' treatment that can be used to stabilize cocaine users in the way that methadone is used for people addicted to heroin. Complete abstinence seems to be the only intervention that is viable. There is considerable interest and investment in the USA in the identification of a pharmacological treatment for cocaine dependence. Several substances have been tried experimentally (Arndt *et al.* 1994, Mello *et al.* 1993), some unsuccessfully (Grabowski *et al.* 1995). However, expanding all approaches to treatment is seen as a priority in the USA (Fulco *et al.* 1995). For the time being, treatment is largely behavioural and supportive. Relapse is high but in some groups long-term abstinence is better than others. As in other dependency treatment outcomes, the older more stable individual with preserved family, social and work contacts recovers more completely (Gold 1997).

Depressants

Benzodiazepines

When the benzodiazepines were initially introduced, the drug companies claimed that they had finally produced a range of anxiolytics and hypnotics that lacked the side effects of the amphetamines and the barbiturates. Benzodiazepines were presented as safe, nonaddictive, and with a low abuse potential, which just goes to show how wrong drug safety studies can be. This group of drugs was introduced as a safe alternative to barbiturates which had been responsible for considerable drug dependency problem in the 1960s.

These drugs are generally used for one of two purposes. Some benzodiazepines are prescribed as tranquillizers aimed at reducing anxiety. These include Valium (diazepam), Xanax (alprazolam), Ativan (lorazepam), Halcion (triazolam), Librium (chlordiazepoxide) etc. and rapidly replaced the role of amphetamines as 'mothers little helper'. The other major medical use of benzodiazepines was to replace the barbiturates as hypnotics for people suffering insomnia. The most common sleepers are Normison (temazepam) and Mogadon (nitrazepam).

After issuing millions of prescriptions for these drugs every year, it eventually became apparent that the benzodiazepines were in fact highly addictive and had a very high abuse potential. All of these substances are both physically and psychologically addictive, and are especially dangerous if mixed with alcohol. Nevertheless, they remain very popular with the hard-core, chaotic drug users who are characteristic of Group B, as discussed above, as well as with alcoholics who do not consider themselves part of the illicit drug subculture.

Benzodiazepines have a tendency to make the user lose control of their faculties, especially if mixed with alcohol. Inhibitions and competence are both lowered, and users stagger around appearing drunk, often getting into very dangerous situations. Benzodiazepines are highly addictive, and mixed with alcohol or other drugs, they have a potentially dangerous cumulative effect. As with barbiturates, convulsions are a serious side effect of withdrawal (Robertson and Treasure 1996, British National Formulary 1997).

Heroin

Heroin has always associated with an outsider subculture, addicts being seen as beyond the pale of the mainstream drug subculture. At the beginning of the 1980s, however, heroin use underwent an enormous process of democratization when there was an enormous influx of the drug that appears to have been linked with the revolution in Iran and the war in Afghanistan. As with cocaine in the late 1980s and early 1990s, heroin went from the margins to the mainstream, replacing cannabis as the drug of choice on council estates all over the UK. Other factors involved here may also be related to the processes through which the new phenomenon of illegal drug use was spreading throughout the community – initially via a cultural and intellectual elite, then snowballing until it eventually makes its way through the whole of society. During the late 1980s, as illicit drug use became less expensive and widely associated with the underclass, there was an increasing tendency in the USA for the more functional members of these elites to give up their use. This process has been particularly evident in the USA in the period between 1960 and the present, but is also true to a lesser extent here in the UK. As a consequence, we are likely to see wide variations between the population of heroin users in the 1960s and the population of users today.

Prior to this, the old British System of attempting to avoid the development of a black market by supplying users with a moderate supply of the drug had been largely successful (Spear 1994). Heroin was rarely available in any serious quantities, and what was available tended to be diverted from pharmacological sources. However, there had been a trend towards abandoning the British system throughout the 1970s, as Drug Dependency Clinics moved away from prescribing heroin, first to injectable methadone and then to oral methadone, and simultaneously, from the use of maintenance prescribing to short-term detoxification (Mitcheson 1994).

Heroin comes in three different forms. Grade III heroin from the golden triangle countries of Burma, Thailand and Laos is a white powder that is very close to pharmacological diamorphine hydro-chloride (Wodak *et al.* 1993). This is rarely seen in the UK, but dominates heroin markets in the East Coast of the USA. 'Tar' heroin comes as a black lump that looks like tar. Produced in Mexico, it is mainly limited to markets on the West Coast and southern states of the USA. The form most commonly found in the UK is the brown 'heroin base' produced in the 'Golden Crescent' countries of the near and middle east – Afghanistan, Pakistan, Turkey, Lebanon, etc. A brown powder, it was initially intended as a product for smoking. However, it is commonly injected after first being dissolved in some form of acid. Vinegar, lemon juice or citric acid are most commonly used for this purpose. Throughout recent years a trend away from injecting heroin has been associated (especially in the USA) with increased occasional use by the middle class population which avoided it as a drug of choice in the 1980s.

Despite its reputation, heroin's major side effect is addiction. There is no evidence that the drug causes any organic damage, even after long-term use. Nevertheless, there are a range of problems associated with any drug that is injected, and novice users and chaotic drug users who mix their use of heroin with other depressants run a serious risk of overdose.

Other drugs used

A wide variety of other substances and compounds are used, falling into several categories. Depressants such as benzodiazepines have already been mentioned, but others such as solvents and gases and alcoholic preparations often assume importance in their abuse poten-tial. Solvents such as butane lighter fuel in aerosols have been shown to be frequently tried by school-aged adolescents and between 1985 and 1991 100 people died from their use (British Medical Association 1997) in the UK. Other opiates used are several including buprenor-phine, dextromoramide, dipipanone, pethidine and others and largely have similar effects to morphine and heroin. Their mode of use, for example by injection, and variety of lengths of action vary and influence their use. Other drugs of varying importance include cyclizine, ketamine, khat, GHB (gammahydoxybutyrate). Anabolic steroids are increasingly used and abused in 'fitness' clubs and injection gives rise to risk of infection. Some authorities consider them to have psychoactive abuse potential.

Conclusion

Drug taking and our understanding of drug taking has, and is, undergoing fundamental changes. A greater range of drugs is being used by a larger sector of the population in many countries. Conventional issues about the damaging effects of drugs are being challenged. The damaging effects of punitive policies towards drug takers are being regarded as much as a cause for concern as the effects of the drugs themselves. More complicated still, the effects that legislation and prohibition have in ever-increasing side effects such as the spread of blood-borne viruses or death from overdose, highlights the need to separate the dangers of drugs from the outcomes which we currently measure.

The effects on healthcare and social care workers are important. The rigid notion of drug takers based on the knowledge of drug type is no longer useful as modes of use change and re-examination of the changes of individual drugs come about. Understanding the social situation as a cause for drug use and an inhibition to recovery must have a fundamental impact on treatment services. As numbers increase, side effects and complications of drug use increase, even rare idiosyncratic reactions become more common and visible when total numbers using the drug or drugs increase.

New patterns of drug taking, increasing numbers and new drugs all challenge treatment services. Multimodal therapy centres have become more common in the USA as the need to sort the needs of those with a variety of drug problems into a variety of types of therapy is required. A better understanding of the complexity of drug types and the problems resulting makes treatment less controversial and hopefully more successful.

Throughout the last century, drug taking policy has been dominated by the need to exert control rather than the need to understand. Legal and political requirements have dominated the agenda often for economic reasons. The results have been a lack of understanding of drugs and why people take them. Drug taking depends upon availability, fashion and social conditions and as seen over several decades less on social approval or constructive legislation. Social trends draw large numbers into new waves of drug taking, and controlling legislation often determines that the mode of use is the most damaging rather than the least damaging. Illegality encourages poor conditions, and in repressive regimes illegal trade flourishes.

The mode of drug taking is frequently connected with its illegal status and precipitates crises like that of HIV in injecting drug users or excessive dance drug use in the 1990s.

Although international upheaval is unpredictable, by its nature out-of-control drugs trade depends upon these other factors, and damaging drug use upon the system in which it exists. A confused, repressive and reactive system based on control and punishment is more likely to create problems than an understanding and knowledgeable system with support for those with problems such as drug dependence.

References

Arndt, I.O., McLellan, A.T., Dorozynsky, L., Woody, G.E., O'Brien, C.P. 1994: Desipramine treatment for cocaine dependence: role of antisocial personality disorder. *Journal of Nervous Treatment Disorders* **182** (3), 151–6.

Berridge, V. 1984: Drugs and social policy: the establishment of drug control in Britain 1900–1930. *British Journal of Addiction* **79**, 18–29.

British Medical Association 1997: *The misuse of drugs.* Harwood Academic Publishers, Amsterdam, pp. 5–35.

British National Formulary 1997 *No.35:151–158.* British Medical Association and Royal Pharmaceutical Society of Great Britain, London.

Cohn, M. 1987: *Narcomania and heroin.* Faber and Faber, London.

Dorn, N., Jepsen, J., Savona, E. 1996: *European drug policies and enforcement.* Macmillan, London, pp. 153–70.

Fulco, C.E., Liveman, C.T., Earlgy, L.E. (eds). 1995: *Development of medications for the treatment of opiate and cocaine addictions: issues for government and private sector.* National Academy Press, Washington, DC, xvii: pp. 110–16.

Gold, M. 1997: Cocaine (and crack): Clinical aspects. In Lowinson, J.H., Ruiz, P., Millman, R.B., Langrod, J.G. (eds). *Substance abuse. A comprehensive textbook,* 3rd edn. Williams & Wilkins, Baltimore, pp. 181–99.

Grabowski, J., Rhoades, H., Elk, R., Schmitz, J., Davis, C., Creson, D., Kirby, K. 1995: Fluoxetine is ineffective for treatment of cocaine dependence or concurrent opiate and cocaine dependence: two placebo-controlled, double-blind trials. *Journal of Clinical Psychopharmacology* **15** (3), 163–74.

Hall, W., Solowij, N., Lemon, J. 1994: *The health and psychological consequences of cannabis use.* National Drug and Alcohol Research Centre Monograph 25. Australian Government Publishing Service, Canberra.

Kerouak, J. 1997: *On the road.* Penguin, London. (First published Viking Press 1955).

Kuhn, T.S. 1970: *The structure of scientific revolutions,* 2nd edn. University of Chicago Press, Chicago.

Leary, T., Burroughs, W.S. 1989: *Flashbacks: a personal and cultural history of an era.* Tarcher, USA.

Mello, N.K., Mendelson, J.H., Lukas, S.E., Gastfriend, D.R., Teoh, S.K., Holman, B.L. 1993: *Harvard Review Psychiatry,* 1 (3), 168–83.

Mitcheson, M. 1994: Drug clinics in the 1970s. In: Strang, J., Gossop, M. (eds). *Heroin addiction and drug policy. The British system.* Oxford University Press, pp. 178–91.

Musto, D.F. 1997: Historical perspectives. In: Lowinson, J.H., Ruiz, P., Millman, R.B., Langrod, J.G. (eds). *Substance abuse. A comprehensive textbook*, 3rd edn. Williams & Wilkins, Baltimore, pp. 1–10.

Nadelmann, E.A. 1993: Progressive legalisers, progressive prohibitionists and the reduction of drug related harm. In: Heather, N., Wodak, A., Nadelmann, E.A., O'Hare, P. (eds). *Psychoactive drugs and harm reduction: from faith to science*. WHURR, London.

Osmond, H. 1973: The medical and scientific importance of hallucinogens. *Practitioner* **210** (255): 112–19.

Robertson, J, R., Treasure, W. 1996: Benzodiazepine abuse – the nature and extent of the problem. *CNS Drugs*, **5** (2), 137–46.

Robins, L.N., Davis, D, H., Goodwin, D.W. 1974: Drug use in US army enlisted men in Vietnam: a follow-up on their return home. *American Journal of Epidemiology* **99**, 235–9.

Robins, L.N., Helzer, J.E., Davis, D.H. 1975: Narcotics use in south east Asia and afterwards. *Archives of General Psychiatry* **32**, 955–61.

Robins, L.N., Helzer, J.E., Hesselbrock, M., Wish, E. 1979: Vietnam veterans three years after Vietnam. In: Brill, L., Winick, C. (eds). *Yearbook of substance abuse*. Human Sciences Press, New York.

Smith, R. 1995: The war on drugs. Prohibition isn't working – some legalisation will help. *British Medical Journal* **311**, 1655–6.

Spear, B. 1994: The early years of 'the British system' in practice. In: Strang, J., Gossop, M. (eds). *Heroin addiction and drug policy. The British system*. University Press, Oxford, pp. 3–27.

Strang, J., Gossop, M. (eds). 1994: *Heroin addiction and drug policy.* The British system. Oxford University Press, Oxford.

Szasz, T. 1987: The morality of drug controls. In: Harmony, R. (ed). *Dealing with drugs: consequences of government control*. Lexington, Lexington, Mass.

Tyler, A. 1996: *Street drugs*. Hodder and Stoughton, London.

United Nations 1990: *A/Res/45/146. Sixty-ninth plenary meeting, December 1990*.

Willis, P. 1976: The cultural meaning of drug use. In: Hall, S., Jefferson, T. (eds). *Resistance through rituals: youth subculture in post-war Britain*. Hutchinson University Library.

Willis, P. 1978: *Profane culture*. Routledge, London.

Wodak, A., Fisher, R., Crofts, N. 1993: An evolving public health crisis: HIV infection among injecting drug users in developing countries. In: Heather, N., Wodak, A., Nadelmann, E.C., O'Hare, P. (eds). *Psychoactive drugs and harm reduction: from faith to science*. Whurr, London, pp. 280–94.

Zimring, F.E., Hawkins, G. 1992: *The search for rational drug control, New York*. Cambridge University Press.

Zinberg, N. 1984: *Drug, set and setting. The basis for controlled intoxicant use*. Yale University, Vail-Ballou Press, New York.

Psychiatric perspective

Eilish Gilvarry

Relationship between psychiatric and psychological disorders and symptomatology

Drug use and misuse, particularly among young people, has been increasing in Britain and many other countries in the last decade. The British Crime Survey (Ramsay and Percy 1996) has shown 45% of 16–19 year olds have used illegal drugs at some time. For some, experimental and recreational use does not represent a long-term problem, though only limited exposure can result in accidents, poisonings, criminal convictions or psychological problems. Research data show a connection between decreased age of initiation and increased use. More variegated patterns of use, and the emergence of polydrug and alcohol use are now the norm.

Psychiatric disorders frequently accompany drug and alcohol use. They can be consequent of substance use, but can precede use, precipitate use and further harmful use, or may share common aetiological pathways with drug use. While drug misusers who develop short-term psychosis which usually resolves with discontinuation of the drug within days to weeks show a good outcome at discharge, the prognosis is poorer for those with coexisting mental illness and continued drug use.

Individuals with associated psychiatric problems and drug use demonstrate more frequent hospitalization, greater use of emergency services, an increased risk of suicidal behaviour and increased aggression, poorer compliance and are more difficult to engage and retain in services. Equally, substance use and use disorders are being increasingly recognized as frequent comorbid disorders that adversely affect the adjustment of persons with severe mental illness. Approximately 50% (Regier *et al.* 1990) of those with severe mental illness will develop alcohol or drug problems at some point in their lives and this rate of comorbidity is even higher among clinical populations. Substance abuse in this population is associated with greater cost to health services, increased hospitalizations, homelessness and disruptive behaviour. It is also associated with more violence and involvement with police. There is some evidence that the association of substance use and mental illness increases psychotic symptoms, and results in greater depression, suicidal behaviour, and social problems, though some demonstrate less negative symptoms, and those who use have better premorbid functioning.

Recent major epidemiological surveys in general populations around the world have noted that alcohol and substance use disorders are among the most common mental health disorders in the community, and are also commonly associated with other forms of mental disorders. Throughout all the studies the substance most frequently associated with abuse and dependence was alcohol followed by cannabis. Other substances had lower rates, though higher prevalence was found in the younger age groups.

Dually disordered patients have been reported as more problematic in terms of assessment, treatment and outcome than those with only one disorder, partly because of the additional complexity that two or more disorders represent, and partly because of the particular relationship between substance use and psychiatric disorder. Substance use may mimic, precipitate, exacerbate, be an effect of, or be independent of non-substance disorder. Such clinical heterogeneity has made initial assessments and subsequent treatments more complex. Moreover, specific patterns may vary even within individuals with the same psychiatric illness or within the same individual over time.

The relationship between drug use and dependence and psychopathology is extremely complex, made more so by the diversity of definitions and differences in conceptual approaches in the literature. Some suggest that psychiatric disorder predates substance use and drugs are used as self-medication. Others see psychiatric disorders as a consequence of drug use either as a direct pharmacological effect, and/or a consequence of the sociocultural effect in the context in which the drug use takes place. Attempts to describe this relationship are fraught with difficulties, as instruments are designed for diagnosis of substance abuse or psychiatric disorder, but not for both simultaneously, or for the interaction between them. Also, psychological symptoms often occur with both intoxication and/or withdrawal from a number of drugs which may complicate the clinical picture. A further complication is the presence of multiple diagnosis and the use of multiple drugs, including alcohol.

Crome (1996) noted the complexity of the relationship between mental disorders and substance misuse:

- substance use and withdrawal may lead to psychiatric syndromes and/or symptoms
- intoxication, excessive use and dependence may produce psychological symptoms
- substance use may precipitate, exacerbate or alter the course of pre-existing mental disorder
- primary mental disorder may precipitate substance use and dependence which in itself may lead to psychiatric symptoms.

Meyer (1986) also described the possible relationships between psychopathology and addictive behaviours. Psychopathology may be a risk factor for addictive behaviours, may modify the course of these behaviours, or psychiatric disorders may emerge during intoxication or withdrawal states.

Much of the literature on comorbidity is primarily from the USA, and only recently has the subject been given importance in the European literature. The research to date deals mainly with the prevalence of substance use and dependence in various psychiatric disorders, and conversely on the prevalence of psychological symptoms and disorder among those who use drugs or present with substance misuse problems. An integrated approach to treatment has been advocated by many, though there is a dearth of evaluative research on outcome and effectiveness of various models of integration.

Comorbidity or dual-diagnosis

For this review comorbidity and dual-diagnosis will be synonymous. The use of the term comorbidity has become increasingly common in reference to mental disorders. The concept has its origins in general medicine, where it is defined by Feinstein (1970) as 'any distinct additional clinical entity that has existed or that might occur during the clinical course of a patient who has an index disease under study'. However, with mental disorders distinctness of coexisting disorders cannot be assumed, because of the substantial overlap in criteria and lack of knowledge regarding phenomenology, and pathogenesis of disorders. The term dual-diagnosis broadly refers to the concurrent existence in an individual of substance misuse and one or more mental disorders.

There is increasing concern regarding dual-diagnosis, both because of the high prevalence of drug use, and its public health implications. Diagnosis of psychiatric disorders is important for a variety of reasons:

- those with dual diagnosis often have more complicating presentations and have a less favourable outcome
- they generally require and use more health and social resources
- they are often more vulnerable and more difficult to engage.

In treatment settings, these patients with dual-diagnosis can be particularly challenging to the clinician, as they may have differing responses to treatment, may relapse more frequently, with greater attrition and readmissions rates, they are more difficult to engage, and may manifest more severe chronic symptoms that appear refractory to treatment.

Psychiatric perspective

In order to understand the complexities of dual-diagnosis and psychological symptoms or disorders it is important to use a diagnostic system. In Europe and the UK, the International Classification of Diseases ICD 10 is used routinely in clinical psychiatric practice. It contains a wide variety of disorders with harmful use defined as a pattern of 'psycho-active substance use causing damage to health, either physical or mental'.

The psychiatric disorders identified to alcohol and drug use are listed below in Table 5.1.

In the USA, the Diagnostic and Statistical Manual DSM-1V is widely used. In the past addictions were generally classified as another form of psychopathology, though now a broad approach adopts a distinction between consumption, dependence and adverse consequences.

The DSM has a multiaxial structure that makes an explicit distinction between clinical syndromes on Axis 1 (schizophrenia, depression, substance abuse and dependence) and personality disorders on Axis 11. It also has inclusion and exclusion criteria for each disorder. These developments are somewhat responsible for the interest in the co-occurrence of clinical syndromes and personality disorders.

However, regardless of these classifications many terms are frequently used to describe the frequency and severity of use such as frequent, severe, chronic, regular and experimental use, abuse, misuse, dependence and addict. However, the boundaries of many of these terms with regard to quantity, frequency and/or consequences

Table 5.1   ICD codes for alcohol and substance use disorders

F10–F19 Mental and behavioural disorders due to psychoactive substance use

F10 – Alcohol
F11 – Opioids
F12 – Cannabinoids
F13 – Sedatives and hypnotics
F14 – Cocaine
F15 – Other stimulants, including caffeine
F16 – Hallucinogens
F17 – Tobacco
F18 – Volatile solvents
F19 – Multiple drug use and use of other psychoactive substances

Mental and behavioural disorders due to drugs

F1x.0 – acute intoxication
F1x.1 – harmful use
F1x.2 – dependence syndrome
F1x.3 – withdrawal state
F1x.4 – withdrawal state with delirium
F1x.5 – psychotic disorder
F1x.6 – amnesic syndrome
F1x.7 – residual and late-onset psychotic disorder
F1x.8 – other mental and behavioural disorders
F1x.9 – unspecified mental and behavioural disorders

Who (1992).

are not always clear. Also, the terminology in DSM and ICD classifications have been adopted for adults with little or no empirical evidence of its appropriateness for children and adolescents.

The psychiatric syndromes and symptoms related to intoxication, harmful use, dependence and withdrawal are well established and have broad agreement across DSM and ICD classifications. The psychological symptoms for intoxication and withdrawal states are operationalized for alcohol and each drug as classified from F10–F19.

Withdrawal states with and without delirium are typically demonstrated in those with alcohol dependence. However, similar reactions likened to the delirium tremens of alcohol withdrawal have been noted from benzodiazepines, chlormethiazole and barbiturates. Withdrawal from opioids is well documented. The cessation of amphetamine and cocaine can induce brief states of dysphoria, low energy and occasional suicidal thoughts and behaviour.

Toxic states and psychoses may arise from drug and/or alcohol use. Sometimes this abnormal mental state is brief as in that due to solvent use lasting up to an hour or a few hours, e.g. lysergic acid diethyl amide (LSD). Very occasionally a psychotic state lasting a few days and mimicking schizophrenia may occur from a single large dose of amphetamine. Cocaine can also produce a brief psychotic state after single dose ingestion.

Longer term psychoses can result from cocaine, ecstasy, amphetamine and other stimulants. Delusions are common, as are many forms of hallucinations with mood alteration, and occasionally aggression and violence can be a feature. Often the user may need acute hospital care with psychotropic medication. Resolution usually occurs with cessation of the drug use.

The presence of more prolonged psychoses in a person who has a history of, or is using drugs does not necessarily imply a causal association. Careful consideration and assessment of past and current drug use as well as its temporal association with onset and continuation of psychiatric symptoms need to be undertaken. It may be that observation over time is necessary to make the diagnosis.

Prevalence

Large scale epidemiological surveys have demonstrated lifetime dual diagnosis rates in both general and clinical populations. Regier *et al.* (1990) analysed the Epidemiological Catchment Area Study (ECA) to give data on substance and mental disorders in general and institutional populations. The lifetime prevalence rates were 22.5% for mental health disorder (other than substance use), 13.5% for alcohol dependence/abuse and 6.1% for other drug abuse/dependence. Almost a third of persons who had a mental disorder had experienced a substance abuse disorder at some point (22% alcohol disorder and 15% drug disorder). Among those with an alcohol problem 37% had a comorbid mental disorder, while of those with a drug disorder (other than alcohol) 53% were found to have a mental disorder.

Individuals in treatment settings, either substance abuse programmes or mental health settings, had significantly higher risk of comorbid disorder. Among those with any mental disorder, the odds ratio of having some addictive disorder was 2.7, with a lifetime prevalence of comorbidity and substance abuse of 29%. Among those with alcohol disorder, the most common mental health disorders coexisting were: anxiety disorder – 19%; antisocial personality disorder – 14%; affective disorder – 13%; schizophrenia – 4%. Among those with drug abuse/dependence the most prevalent were: anxiety disorder – 28%; affective disorder – 26%; antisocial personality disorder – 18%; schizophrenia – 7%. Of considerable concern is the high prevalence of addictive and mental health disorder in the prison population.

In the UK, the prevalence of alcohol dependence in the general population has been estimated to be 4.7%; drug dependence, 2.2%; neurotic illness, 14%; while that for psychotic illness was 0.4% (Mason and Wilkinson 1996). The British Psychiatric Morbidity Survey (Meltzer *et al.* 1996) found moderately higher rates of alcohol and drug dependence among those with mental disorders.

Menezes *et al.* (1996) noted high rates of comorbid alcohol and drug disorders among those with severe mental illness. Of 171 subjects with psychotic illness, the one-year prevalence rate for any substance problem was 36.3%; for alcohol problems it was 31.6% and for drug problems 15.8%. Young males were at higher risk of substance use. Moreover, those with substance use problems had spent twice as long in hospital with obvious resource implications. Gill *et al.* (1996) noted in a survey of homelessness high rates of heavy drinking and drug use; a 50% prevalence of alcohol dependence; up to 46% of people using drugs, and a high level of comorbid mental disorder.

Also of importance in homeless individuals is the increased risk of HIV transmission. Susser *et al.* (1996) noted a high lifetime risk of injecting drug use in a homeless group with mental illness. The men who injected drugs showed little awareness of safe injecting and sexual practices. This group is particularly important to engage with, and demonstrates the need to deploy prevention efforts.

Hendricks (1990) noted in those attending a detoxification centre that 80% of the sample had at least one recent psychiatric disorder as well as substance abuse. The most common were antisocial personality disorder, depressive disorder and anxiety-related disorder; these were commonly diagnosed in combination.

Substance use and affective disorder

Several studies have demonstrated an association between substance abuse and bipolar affective disorder (manic depression). This association is evidenced both from general populations studies and clinical populations of bipolar patients and those with substance abuse/dependence. In particular cocaine and alcohol dependence is far more common in bipolar affective disorder populations than the general population. Prevalence rates from the ECA study indicate that bipolar affective disorder is the Axis 1 disorder most likely to be associated with some form of substance abuse/dependence. It showed 60% of the bipolar 1 group had any drug or alcohol problem, with 46% having an alcohol problem and 40% a drug abuse/ dependence diagnosis. The rates of substance abuse and dependence were significantly higher among those with bipolar disorder than those with unipolar depression. While many have noted the association there is less information of the effect of substance abuse on the course and outcome of comorbid mood disorder. There is some evidence that bipolar patients with coexisting substance abuse have a worse course of illness. Sonne *et al.* (1994) noted that those with bipolar disorder and comorbid substance abuse were more likely to have more hospitalizations, a higher incidence of dysphoria, mania and earlier onset of mood problems. Equally diagnosis of bipolar disorder with substance use can be fraught with difficulties as drug use and its effects may mimic most psychiatric disorders. This is particularly true with use of stimulants where mania may be mimicked by intoxication and substantial depressive symptoms emerge during withdrawal.

There is an important association between substance use/misuse and suicide and deliberate self-harm. Kjelsberg *et al.* (1995) noted risk factors for suicide victims with histories of substance misuse of psychoses, suicidal ideation, somatization disorder and a history of failed treatment. Psychological autopsies have also demonstrated the link of suicide and substance abuse; 60% were reported to have had a drug use disorder. Suicide accounts for 35% of deaths of intravenous drug users (Frischer *et al.* 1993), a rate 30 times that of the general population. Substance misuse is associated with a seven times increased risk of attempted suicide. However, studies do not always specify the nature of the substance use, whether misuse or dependence, alcohol and/or other drugs, and there is concern that suicide and deliberate self-harm among drug users are underrepresented among official statistics. This important link demonstrates the need for active preventive strategies, e.g. awareness of and identification of risk factors, as well as identification of depression and its appropriate treatment.

Schizophrenia and substance use

Estimates of the prevalence of substance abuse disorders in schizophrenia have ranged from 10% to over 65% during a lifetime. This wide range is accounted for variations in assessments, definitions, populations sampled and other methodological problems. Nevertheless, it is apparent from most studies that substance abuse in schizophrenic patients is a common problem. Alcohol is consistently the most commonly abused substance, though there is a close link with other drug use particularly cannabis and stimulants. The ECA study noted that 16.7% of the general population had a history of substance abuse disorder, compared with 47% of the schizophrenic patients. Demographic and clinical predictors of substance use in schizophrenia include younger age, male, early onset of illness, lower education, good premorbid social adjustment though poor treatment compliance, a high relapse rate and higher levels of suicidality.

Substance use in schizophrenia has been linked with a more severe course, worse symptomatology and an increased rate of hospitalization.

Anxiety disorders

Again an association is often made, though there is a diverse prevalence ranging from 8–50% for generalized anxiety, 2–40% for agoraphobia and similar ranges for social phobia and 3–10% for obsessive compulsive disorder. Generalized anxiety disorder stands out in studies as being particularly associated with substance use disorders, especially alcohol dependence. Wittchen (1988) noted that about 40% of persons with panic disorders or agoraphobia had a lifetime risk for substance abuse disorders, particularly sedative abuse. While comparisons across studies are difficult to make, findings suggest a consistent and diagnosis-specific association of many anxiety disorders with substance disorders. Many with substance abuse/ dependence present with psychological distress and somatic symptoms evident clinically and by rating scales. These symptoms of distress, largely mixed symptoms of dysphoria, anxiety, mood alteration, panic and sleep disturbances are common as patients enter treatment, though these symptoms quickly subside. Authors have demonstrated a reduction in these symptoms, sometimes up to 3 months after detoxification. It is therefore important that diagnosis should be clear before specific treatment either pharmacological or psychological is initiated for anxiety or depression.

Eating disorders

Bulimia nervosa is often concomitant with alcohol and other drug abuse, with rates of comorbid substance abuse varying from 9% to 55%. Garfinkel et al. (1995) found a significantly higher lifetime rate of alcohol dependence in bulimics (31%) as compared with subsyndromal bulimics (9%) and controls (3%). A significantly higher rate of alcohol abuse was also found in the parents of bulimics (42%), compared with the other two groups. Other studies have noted similar results (Herzog et al. 1991, Kassett et al. 1989).

Bulik (1987) noted the most frequently diagnosed disorders were major depression, alcohol/drug dependence and suicide attempts among a sample of bulimic females. Also, their 1st and 2nd degree relatives were more likely to have alcohol/drug dependency and psychopathology. Walfish et al. (1992) noted an incidence of 14% concurrent eating disorder in a residential substance treatment centre. The highest incidence was for cocaine dependence followed by alcohol abuse. This suggests the need for those in treatment programmes for alcohol and drugs to have assessment for the presence of eating disorders.

Some authors suggest a poorer outcome if eating disorder and substance use coexist, though research has not always demonstrated this link. Mitchell *et al.* (1991) observed that bulimia nervosa and anorexia nervosa may share common behaviours that resemble addiction: craving, lack of control, denial, impairment of functioning. They cautioned against the interpretation that eating disorders are variants of addictions.

Personality disorders and substance use

The concept of personality disorder in drug users, while relevant to clinical management is often misused, unscientifically applied to a range of behaviours resulting in wide interpretations, is seen as judgmental and pejorative, and arouses much suspicion among drug workers who may not see the concept as helpful or relevant to clinical management. Nevertheless, personality disorder can be associated with a range of negative outcomes and presents real challenges to the worker. Personality disorder (PD) refers to attributes and behaviours that cause distinct and significant impairment in functioning.

Both the international classification of mental disorders (largely used in the UK) and the American Psychiatric Association DSM-IV have included personality disorder. The DSM-IV definition is more exactly defined as 'an enduring pattern of inner experience and behaviour that deviates markedly from the expectations of the individual's culture, . . . is inflexible and pervasive across a broad range of personal and social situations, leads to clinically significant distress or impairment, . . . is stable and of long duration and its onset can be traced back at least to adolescence or early adulthood'.

There are a range of personality disorder types described in both classifications that are essentially similar (Table 5.2).

Verheul *et al.* (1995) in a comprehensive review of the relationship of substance use and personality disorder noted that the best estimate of overall prevalence ranges from 44% among alcohol dependence to 79% among opiate addicts. Most of the studies of prevalence rates of PD in substance users were in clinical populations. Variation in rates for specific personality disorders is considerable, due in part to difficulties in distinguishing behaviours inherent in drug misuse and those which are part of personality disorder, and to variations in rating instruments and clinical settings. Those with alcohol dependence show lower prevalence rates than do drug abusers, while in-patient samples had the highest prevalence ranges. Up to two-thirds of drug users had evidence of personality disorders with antisocial

Table 5.2 DSM-IV Personality disorder categories

Types	Main features
Cluster A	
Paranoid	Distrust, suspiciousness
Schizoid	Isolation, detachment, coldness
Schizotypal	Eccentricity, social unease
Cluster B	
Antisocial	Criminality, aggressiveness, impulsiveness
Borderline	Instability, self-harm
Histrionic	Attention-seeking, emotional liability
Narcissistic	Self-importance, exploitation of others
Cluster C	
Avoidance	Social anxiety, hypersensitivity
Dependent	Dependence on others, submissiveness
Obserssive–compulsive	Pre-occupation with orderliness, inflexibility

Source: adapted from Sieveright and Daly (1997)

personality disorder (ASPD) being the most frequent. Detected rates of ASPD ranged from 7–60%

Conversely, rates of PD in those with psychiatric disorders, mostly anxiety, depression and other neurotic disorders, have been found to be much higher than rates in the general population; 20–40% in out-patient and even higher in in-patient settings.

The importance of PD among drug users lies in its association with a range of negative outcomes, such as poor social functioning, early relapse and drop-out from treatment, psychiatric problems and increased HIV risk behaviours and infection rates. Brooner *et al.* (1993) noted in 100 intravenous drug users with ASPD higher rates of sharing injecting equipment, and frequency of sharing, and higher rates of infection than those without ASPD.

The relationship between crime, substance abuse and mental disorders is of particular importance. Many offenders commit crimes while intoxicated with alcohol or drugs. Much acquisitive crime in particular is committed by drug users to finance their lifestyles, though drug users are also involved with violent crimes and homicides. Many violent crimes are preceded by heavy alcohol use. Lindqvist (1991) noted that homicides committed by abusers of illicit drugs were characterized by less intimacy, and the offenders were considerably younger than their victims. Almost all the perpetrators had a record of juvenile delinquency and all abused multiple drugs.

The importance of comorbidity of substance use and personality and/or other mental health disorders is particularly relevant to the concept of dangerousness and forensic assessment of responsibility and diminished responsibility. Many demonstrate a substance abuse disorder. In a study by Dittmann (1996) only 23% of offenders showed one diagnosis, 38% two, 29% three and 10% more than four diagnoses.

In the UK, addiction and intoxication alone generally are not accepted as an excuse from criminal responsibility. However, the presence of coexisting other mental illness makes it crucial that careful and comprehensive assessment of this comorbidity is undertaken.

Several studies have shown that co-occurring substance abuse in those with other mental disorders increases rates of delinquent behaviour, especially violent crimes significantly. Offenders with comorbidity of substance use and ASPD tend to be more criminally active, more dangerous and have a poorer outcome after treatment. Close collaboration between forensic and addiction specialists, both in clinical management and research is required.

Post-traumatic stress disorder

In the few studies that assessed post-traumatic stress disorder (PTSD), it has emerged as a relatively common co-occurrence among substance abusers. The self-medication hypothesis postulates that substance use is a means of achieving symptom control. However, some studies have noted that the onset of substance use predates the onset of PTSD symptoms. The literature provides evidence that the presence of PTSD has a deleterious effect on treatment outcome for substance abuse.

Young people

Adolescence is a critical developmental period for the onset and recognition of psychiatric disorders which includes psychoactive substance abuse disorders. Here however, it is important to recognize the variations in definitions and terminology, the public concern at present of drug use among young people, the increased prevalence of drug use, the importance of antecedent risk factors, the context of drug use and its consequences. Most young people will not develop dependence, though may suffer adverse consequences related to intoxication and excessive use. The importance of psychological and psychiatric factors, either directly related to drug use, e.g. dysphoria, for stimulant use and its implications for assessment and care planning cannot be overemphasized.

The co-occurrence of psychoactive substance disorder (PSUD) with other psychiatric disorders is high and has important clinical, public health and research implications. Psychoactive substance disorder, regarded as different from substance use (meaning non-pathological use or experimentation), refers to pathological use of a drug that has become a regular feature in the lifestyle and includes abuse and dependence according to DSM-IV. In this chapter the terms 'abuse' and 'misuse' are used. This co-occurrence of disorders is seen in a variety of settings. Research findings have suggested a major role for substance use in the aetiology and prognosis of psychiatric disorders such as affective disorders, conduct disorder, attention deficit hyperactivity disorder and anxiety states. Likewise, psychiatric disorders play an important role in the aetiology and vulnerability to substance use disorders.

One of the primary obstacles blocking research into comorbidity is the lack of valid and reliable criteria for diagnosis of substance abuse. Many of the definitions have been adapted from adults, with little or no empirical evidence for their appropriateness for adolescents. Lack of clarity and standardization of terminology used for substance use disorders in general has added to the confusion. This inconsistency is probably related to the wide variety and array of concepts and terms that are actively used by the numerous professionals in the field, with much disagreement among the many disciplines. Likewise the state-of-the-art in child psychiatric nosology can be equally confusing in terms of the validation of diagnostic entities that can be truly distinguished from each other. For example, the high level of comorbidity that exists between attention deficit hyperactivity disorder (ADHD), conduct disorder and oppositional defiant disorder (ODD) has been noted and has led many to speculate that there exists a single unitary disruptive behaviour disorder that manifests itself with slightly different characteristics at different developmental states.

Community surveys of the prevalence of psychiatric disorders in children and young people have generated estimates of 14–20% for moderate to severe disorders. In general the following prevalence rates occur for particular conditions:

- emotional disorders – depression and anxiety and conduct disorders (e.g.stealing, aggression delinquency) in children: 10%
- emotional and conduct disorders in adolescents: 20%
- major depression in mid-childhood: 0.5–2.5%
- major depression in mid-adolescent: 2–8%
- anorexia nervosa in 15–19 year olds females: 1%
- in age group 15–19, approx. 400 per 100 000 attempt suicide and 7–8 complete suicide.

Verhulst *et al.* (1997) estimated the prevalence of psychiatric disorders among Dutch adolescents to be approx. 21%. The most frequent disorders were simple phobia, social phobia and conduct disorder. The prevalence of two or more diagnoses was 3–5%. Those with multiple diagnosis were regarded as more disturbed by the interviewers. Substance use and ADHD were seldom diagnosed in those who did not meet criteria for other diagnosis. Reinherz *et al.* (1993) in a community sample of older adolescents noted a lifetime prevalence rate of 32.4% for alcohol abuse/dependence; followed by phobias at 22%; major depression, 9%; drug abuse/dependence, 9.8%; and less commonly post-traumatic stress disorders and obsessive compulsive disorders. Adolescents with specific psychiatric disorder had significantly poorer functioning on measures of behavioural problems, interpersonal problems, self-esteem and school performance. This suggests both the need to identify concurrent psychiatric disorder in adolescents and for prompt treatment and prevention strategies.

A pivotal source for the prevalence of psychiatric disorders, alcohol and substance misuse in the community is the ECA study. The rates of anxiety disorders, major depression and substance use disorders were high in the age group 18–24 years. Rohde *et al.* (1996) looked at psychiatric morbidity and problematic alcohol use in high school students. Increased alcohol use was associated with the increased lifetime occurrence of depressive disorders, disruptive disorders, drug and tobacco use. More than 80% of those with alcohol abuse/dependence had some form of additional psychopathology. Comorbidity was associated with an earlier age of onset of alcohol abuse and with a greater likelihood of mental health service utilization. The likelihood of another psychiatric disorder in the presence of problematic alcohol use often appeared to be dose-related, systematically increasing with increased consumption of alcohol. Consistent with problem behaviour theory, the strongest association was seen between alcohol abuse and that of illicit drug use and delinquent type behaviours.

Comorbidity research has mainly focused on clinical populations. Among adolescents with severe emotional disorders, the risk of comorbid substance use disorder has been considered to be substantial, though much further research needs to be conducted. Eliott *et al.* (1989) found that adolescents with serious emotional disorders tended to have higher prevalence rates of problem substance use, and greater mental health utilization. The highest prevalence of alcohol and problem substance use was found among adolescents with both delinquency and emotional problems. Greenbaum *et al.* (1991) in a study of those with serious emotional disorder noted prevalence rates for substance use disorders were 21% and 18% at mild/moderate and severe levels respectively.

Other authors have examined the prevalence of psychiatric disorder in those with substance abuse. Hovens *et al.* (1993) looked at the co-occurrence of psychiatric disorders in a group of substance abusers and 23 non-substance abusing adolescents with conduct disorder admitted to the same in-patient facility. Excluding CD and ODD, 85% of the substance abusers had other psychiatric disorders. Substance abusers had a higher incidence of dysthymia, major depression and social phobia than did the comparison group in which conduct disorder and ADHD prevailed.

Depression is common among young people with both conduct disorder and substance problems. Riggs *et al.* (1994) studied depression among youths with both conduct disorder and substance problems. The prevalence of depression in referred groups of children and adolescents with conduct disorder is 15–24%. Depressed delinquents had more substance problems tended to initiate behavioural problems at an earlier age, had increased anxiety and attentional problems than non-depressed delinquents.

Relatively few adolescents with serious emotional disturbances have substance use problems in isolation from other psychiatric disorders. Substance use represents a major component of the clinical profile, characterizing adolescents with psychiatric disorders and should be addressed concurrently among those who have serious emotional disorders, particularly conduct disorder and depression.

A comorbid pattern of substance use disorder is not equally likely among all core psychiatric disorders. The main associations for comorbid patterns are for conduct disorder and depression. Attention deficit disorders also tend to be associated with substance use disorder, but do not represent unique variance.

There are a number of implications:

- among those with conduct disorder or depression assessment of substance use and abuse is recommended
- when such assessments indicate comorbidity, the provision of combined mental health and substance abuse treatment seems appropriate
- even for those without positive confirmation of concurrent substance use clinicians should be sensitive to the high vulnerability of young people with conduct disorder and depression to develop substance use disorders
- early intervention programmes have an important place to play in prevention of these coexisting disorders. This has also significant policy implications in wider prevention programmes for this age group.

Conduct disorder and anti-social personality disorder have long been associated with substance abuse. This relationship can take several forms:

- antisocial behaviour as an antecedent to substance use and abuse
- antisocial behaviour or substance use modifying the course of the coexistent disorder
- substance use as a risk factor in the development of conduct disorder.

While substance abuse occurs frequently among those with problematic alcohol use in the ECA study, this association may be due in part to the fact that substance abuse is one of the diagnostic criteria for ASPD. Additionally, intoxication leads to behavioural disinhibition, thus lowering the threshold for antisocial behaviour.

Whether hyperactivity disorder (ADHD) is an independent risk factor for illegal drug use remains controversial. Although most studies report that grown-up ADHD children are at greater risk of substance abuse than controls, the differences between groups are small and not statistically significant in most studies. The existing literature suggests that for the child with ADHD, the risk of substance use disorders is mediated by comorbid conduct disorder and is not a direct complication of ADHD. A further issue relevant to risk of substance abuse in children with ADHD is that psychiatric morbidity in ADHD is not limited to conduct disorder but extends to mood and anxiety disorders as well. Horner and Scheibe (1997) reviewed the prevalence of ADHD in adolescents attending drug treatment programmes. Up to half met the criteria for ADHD diagnosis. These young people began drug use at an earlier age, had more severe substance use, more negative self-image that improved with drug use. They also experienced more negative affective responses related to substance use, more craving and attentional difficulties in treatment than controls. These results support the suggestion of a substantial comorbidity of ADHD among adolescent substance abusers. They indicate the need for counselling for ADHD and perhaps specific medication may be indicated to improve treatment outcome and future functioning.

Adolescents in treatment for substance use and abuse should be carefully screened for ADHD. Treatment planning needs to take into account the impulsivity, inattention and restlessness that typify these young people. This is particularly important as drug use may mimic this impulsivity and restlessness. Counselling concerning the effects of ADHD should be an additional focus of substance use treatment. These adolescents may also require pharmacological intervention. This needs to be carefully administered and monitored to avoid further substance abuse.

Suicide

In childhood and early adolescence, suicides are infrequent with no gender difference. However, the incidence in males increases throughout adolescence most rapidly after the age of 16. This rate among males, particularly in the age group 16–24 years has shown a significant increase since the 1970s. Alcohol and drug use are significant risk factors for a wide range of health and social problems including a precipitant both for suicide and deliberate self-harm. A review by Shaffer *et al*. (1996) of psychological autopsies demonstrated a significant link between substance and/or alcohol abuse and suicide. However, they noted that the diagnosis of substance abuse disorder was almost invariably present with another diagnosis, most commonly disruptive or mood disorder. Shaffer concluded that a limited range of diagnoses, most commonly a mood disorder alone, or in combination with conduct disorder and/or substance abuse characterized most adolescent suicides. Similarly Brent *et al*. (1993) noted the most significant risk factors for suicide were major depression, bipolar mixed states, substance abuse and conduct disorder. Substance abuse was a more significant risk factor when comorbid with a mood disorder than when alone. However, the rates of comorbid diagnosis occurring with substance misuse ranges from 44% to 100%.

Equally, the link between substance misuse and parasuicide has received much attention. The rates of substance misuse varies from 13% to 44% depending on the sample and the definition of substance abuse, misuse or dependence. Importantly, Hawton *et al*. (1993) also noted that the best predictor of completed suicide among those with a history of deliberate self-harm was substance misuse.

This important link highlights the need for an active prevention strategy, particularly among young people. This will include assessment and treatment if required of mood disorder, identification of co-occurring mental illness or behavioural disorder, and a wide education programme to healthcare workers about the association of substance use and suicidal behaviour. Williams and Morgan (1994) suggested the need for 'appropriate preventive strategies as well as effective, well coordinated secondary care services'. The same report also suggested that 'focusing on drug and alcohol abuse would have a greater impact on adolescent suicide rates than any other primary prevention programme'.

Alcohol and drug use that is problematic in adolescents usually occurs within a comorbid diagnosis. Although the existence of psychiatric comorbidity is generally accepted, there are unresolved issues about its validity and significance. Because adolescents with substance abuse are at high risk for other forms of psychopathology, they need to be carefully evaluated for psychiatric comorbidity to provide them with a comprehensive treatment plan. Integrated models of care that include interventions, not only for substance abuse but also treatment of the psychiatric disorder, e.g. pharmacological treatment for ADHD, but also parent training and social skills training, is essential.

Issues for psychiatric services

Psychiatric aspects of drug use have received much attention in the USA for some time and more recently in Europe and the UK in the last decade. This increasing concern centres in particular on the increased prevalence of drug use and misuse among those with severe mental illness, the recognition of comorbidity of mental illness and addiction regardless of the aetiological pathways, the possible poorer prognosis for those individuals, the increased utilization of health and social care, and its cost implications, and the problems of effective and appropriate service provision for those with psychiatric and drug use problems.

One of the challenges posed by those with psychiatric disorder and substance abuse is that they are seen in their respective settings, i.e. mental health hospitals/community teams and drug services. This compartmentalization of services has led to separate services being developed by different staff with widely differing skills. The ethos of each is often strikingly different, with different approaches to assessment, responsibility, definition of the problem, with interventions spanning a harm reduction approach to abstinence. The programmes based on the 12-step approach incorporating Alcoholics Anonymous (AA) and Narcotics Anonymous (NA) are often confrontatory and practise a total drug-free state, including prescribed psychotropic medication. There are also major differences in different addiction services, not only that of the 12-step approach. Many agencies will not use conventional diagnoses in their assessment and management of clients, but rather a problem-orientated approach. This may be appropriate, though assessment of mental state and identification of treatable psychiatric disorders may be either inadequate or services lack the skills to assess and treat correctly. Even in services where these skills exist, there is both a lack of recognition of coexisting or consequent psychiatric disorder in those with alcohol and drug problems as well as no formal system or procedure for diagnosis and appropriate referral.

Psychiatric settings conversely may ignore the substance use or minimize its importance both in symptom formation and relapses. Skills in assessment of drug and alcohol use, and its importance and relevance to the psychiatric state, may be missing or inadequate. In particular those with personality disorders who use drugs and alcohol are seen with low expectations, in that there are no effective treatments or appropriate healthcare responses available. Equally those with drug and alcohol use in psychiatric settings are often not seen as having a psychiatric illness and project disillusionment and anger through staff.

Both settings operating independently may in fact be counterproductive to the person with dual difficulties. There is often poor continuity of care, boundary disputes between the services, with lack of skills and confidence in both management of substance use and psychiatric disorder in the respective settings. A further issue is the prioritization of problems. A person with schizophrenia whose cannabis use may be significantly interfering with mental state and compliance of treatment may be referred to addiction services. However, the cannabis use in addiction services may not be regarded as high priority or indeed recognized as a problem.

Several impediments exist for the successful management of the patient with psychiatric illness and substance use and misuse:

1 Individuals with dual diagnosis and multiple problems often fall between the traditional boundaries of services and are 'lost'.

2 Those with problems such as homelessness are particularly at risk.

3 Skills of workers are often attributable to either substance use or psychiatric disorder though rarely to both.

4 Management of the aggressive person, the intoxicated or those with behavioural disorder remains problematic with often punitive responses and discharge from services.

5 Residential placements are few.

6 There is a lack of procedures for assessment and treatment in both settings.

7 Shared care arrangements are often *ad hoc*, demonstrate boundary disputes and exacerbate poor continuity.

8 Children with both substance use and behavioural problems often 'fall between the stools'. An integrated model of service delivery with child services is warranted.

Assessment

Given the high prevalence of drug use in the general population and especially in clinical populations, consideration of substance use and misuse should be routinely conducted on all psychiatric patients rather than only exceptional cases. The reverse also holds true, in that for those who use and/or misuse substances assessments of psychological state should be conducted with appropriate intervention if required.⁾

Use of substances can mimic most psychiatric disorders. Withdrawal from alcohol or benzodiazepines can cause hallucinations and delirious states. Amphetamine and other stimulant drugs may cause paranoia and temporary psychotic states. Use of cannabis can also cause paranoia and panic states. It is imperative that substance use is considered in all those presenting with severe mental illness, and that hasty diagnoses of disorders such as schizophrenia are not made.

Assessment is often rendered difficult by the broad impact of disorders such as depression on the psychosocial functioning of the individual. Many people with psychiatric disorders who use and abuse drugs may have complex needs. They may be highly mobile, difficult to engage with services, often presenting only in crises, demonstrate poor compliance with treatment services and 'do not fit' into the general pattern of service provided. Attention needs to be paid to their social support and to their accommodation.

Given the high rates of co-morbidity in those who misuse drugs and alcohol, careful and thorough assessment regarding other forms of current and antecedent psychopathology needs to be carefully conducted. Assessment must consider the individual differences both in substance use and in psychiatric disorders. Patients differ in substances used, the frequency and degree of use which may range from recreational use to dependence, as well as in the multiple reasons for initiation and continued use of drugs.

A comprehensive, methodical and objective evaluation of substance use and abuse is necessary for the development of an effective treatment or management plan. A detailed assessment of the person as well as relevant carers or partners is important in order to understand the functioning of the person in their environment.

The assessment may take time and can be conducted in various settings. A general format could take the following steps:

- general assessment; to include presenting problem and stage of change
- alcohol and drug history; frequency and pattern, route of use, context of use, level of problematic use and its consequences, e.g. tolerance, dependence
- social context; educational and occupational performance, quality of family functioning and social supports, issues such as accommodation, finances, legal or police involvement, use of time

- physical health; consequences of drug use, nutritional status, infectious diseases, pregnancy, sexuality and contraception
- mental health; past or current behavioural problems, subjective distress, self-injurious or suicidal behaviour, interpersonal relationships, possible past or current physical, sexual or emotional abuse
- treatment considerations; previous episodes of substance use and/or psychiatric problems and response to intervention
- for the young person presenting with substance use, the competence and developmental maturity of the child needs to be assessed. His/her wish for confidentiality needs to be balanced against the needs and complexity of the problems, as well as the young person's ability to understand the issues involved.

It is important that a physical examination and laboratory work are incorporated into the assessment process. Detailed corroborative information from relatives and/or significant others is important. The use of laboratory drug screening can be useful to confirm self-reports independently, and to monitor objectively the presence or maintenance of a drug-free state. However, care must be taken when interpreting the results both in terms of varying half-lives of different drugs as well as the reliability if drug use is intermittent. Hair analysis may provide more accurate assessment of recent drug use, though it takes time and is expensive. Further analyses of some import in assisting accurate diagnosis are the presence of markers of alcohol use, e.g. elevated levels of gamma glutamyltransferase and mean corpuscular volume (MCV), antidepressant levels, hepatitis screen, breath alcohol level, and other liver and blood function tests.

While accurate diagnosis of substance use and misuse in those with psychiatric disorder is often difficult, the use of more than one measure, including a reliable structured interview, enhances the ability to diagnose accurately. To aid accurate diagnosis, there are a number of tools in common use, mainly structured interviews, semi-structured interviews and self-report questionnaires.

A structured interview (Diagnostic Interview Schedule [DIS]) has been used particularly in epidemiological studies. It assesses drug, alcohol and mental disorders and reflects the ICD-10 and DSM-IV diagnostic classifications. The standardized clinical interview for DSM (SCID) questions the role of drug use in symptom formation. A wide range of semi-structured interviews is available, including the Schedule for Affective Disorders and Schizophrenia (SADS-L), and Structured Interview for Disorders of Personality (SIDP). There is also a large range of instruments to measure alcohol and drug use and dependence. Examples include Audit, Severity of Opiate

Dependence Questionnaire and the Leeds Dependence Questionnaire (LDP).

Some screening instruments have been specifically designed for adolescents, such as the Chemical Dependency Assessment Scale (CADS), which is widely used. Diagnostic instruments in child and adolescent psychiatry are also designed to diagnose substance use disorders, and are reasonably able to differentiate use from abuse, and to diagnose comorbid psychiatric disorders. Some rating scales include: the Diagnostic Interview Schedule for Children – Revised (DISC–R) and the Kiddie Schedule for Affective Disorders and Schizophrenia (K–SADS). Other aspects of assessment of drug users are discussed in Chapter 8.

Treatment

Drug and alcohol use and abuse in those with psychiatric disorder is one of the most pressing concerns in mental health services. Conversely psychiatric symptomatology in those who use and abuse drugs needs special consideration. Many have advocated the need for special programmes that integrate both psychiatric and substance use treatment.

Osher and Kofoed (1989) put forward a four-staged process of treatment: (a) engagement of the patient in treatment; (b) persuasion to accept long-term abstinence as a goal; (c) active treatment which includes pharmacotherapies, social skills training, community reinforcement, etc.; and (d) relapse prevention.

Drake et al. (1993) outlined nine principles of treatment of substance abuse in those with severe mental illness. These principles could equally apply to those presenting with primary substance use/ abuse with psychiatric symptomatology.

1 **Assertive outreach:** people with dual diagnosis may appear only in crises, may be difficult to engage, and demonstrate poor compliance with treatment. Intervention needs to prioritize engagement in services, that is flexible and appropriate to the needs of the person at the time. Those appearing unmotivated need to be encouraged rather than rejected or discharged from services. In some areas, interdisciplinary teams explicitly focus on engagement and maintenance of stability of both mental state and psychosocial functioning. This assertive outreach philosophy fits well with the substance abuse field which promotes outreach and service retention as a harm reduction approach.

2 **Close monitoring:** this is often intensive with use of involuntary methods (e.g. Mental Health Act) to aid compliance depending on the level of disability, and functioning of the person. In England and

Wales, the Mental Health Act 1983 allows for compulsory detention of those with mental disorder in certain defined circumstances, though dependence on alcohol and or drugs alone even if diagnosable under ICD-10 or DSM-IV criteria does not allow compulsory detention.

3 Integration: as noted traditionally addiction services and psychiatric services have developed separately with different ethos and philosophies governing treatment. the person with multiple disorder often 'falls between the stools'. Integration of treatment programmes can be at several levels, from super-speciality services for those with dual diagnosis as advocated by some, to more modest integrated models of sharing skills and staff between addiction and psychiatric services. Hall (1997) has suggested the creation of these super specialities centres to be limited to research centres initially until their effectiveness have been demonstrated.

4 Comprehensiveness: this calls for a broad-based approach that incorporates both the elements of substance abuse treatment and psychiatric interventions. Issues of accommodation, social skills, relationships, occupation and social networks all need to be addressed. Comprehensiveness also includes the range of professionals that may need to be involved from housing associations to befriending and self-help groups.

5 Stable living conditions: those with dual diagnosis are often mobile, live in temporary accommodation whose environment renders them more vulnerable to relapses and further drug use. Supportive housing may be necessary, but often their continued drug use makes them less acceptable to their neighbours; this may need to be addressed.

6 Flexibility and specialization – both of programmes and clinicians: this is important for both professionals in the addiction field and mental health fields. A new knowledge and perhaps modification of approach needs to be gained by both sides, for example the role of psychoactive drugs, harm reduction, management of detoxification. Rather than creating new teams or new services the prospect of an exciting new collaboration exists. For example, with young people who have multiple problems both antecedent and consequent to drug misuse, one option is of exploiting the potential for expanding the scope of specialists agencies by invigorating collaboration between existing drug and alcohol agencies, community child health mental health services, social and educational services and youth agencies. This collaboration should increase awareness skills and enhance identification of both substance use and psychiatric disorder. However, whatever model is adopted, rigorous evaluation is required.

7 Stages of treatment: the Proschaska and Diclemente model of change is a common model adopted in the addiction field. It is important that treatment is matched to the person's stage of change.

8 Longitudinal perspective: treatment is required over many years for those with severe mental illness and drug and alcohol use rather than simply during crises.

9 Optimism: patients with drug and alcohol use, particularly in psychiatric settings, are often viewed as unmotivated and hopeless, with staff taking a rejecting attitude to them. Morale of staff needs to be encouraged, and a range of harm reduction strategies provided that is matched to the person's stage of change.

Treatment models

Descriptive accounts of differing models of specialist service have appeared for those in particular with severe mental illness and drug use and misuse. Most authorities advocate the integration of addiction and general psychiatric services to provide the multiple levels of care needed for those with often very different levels of functioning.

Galanter *et al.* (1994) described a model treatment system in New York composed of three complementary units; a locked ward, a half-way house and an out-patient programme. The ward offers conventional psychiatric treatment in addition to relapse prevention, and educational programmes related to substance misuse, such as AIDS education and infectious disease counselling. The addiction model is that of the 12-step programme with daily AA and NA meetings. The half-way house and outpatient programme are also adapted from a drug-free therapeutic community with emphasis on social rehabilitation.

Rosenthal *et al.* (1992) noted the difficulty especially of provision of services for those with schizophrenia and substance use; treatment programmes are ill-defined, there is limited outcome data on programmes, those with schizophrenia may have difficulty reconciling the different ethos of separate services, with different priorities being put on needs by different services. He proposed an out-patient integrated model of care – the Combined Psychiatric and Addictive Disorder (COPAD). Components include supportive group therapy, education about mental illness, drug and alcohol use, peer group support monitored by staff, attendance at AA and NA encouraged, regular medication review and random urine screens. Unlike most programmes, this does not demand a drug-free state as a prerequisite for attendance.

Other models in the US include the 'Continuous Treatment Teams'. They work only with those with dual diagnosis, have small caseloads, provide a 24-hour service with assertive outreach and engagement of the client a priority. Therapies also include motivational work, general support and relapse prevention. Preliminary research findings are encouraging with fewer hospitalizations, less drug use and improved functioning.

In the UK there is limited development of joint working between addiction and general psychiatry. Joint working could maximize resources, reduce boundary disputes and increase informal training and support. However, it is time consuming to organize, and prioritization of patients remains problematic. For example, a person with schizophrenia who is smoking cannabis only may not be a priority for addiction services. However, his drug use may worsen his mental state, and affect his compliance both with attendance and medication making him/her particularly problematic to manage for the psychiatric team.

Several models of service organization could be instigated. These could include:

- an addiction worker attached to each community mental health team to improve identification and referral procedures
- training of all mental health care staff in addiction therapies, which could be costly and numbers involved could make it unrealistic
- attachment of a 'dual trained' specialist to mental health teams.

However, the most practical solution at present would be to increase the ability of both generic mental health teams and substance use services in recognition and assessment of substance use and psychiatric disorder. This could include some joint working with joint assessment clinics and linked staff both to addiction and psychiatric service with integrated management structures. Assertive outreach and more active engagement in services could be addressed.

Coordination of services and treatment philosophies and timing of the intervention may prove more important than integration of staff themselves. All models of service delivery and treatments offered need to be evaluated.

However, services at primary care level need to address the co-occurrence of psychiatric disorder and substance use and misuse. This includes both the short and long-term psychological effects directly related to drug use, and the effects of drugs on symptoms, outcome, and compliance in those with diagnosable mental disorder. These services have an important role in identification of symptoms, attribution of those symptoms, early treatment, communicating accurate information, and giving support and information to carers and parents. They could also consider using outreach techniques in their practice to improve accessibility, and to detect vulnerable people, especially young people. They may offer counselling, assistance in crises, maintain awareness of appropriate referrals, and continue to play a role in shared care arrangements of those with more complex needs.

Summary and recommendations

1 Commissioners should have adequate and clear arrangements for treatment for those with dual diagnosis.

2 Procedures for assessment need to be addressed by both primary workers and specialist staff in addiction centres and psychiatric settings.

3 Standardization of definitions and terminology would be welcomed by clinicians.

4 There needs to be greater recognition of psychiatric problems and comorbidity by all professionals, both generic and specialist.

5 Training needs to address all aspects of drug use and psychological problems, both antecedent and consequent to drug use. This training needs to be appropriate to the level of intervention.

6 All pilot or new service needs to be carefully evaluated.

References

Brent, D., Perper, J., Moritz, G., Allman, C., Friend, A., Roth, C., Schweers, J., Balach, L., Baugher, M. 1993: Psychiatric risk factors for adolescent suicide: a case control study. *Journal of American Academy Child Adolescent Psychiatry* **32**, 3 May.

Brooner, R.K., Greenfield, L., Schmidt C., Bigelow, G.E. 1993: Antisocial personality disorder and HIV infection among intravenous drug abusers. *American Journal of Psychiatry* **150**, 53–8.

Bulik, C. 1987: Drug and alcohol abuse by bulimic women and their families. *American Journal of Psychiatry* **144**, 1604–606.

Crome, I. 1996: In: Franey, C. Dual diagnosis. *Newsletter of the Psychology Special Interest Group in Addiction* edition 5, Spring 1997.

Diagnostic and Statistical Manual 1994: American Psychiatric Association.

Dittmann, V. 1996: Substance abuse, mental disorders and crime: comorbidity and multi-axial assessment in forensic psychiatry. *European Addiction Research* **2**: 3–10.

Drake, R., Bartels, S., Teague, G., Noordsy, D., Clark, R. 1993: Treatment of substance abuse in severely mentally ill patients. *Journal of Nervous and Mental Disease* **181** (10), 606–11.

Elliott, D., Huizinga, D., Menard, S. 1989: *Multiple problem youth: delinquency, substance use, and mental health problems.* Springer-Verlag, New York.

Fairburn, C.G., Kirk, J., O'Connor, M., Anastasiades, P. 1987: Prognostic factors in bulimia nervosa. *British Journal of Clinical Psychology,* **26** 223–4.

Feinstein, A.R. 1970: The pre-therapeutic classification of comorbidity in chronic disease. *Journal of Chronic Disease,* **23**, 455–68.

Frischer, M., Bloor, M., Goldberg, D. 1993: Mortality among injecting drug users; a critical appraisal. *Journal of Epidemiology and Community Health,* **47**, 59–63.

Galanter, M., Egelko, S., Edwards, H., Vergaray, M. 1994: A treatment system for combined psychiatric and addictive illness. *Addiction* **89**, 1227–35.

Garfinkel, P.E., Lin, E., Goering, P., Spegg, C., Goldbloom, D.C., Kennedy, S., Kaplan, A.S., Woodside, D.B. 1995: Bulimia nervosa in a Canadian sample: Prevalence and a comparison of subgroups. *American Journal of Psychiatry* **152** (7), 1052–8.

Gill B., Meltzer, H., Hinds, K., Petticrew, M. 1996: *Psychiatric morbidity among homeless people.* OPCS Surveys of Psychiatric Morbidity in Great Britain, Report 7. HMSO, London.

Greenbaum, P., Prange, M., Friedman, R., Silver, S. 1991: Substance abuse prevalence and comorbidity with other psychiatric disorders among adolescents with severe emotional disturbances. *Journal of American Academy Child Adolescent Psychiatry* **30**, 4 July.

Hall, W. 1997: Evidence based treatment for drug misuse: bridging the gap between aspiration and achievement (editorial). *Addiction,* **92** (4), 373–4.

Hall, W., Farrell, M. 1997: Co-morbidity of mental disorder with substance misuse. *British Journal of Psychiatry* **171**, 4–5.

Hawton, K., Fagg, J., Platt, S., Hawkins, M. 1993: Factors associated with suicide after parasuicide in young people. *British Medical Journal,* **306**, 1641–4.

Hendricks V 1990: Psychiatric disorders in a Dutch addict population: rates and correlates of DSM-III diagnosis. *Journal of Consulting and Clinical Psychology* **58** (2), 158–65.

Herzog, D.B., Keller, M.B., Lavori, P.W., Bradburn, I.Z. 1991: Bulimia nervosa in adolescence. *Journal of Development Behavioural Paediatrics* **12** (3), 191–5.

Hovens, J., Cantwell, D., Kiriakos, R. 1993: Psychiatric comorbidity in hospitalized adolescent substance abusers. *Journal of American Academy Child Adolescent Psychiatry* **33**, 4, May.

Kassett, J.A., Gershon, E.S., Maxwell, M.E., Guroff, J.J., Kazuba, D.M., Smith, A.L., Brandt, H.A., Jimerson, D.C. 1989: Psychiatric disorders in the first-degree relatives of probands with bulimia nervosa *American Journal of Psychiatry* **146** (11), 1468–71.

Kjelsberg, E., Winther, M., Dahl, A. 1995: Overdose deaths in young substance abusers; accidents or hidden suicides? *Acta Psychiatrica Scandinavica,* **91**, 236–42.

Lindqvist, P. 1991: Homicides committed by abusers of alcohol and illicit drugs. *British Journal of Addiction* **86**, 321–6.

Mason, P., Wilkinson, G., 1996: the prevalence of psychiatric morbidity OPCS survey of psychiatric morbidity in Great Britain. *British Journal of Psychiatry* **168**, 1–3.

Meltzer, H., Baljit G., Petticrew, M., Hinds, K. 1996: *OPCS surveys of psychiatric morbidity in Great Britain. Report 2. Physical complaints, service use and treatment of adults with psychiatric disorders.* HMSO, London.

Menezes, P., Johnson, S., Thornicroft, G., Marshall, J., Prosser, D., Bebbington, P., Kuipers, E. 1996: Drug and alcohol problems among individuals with severe mental illness in South London. *British Journal of Psychiatry* **168**, 612–19.

Meyer, R.E. 1986: *Psychopathology in addictive disorders.* Guildford Press, New York.

Mitchell, J.E., Specker, S.M., DeZwann, M. 1991: Comorbidity and medical complications of bulimia nervosa. *Journal of Clinical Psychiatry* **52**, 13.

Osher, F., Kofoed, L. 1989: Treatment of patients with psychiatric and psychoactive substance abuse disorder. *Hospital and Community Psychiatry* **40**, 1025–30.

Ramsay, M., Percy, A. 1996: *Drug misuse declared: results of the 1994 British Crime Survey.* Home Office, London.

Regier D.A., Farmer, M.E., Rae, D.S. 1990: Comorbidity of mental disorders with alcohol and other drug abuse: Results from the epidemiological catchment area (ECA) study. *Journal of the American Medical Association* **264**, 2511–18.

Reinherz, H., Giaconia, R., Lefkowitz, E., Pakiz, B., Frost, A. 1993: Prevalence of psychiatric disorders in a community population of older adolescents. *Journal of American Academy Child Adolescent Psychiatry,* **32**, 2 March, 369–77.

Riggs, P., Baker, S., Mikulich, S., Young, S., Crowley, T. 1994: Depression in substance dependent delinquents. *Journal of American Academy Child Adolescent Psychiatry* **34**, 6 June.

Rohde, P., Lewinsohn, P., Seeley, J. 1996: Psychiatric comorbidity with problematic alcohol use in high school students. *Journal of American Academy Child Adolescent Psychiatry* **35**, 1 Jan.

Rosenthal, R., Hellstein, D., Miner, C. 1992: A model of integrated services for outpatient treatment of patients with comorbid schizophrenia and addictive disorders. *American Journal on Addictions* **1** (4), Fall.

Shaffer, D., Gould, M., Fisher, P., Trautman, P., Moreau, D., Kleinman, M., Flory, M. 1996: Psychiatric diagnosis in child and adolescent suicides. *Archives of General Psychiatry* **53**, April, 339–48.

Sieveright, N., Daly, C. 1997: Personality disorder and drug use: a Review. *Drug and Alcohol Review* (in press).

Sonne, S., Brady, K., Morton, W. 1994: Substance abuse and bipolar affective disorder. *Journal of Nervous and Mental Disease* **182** (6), 349–52.

Susser, E., Miller, M., Valencia, E., Colson, P., Roche, B., Conover, S. 1996: Injecting drug use and risk of HIV transmission among homeless men with mental illness. *American Journal of Psychiatry* **153** (6), 794–7.

Verheul, R., van den Brink, W., Hartgers, C. 1995: Prevalence of personality disorders among alcoholice and drug addicts; an overview. *European Addiction Research* **1**, 166–77.

Verhulst, F., van der Ende, J., Ferdinand, R., Kasius, M. 1997: The prevalence of DSM-III-R. Diagnosis in a national sample of Dutch adolescents. *Archives of General Psychiatry* **54**, April.

Walfish, S., Stenmark, D., Sarco, D., Shealy, S., Krone, A. 1992: Incidence of bulimia in substance misusing women in residential treatment. *International Journal of the Addictions* **27** (4), 425–33.

Williams, R., Morgan, H. 1994: Suicide prevention – the challenge confronted. NHS Health Advisory Service, HMSO, London.

World Health Organization 1992: *International statistical classification of disease and health related problems*, 10th revision. WHO, Geneva.

6 Medical complications of drug taking

Alex Wodak

Introduction

Illicit drug use is associated with a multitude of serious adverse health, social and economic consequences. Consideration of the health sequelae of illicit drug use requires some thought about social and economic complications of drug use, as these considerably influence health costs and are also considerably influenced by them. Health complications of injecting drug use threaten individual drug users, their partners and families. In the case of HIV, complications of injecting drug use also threaten the general community.

It is difficult to separate the direct health consequences of illicit drugs from the effects of widely adopted law enforcement policies which are intended to diminish illicit drug use. For example, there is an appreciable risk of death from drug overdose when street heroin is consumed (especially if this is administered by injection). However, the risk of drug overdose when heroin is prescribed medically is very low. In the 1146 patients prescribed heroin in a recent large but uncontrolled study in Switzerland, there were no drug overdose deaths during the 18 months of follow-up (Uchtenhagen *et al.* 1996).

It is hard to escape the conclusion that most of the adverse health, social and economic costs of currently illicit drug use at present are the inadvertent results of policies intended to minimize the number of persons who use these drugs. Only some of the health (and other complications) can be explained entirely by the pharmacological properties of illicit drugs. Complications of drug use may be due to particular pharmacological properties of a drug being consumed, related to the method of administration or caused by associated factors such as contamination or combination with other mood altering substances taken at the same time. The sedative effect of opioids (such as heroin or morphine) which can cause death from respiratory depression is an example of a drug-specific complication. Amphetamine and cocaine, which are both stimulants, can induce a temporary psychotic state. Benzodiazepines and barbiturates cause sedation and sometimes during withdrawal rebound hyperactivity including convulsions can occur.

The transmission of blood-borne viruses (such as HIV or hepatitis B and hepatitis C) associated with drug injecting (and sharing of needles and syringes) is an example of a complication due to the route of administration of the drug. This complication can occur with any kind of injected drug. Nasal septal perforation associated with cocaine snorting is another example of a complication linked to a particular route of administration.

The physical complications of illicit drug use can be irreversible, disfiguring and debilitating. It is critical that all efforts are made to prevent the occurrence of these complications, because most drug users sooner or later decide that the negative aspects of drug use outweigh any benefits. If they have not sustained any serious and irreparable health, social or legal complications, integration back into mainstream society is relatively straightforward.

Treatment providers have to accept the goals of the patient as they are at the time. Support must be sustained over sometimes lengthy periods. Often eventual recovery includes more than one relapse. If these limitations are accepted, results of interventions over time are usually very rewarding.

Most of the existing literature on illicit drug users refers to individuals well known to health and law enforcement authorities. It has long been suspected that there are many other individuals who use illicit drugs, but who manage to evade the attention of authorities, keeping their illicit drug use discreet and undetected. These individuals have stable employment, residence and social relationships and remain in good health. Some studies even suggest that there may be many more functional drug users than the variety so well known to health and law enforcement authorities and drug researchers (Eisenhandler and Drucker, 1993).

In many countries, spread of HIV among and from injecting drug users has had a dramatic impact on HIV spread in the general population, out of all proportion to the number of injecting drug users. For this reason, HIV/AIDS is discussed separately in Chapters 7a and 7b.

Until the 1980s, little was known (or suspected) of injecting drug use in developing countries. It is now estimated that there is a global population of eight million drug injectors in over 120 countries (Stimson *et al.* 1996). Most of the recent increase in drug injecting around the world has occurred in developing countries. It should not be assumed that the adverse consequences of illicit drug use are the same in developing and developed countries. Much less is known of the health and other consequences of illicit drug use in developing countries compared with developed countries. While a stabilization of drug use and a trend away from injecting to non-injecting routes of administration is evident in many developed countries, the opposite is the case in many developing countries. Because polydrug use is rapidly replacing the previous pattern of single drug use, health effects of injecting drug use now need to take increasingly into consideration a pattern of consumption involving multiple drugs.

Health outcomes

Mortality rates

The pooled Standardized Mortality Rate of injecting drug use was estimated in 12 studies from several developed countries carried out between 1968 and 1993 to be 13.2 (English *et al.* 1995). This means that the mortality rate observed among injecting drug users is about 13 times higher than expected for age and sex matched peers with no history of injecting drug use. In parts of the world where the prevalence of HIV infection among injecting drug users is still low, the mortality of injecting drug use is about 1% per annum. For example, a survey of an Edinburgh general practice with 18 000 patients found a mortality rate of 9.7 per 1000 person years among past and present heroin users (Bucknall and Robertson, 1986). Most deaths among injecting drug users occur from a condition known as 'drug overdose'. Infections, suicide and violence also claim many young lives.

When HIV enters drug injecting populations, HIV-related medical complications soon come to dominate the clinical picture. The mortality rate increases within a few years and deaths from HIV/AIDS then become even more common than deaths from drug overdose.

Simple estimation of mortality rates fails to convey the magnitude of the impact of illicit drugs on the health of populations because these deaths occur at a relatively early age. Although illicit drugs were estimated to account for only 0.4 % of all deaths in Australia in

1992, these deaths amounted to 2.4% of person years of life lost due to all causes before the age of 70 years. Illicit drug deaths occurred at an average of 36.7 years of life lost per death compared with 4.7 years for cigarette smoking and 15.2 years for hazardous and harmful alcohol consumption (English *et al.* 1995). Cigarette smoking accounted for 38 times and hazardous and harmful alcohol consumption for 7.5 times as many deaths, but cigarettes accounted for only 4.9 and hazardous and harmful alcohol consumption for only 3.0 times as many person years of life lost before the age of 70 years.

Morbidity

Injecting drug use is also associated with considerable morbidity. Most of the morbidity is indirectly related to drug injecting. Injecting drug use is often accompanied by hazardous consumption of other legal and illegal drugs including alcohol, cigarettes, benzodiazepines, barbiturates, amphetamine, cocaine and cannabis. Illicit drug use is also often associated with other factors which independently contribute to excess morbidity (and mortality) including low socio-economic status, squalid living conditions, an inadequate and irregular diet, limited education, high rates of unemployment, a history of incarceration, significant debt and membership of a minority ethnic group.

Injecting drug users often have limited access to medical care. In countries without universal health care, such as the United States and developing countries, limited utilization of health care probably contributes to poorer outcomes among injecting drug users.

Morbidity is more difficult to measure than mortality. Hospital bed utilization is often accepted as a reasonable quantitative marker of morbidity. Illicit drugs were estimated to result in 0.2 % of all hospital episodes and 0.3% of all hospital bed days in Australia in 1992 (English *et al.* 1995). Common complaints among injecting drug users include skin diseases, gynaecological complaints, respiratory conditions (linked to smoking) and chronic hepatitis.

Specific health problems

Drug overdose

'Drug overdose' is the major cause of death among injecting drug users in parts of the world where the prevalence of HIV infection in this population is still low. Nevertheless, it is a very poorly understood condition. 'Drug overdose' is the major cause of death among injecting drug users and the second most common cause of death after AIDS in countries where HIV is prevalent among injecting drug users. Experience of non-fatal drug overdose is very common. Even after a short period of injecting drug use, most injecting drug users have witnessed a non-fatal or even a fatal overdose and many will have had personal experience of a non-fatal drug overdose. The number of deaths from drug overdose has been increasing alarmingly in many countries of the world in recent years. It is not clear why these deaths are increasing. An increase in the population at risk because of illicit drug use (especially drug injecting) is likely to be a most important factor in many countries.

Drug overdose often occurs following ingestion of multiple substances. A common combination in fatal overdoses is heroin accompanied by other central nervous system depressant drugs, especially alcohol and benzodiazepines. Respiratory depression results from each drug and the result of consuming a combination of depressant drugs is additive. Inhalation of vomitus sometimes occurs as a terminal event. Barbiturates have an even smaller margin of safety then other depressant drugs. A poor correlation has been reported in many studies between the blood or biliary level of morphine (as a marker of heroin) and fatal outcome. This has led many to conclude that heroin exposure is not the only determinant of outcome.

Loss of tolerance to opioids and subsequent relapse to heroin injecting is particularly risky. The risk of overdose is even higher than usual immediately following release from prison because opioid tolerance is low and exposure to heroin extremely common. Although many have attributed the recent increase in heroin overdoses in a number of countries to a widespread increasing purity of street heroin, this seems unlikely to be the sole explanation. Heroin overdose is more common among persons who inject the drug rather than those who use non-parenteral routes such as inhaling the vapour ('chinesing' or chasing the dragon). In countries where cocaine use is prevalent, deaths from cocaine overdose are also common.

It is generally accepted that the majority of drug overdose deaths are unintentional and do not represent successful attempts at suicide. Attempts to achieve temporary chemical oblivion are inherently risky. This is even more so when the most potent mood altering substances available are illegal and therefore of uncertain concentration.

The net risk of fatal overdose decreases by as much as 75% following entry to a methadone maintenance programme. However, methadone itself has also been implicated in some overdose deaths. Criteria for attributing death to methadone alone or in combination with other drugs have not been specified. Many such deaths have been attributed to methadone in the presence of very high concentrations of other depressant drugs. Several studies suggest that methadone-related deaths have increased at approximately the same rate as heroin-related deaths (Neeleman and Farrell 1997, Shishodia *et al.* 1998). Recruitment and retention into other forms of treatment is likely also to reduce overdose deaths, but treatment modalities other than methadone have only modest success in attracting and retaining drug users.

Naloxone, a parenteral short-acting opioid antagonist, is effective in resuscitating heroin injectors found soon after the event. Fatal overdoses have not occurred in legally sanctioned injecting rooms in several cities in Switzerland after more than a decade of operation. Patients who lose consciousness are rapidly revived with oxygen. Naloxone is no longer used in these settings.

Hepatitis

HIV, hepatitis B and hepatitis C are spread by blood–blood contact while HIV and hepatitis B are also transmitted by sexual contact. The spectacular impact of HIV spreading among and from injecting drug users has overshadowed the global epidemic of overdose deaths and rampant infection with hepatitis B and hepatitis C in this population. Coinfection with hepatitis B and C is common and carries a worse prognosis than either infection on its own. Consumption of considerable quantities of alcohol over time in the presence of chronic hepatitis B or hepatitis C is associated with poorer outcomes. There is no known threshold below which alcohol consumption is 'safe' in the presence of chronic hepatitis B or hepatitis C infection.

One case control study showed a nine-fold elevated increased risk of hepatitis A among injecting drug users. Hepatitis A, which spreads by the oral–faecal route, is more common among injecting drug users because of unsanitary living conditions. A safe and effective hepatitis A vaccine is now available but is still quite expensive. Ideally, individuals with hepatitis B or hepatitis C infection should be vaccinated against hepatitis A and those with hepatitis C should also receive hepatitis B vaccine.

In developed countries, injecting drug use is a relatively important mechanism for spread of hepatitis B and hepatitis C, although other transmission factors have also been well described. In developing countries, injecting drug use is usually overshadowed as a transmission factor for hepatitis B and hepatitis C. Although a safe, effective and (recently) inexpensive vaccine for hepatitis B has been in existence for more than 15 years, only a tiny minority of injecting drug users have been vaccinated against hepatitis B, even in industrialized countries where resources are relatively plentiful. Vaccination of injecting drug users against hepatitis B has been demonstrated to be logistically feasible and achieves acceptable antibody levels.

In many countries, as many as a third of drug injectors are infected with hepatitis C within 3 years of commencing drug injecting and two-thirds within 5 years. Even higher rates have been reported in some countries. Hepatitis C infection is universally more prevalent among injecting drug users than hepatitis B which is generally more common than HIV. Even in countries where there is a high prevalence of HIV among injecting drug users, hepatitis B and C infection are almost always more common. Hepatitis B and C infection from blood–blood contact appears to occur following relatively minor breaches of infection control guidelines compared with HIV. In countries like Australia where sterile injection equipment is readily available and sharing of injection equipment has decreased markedly over the last decade, hepatitis C continues to spread rapidly, although HIV infection is uncommon. The risk of infection following a needle stick injury in occupational settings has been estimated to be 30% following exposure to HBeAg positive blood, 5% following HBsAg blood, 3% following hepatitis C antibody positive blood and 0.3% following HIV positive blood (Gerbeding 1995) The risk of HIV infection following sharing of a needle and syringe has been estimated at 0.67% (Kaplan and Heimer 1994).

Infection with hepatitis B in adulthood, as among injecting drug users, causes fewer health problems than infection during infancy. Chronic active hepatitis, cirrhosis (with subsequent development of liver failure or hepatocellular carcinoma) are potential complications of hepatitis B and C.

Debilitating lethargy is very common in chronic hepatitis C infection, including persons who have not yet developed cirrhosis. It is estimated that 20 to 25% of individuals with chronic hepatitis C develop cirrhosis within 20 years and perhaps 10% will ultimately succumb from liver failure or hepatocellular carcinoma. While the proportion succumbing to fatal complications is much lower and over a longer time course than for HIV, the very high prevalence of hepatitis C among injecting drug users world wide suggests that this epidemic will result in an immense and growing health and economic burden. The annual incidence of hepatitis C among injecting drug users has been estimated at 15% in Australia (Crofts et al. 1997).

Although harm reduction measures such as peer-based, explicit education, needle exchange and methadone programmes have been demonstrated convincingly to avert HIV epidemics among injecting drug users and even restore control if introduced early and vigorously, their impact on hepatitis B and hepatitis C transmission seems much more modest. Bleach decontamination of injecting equipment may have some effect on reducing transmission of HIV, but no such effect has yet been demonstrated for hepatitis B or hepatitis C. Current treatment for chronic hepatitis B and hepatitis C infection is expensive, only moderately effective and is accompanied by not inconsiderable side effects. However there is considerable confidence that the effectiveness of treatments for these conditions will improve in the near future.

Sexually transmissible infections and gynaecological complaints

Although a history of sexually transmissible infections is very common among injecting drug users, it is hard to know which group they should be compared with. Experience of engaging in prostitution is common, especially among female injecting drug users. This may account for the increased risk of sexually transmissible infections and pelvic inflammatory disease (and also to some extent for the increased risk of hepatitis B). Crack cocaine use is associated with an increased risk of unsafe sexual practices especially in 'sex for drugs'. This practice has been linked to high rates of sexually transmissible infections including HIV.

Menstrual irregularities including amenorrhoea are common among female injecting drug users. These problems usually resolve after enrolment in methadone programmes, presumably reflecting improved nutritional status and a more stable life.

Bacterial infections

Bacterial complications of injecting drugs include infection with the agents which causes tetanus and botulism. The former was one of the first serious complications described as far back as the 1880s (Selwyn 1993). More recently outbreaks of botulism, a serious disease causing muscle paralysis and possible death, have been linked to the use of heroin known, because of its appearance, as Black Tar Heroin. The infection occurs because of the contamination of the drug with plant material and dirt in which these organisms dwell. It is not therefore necessarily related to sharing injecting equipment. The infection occurs when the drug is injected subcutaneously into the skin rather than into the bloodstream. As there is oxygen in the blood these organisms do not grow when injected intravenously but multiply in the subcutaneous tissues. The result is a lethal flaccid paralysis eventually affecting breathing (Passaro et al. 1998).

Tetanus was the first infection ever reported to be associated with illicit drug injecting. Local and distal bacterial infections may have become less common since sterile injecting equipment has become readily available in many countries. Before the HIV/AIDS epidemic, authorities in most countries restricted access to sterile injecting equipment in the mistaken belief that this would act as a deterrent to drug injecting. Cellulitis and local abscesses around injecting sites were common and these sometimes resulted in the development of large necrotic ulcers.

Distal bacterial infection can result in septicaemia, endocarditis, lung, brain and joint abscesses. These were also probably more common in the era before needle exchange. Bacterial (or fungal) endocarditis resulting from drug injecting is said to be more common on the right side of the heart (especially tricuspid regurgitation). Injecting drug use accounts for an estimated 14% of all cases of endocarditis (English *et al.* 1995).

Violence

Injecting drug users are often injured or killed by violent means. Some injuries and deaths result from territorial disputes between drug trafficking gangs. Violence appears to be more often associated with consumption of cocaine than heroin. There is a stronger association between the consumption of alcohol and becoming a victim or perpetrator of violence. Illicit drug use appears to contribute little to road crash injuries or fatalities. There may be some cross substitution between alcohol and cannabis consumption. When the minimum drinking age was raised from 18 to 21 in the United States in the 1980s, a significant net reduction in road crash fatalities occurred in this age group associated with reduced alcohol consumption and increased cannabis consumption. There appears to be an increased incidence of violence among injecting drug users who also have a psychiatric condition.

Fungal infections

Candidal and other fungal endophthalmitis occurs among injecting drug users (Servant *et al.* 1985). Aspergillis endophthalmitis has been linked to contamination of lemon juice containers used to acidify street heroin to facilitate the drug going into solution.

Tuberculosis

After several decades of declining incidence and prevalence, tuberculosis is once again emerging as an international problem. Tuberculosis is more common in HIV infected injecting drug users. The increasing incidence of tuberculosis linked to HIV infected injecting drug users became a public health problem in the United States during the 1980s and 1990s.

Parasitic infections

Malarial outbreaks linked to injecting drug use and sharing of injecting equipment have been detected in temperate climates.

Venous and arterial problems

Damage to veins occurs from repeated venipuncture, often with blunt, previously used needles. Chemical phlebitis results from adulterants commonly found in street drug samples such as talc used to dilute street heroin or from injection of methadone syrup (which is very viscous). A methadone syrup formulation is used in some countries to discourage injection. Some injecting drug users also grind up and inject tablets including benzodiazepines, buprenorphine and other opioids.

Accidental injection into arteries sometimes occurs when drug injectors have used up all available superficial veins and begun to inject into deep veins such as the jugular or femoral. Injection into arteries can cause arterial spasm, damage to arterial walls or thrombosis with gangrene of distal extremities a possible end result (Blair et al. 1991).

Dental problems

Accelerated dental decay is common among injecting drug users due to a combination of factors. Poor dental hygiene is common among drug injecting populations. Opioid drugs (including heroin and methadone) decrease salivary flow and therefore increase the rate of dental caries. Long duration of enrolment in higher dose methadone programmes is associated with improved outcomes generally, but carries an increased risk of advanced dental decay. Poor dental health makes it more difficult to eat a healthy diet.

Respiratory disease

Respiratory symptoms are common among drug injectors and are usually due to tobacco smoking, an almost universal phenomenon in this population. Acute pulmonary oedema is often found at post mortem in individuals who are believed to have died from a heroin overdose. The mechanism is uncertain. It may be an allergic phenomenon.

Cardiovascular problems

Arrhythmias and myocardial infarction are known but unusual complications of cocaine use. Cocaine use is also associated with hypertension which can result in cerebrovascular accidents or epileptic seizures.

Mental illness

A high prevalence of a variety of mental illnesses have been repeatedly found in studies of injecting drugs users. It is difficult to distinguish psychiatric conditions which have contributed to the initiation of drug injecting from those which have resulted from this practice. Anti-social personality disorder is a particularly common finding, but there is clear overlap in the criteria used to diagnose this condition and injecting drug use. Affective disorders are also extremely common. However, many of the symptoms and signs used to diagnose affective disorders may be associated with drug using lifestyles or replicated by drug withdrawal. It is therefore difficult to establish the nature of these associations. It is believed that some individuals with a mental illness consume mood altering drugs to reduce the symptoms of mental illness to a more tolerable level. A history of childhood sexual abuse is common among injecting drug users and mental illness is sometimes attributed to this traumatic experience.

Use of amphetamine and cocaine has been linked directly to acute paranoid psychosis. There is some evidence that cannabis exacerbates pre-existing mental illness, but this remains controversial. It is generally accepted that cannabis does not initiate chronic psychotic disorders. The diagnosis of psychosis in a person taking drugs should be made with great caution as the label can often have profoundly negative long-term effects.

Social sequelae

Unemployment

Unemployment is very common among injecting drug users. Periodic intoxication is not conducive to steady employment, but some drug users do manage to hold down a steady job. Although some countries maintain a strong social net to ensure acceptable standards of health for all citizens, this is far from universal even in industrialized countries. Social nets are declining in developed countries and do not exist in developing countries. Direct adverse health consequences of unemployment have been identified.

Incarceration

A history of imprisonment is very common among (especially male) drug injectors. Incarceration is not conducive to sound mental health and in some countries is a good predictor of HIV infection. HIV infection has been reported in long-term inmates incarcerated continuously from before AIDS was recognized. An HIV outbreak has been reported in a prison in Scotland (Taylor *et al.* 1995). There may also be an increased prevalence of hepatitis B and hepatitis C among inmates and ex-prisoners. An experience of incarceration of injecting drug users is common because property crime is the major means of funding purchase of expensive street drugs. Imprisonment for injecting drug users often involves multiple entries for short periods in comparison with fewer entries for longer periods for non-drug related offenders. The dynamic movement between prison and the community and the rapid movement between and within prisons has important public health implications as this sets up a pattern of random mixing between inmates. This pattern of mixing increases the dissemination of infections, especially as scarce and extensively worn injecting equipment is usually shared repeatedly between numerous partners in jail.

Living conditions

Injecting drug users often live in temporary and sometimes chaotic accommodation. Homelessness is a common experience of injecting drug users in some countries. Living conditions of injecting drug users are generally conducive to poor health.

Crime

Although many injecting drug users have a criminal record which precedes their drug use, it is generally accepted that drug use tends to intensify and prolong criminal activity. Property crime is often committed to generate income to pay the inflated black market prices of street drugs (which include a premium on risk of arrest). The cycle of drug use, crime, imprisonment, release and return to drug use worsens already poor health outcomes.

Economic factors

Most illicit drug users are substantially in debt for the majority of their drug using careers. Weekly expenditure on drugs of $ US 1500 is not uncommon. Earnings from property crime, fraud, prostitution, welfare and selling drugs never quite match outgoings. A life of chronic poverty has an independent impact on health.

Factors affecting adverse consequences of illicit drug use

The adverse consequences of illicit drug use are largely determined by the route of administration of the drug, the nature, extent and patterns of drug use, the prevalence of blood-borne viruses among other injecting drug users, life style factors associated with drug use, the drug policy environment and the characteristics of the healthcare system.

Drug injecting is associated with higher risks of dependence than sniffing (inhalation or 'chasing the dragon'), snorting or swallowing drugs. Snorting cocaine is associated with some risk of hepatitis C transmission through sharing of straws, nasal ulceration and bleeding, but risks of serious infection are otherwise restricted to drug injecting or relapse from other routes of administration back to injecting. Use of depressant, stimulant and hallucinogenic drugs is associated with different kinds of physical and psychiatric complications. The duration of drug consumption, quantity consumed and pattern of consumption are important predictors of outcome. The risk of blood-borne viral infection is determined by injection practices, infectivity of the particular virus (including duration of infectivity) and the prevalence of infection among other drug injectors. Many of the health consequences of injecting are in fact due to lifestyle factors such as poor diet and squalid living conditions. In environments where considerable emphasis is given to illicit drug law enforcement, higher health costs are often seen. Somewhat harmful drugs consumed by inhalation, snorting or swallowing are replaced by more concentrated forms of these drugs administered by injection with more serious adverse health consequences. Public health measures to prevent spread of blood-borne viral infections, such as needle exchange, are often obstructed. Shooting galleries, only found in countries with drug policies which rely almost entirely on illicit drug law enforcement, are associated with much higher rates of spread of HIV (Des Jarlais et al. 1991). Universal healthcare ensures a reasonable basic level of primary healthcare which is critical for disadvantaged groups like injecting drug users.

Improving the health of injecting drug users

Minimizing the number of individuals who consume illicit drugs has been the mainstay of drug policy in most countries for most of the 20th century. The epidemic of HIV ensured that the nature of drug taking would never be the same again. Many countries recognized the momentous implications for public health of a mismanaged HIV epidemic among injecting drug users, and implicitly or explicitly accepted a harm reduction framework. This meant that reducing the adverse consequences of drug use became the pre-eminent focus of policy and reducing illicit drug consumption became a possible means to this end rather than an end in itself.

Several clear conclusions are now evident. First, that outcomes of injecting drug users not in treatment are usually poor and often improved by attraction and retention in treatment. Second, that pharmacological treatments, especially methadone maintenance, are far more successful in attracting and retaining drug users in treatment and better supported by evidence of benefit than all other drug treatment modalities. Third, that not all who might benefit from drug treatment are currently attracted or retained in treatment and not all who are attracted or retained in treatment benefit from enrolment. Fourth, that outcomes are much improved if injecting drug users are also provided with quality primary health care. Fifth, that there is ample evidence that hepatitis B vaccination should be provided to all injecting drug users at no or little cost. Sixth, that harm reduction strategies such as user groups, explicit peer-based education, needle exchange and methadone maintenance, are effective in slowing the spread of HIV among and from injecting drug users. Seventh, that hepatitis C continues to spread rapidly in the presence of drug injecting notwithstanding these measures, and will result in considerable health and economic costs in the future. Finally, that more effective policies are required in response to illicit drug use to diminish the unacceptably high health, social and economic costs of consuming these drugs to individual drug users and their communities.

References

Blair, S.D., Holcombe, C., Coombes, E.N., O'Malley, M.K. 1991: Leg ischaemia secondary to non-medical injection of temazepam. *Lancet* **338**, 1393–4.

Bucknall, A.B.V., Robertson, J.R. 1986: Deaths of heroin users in a general practice population. *Journal of the Royal College of General Practitioners* **36**, 120–22.

Crofts, N., Jolly, D., Kaldor, L., van Beek, I., Wodak, A. 1997: The epidemiology of hepatitis C virus infection among injecting drug users in Australia. *Journal of Epidemiology and Community Health* **51** (6), 692–7.

Des Jarlais, D.C., Quader-Abdul, A., Minkoff, H., Holgsberg, B., Lauderman, S., Tross, S. 1991: Crack use and multiple AIDS risk behaviours. *Journal of Acquired Immune Deficiency Syndrome* **4**, 446–7.

Eisenhandler, J., Drucker, E. 1993: Opiate dependency among the prescribers of a New York area private insurance plan. *Journal of the American Medical Association* **269** (22), 2890–91.

English, D.R., Holman, C.D.J., Milne, E., Winter, M.G., Hulse, G.K., Coddle, J.P., Bower, C.I., Corti, B., de Klerk, N., Knuiman, M.W., Kurinczuk, J.J., Lewinm, C.E., Ryan, C.A. 1995: *The quantification of drug caused morbidity and mortality in Australia, 1995* edn. Commonwealth Department of Human Services and Health, Canberra.

Gerbeding, J.L. 1995: Drug therapy: management of occupational exposures to blood-borne viruses. *New England Journal of Medicine* **332**, 444–51.

Kaplan, E.M., Heimer, I.T. 1994: HIV incidence among needle exchange participants: Estimates from syringe tracking and testing data. *Journal of Acquired Immune Deficiency Syndrome* **7**, 182–9.

Neeleman, J., Farrell, M. 1997: Fatal methadone and heroin overdoses: time trends in England and Wales. *Journal of Epidemiology and Community Health* **51** (4), 435–7.

Passaro, D.J., Werner, B., Mcgee, J., MacKenzie, W.R., Vulgia, D.J. 1988: Wound botulism associated with black tar heroin among injecting drug users. *Journal of the American Medical Association* **297**, 859–63.

Selwyn, P.A. 1993: Illicit drug use revisited: what a long strange trip its been. *Annuals of Internal Medicine* **119**, 1044–46.

Servant, J.B., Dutton, G.N., Ong-Tone, L., Barrie, L., Davey, C. 1985: Candidal endophalmitis in Glaswegian heroin addicts: report of an epidemic. *Transcripts of the Ophthalmological Society* **104**, 297–308.

Shishodia, P., Robertson, J.R., Milne, A. 1998: Causes and frequencies of deaths in injecting drug users between 1981 and 1997 in a general practice in Edinburgh. *Health Bulletin, Scottish Office* **56**(2), March 1998.

Stimson, G.V., Adelekan, M., Rhodes, T. 1996: 'The diffusion of drug injecting in developing countries.' *International Journal of Drug Policy* **7** (4), 245–55.

Taylor, A., Goldberg, D., Emslie, J., Wrench, J., Gruer, L., Cameron, S., Black, J., Davis, B., McGregor, J., Follet, E., Harvey, J., Basson, J., McGavigan, J. 1995: Outbreak of HIV infection in a Scottish prison. *British Medical Journal* **310**, 289–92.

Uchtenhagen, A., Dobler-Mikola, A., Gutzwiller, F. 1996: Medical prescription of narcotics. Background and intermediate results of a Swiss national project. *European Addiction Research* **2**, 201–207.

HIV/AIDS – infection

Marco Rizzi

Caring for HIV infected drug users

As discussed above, there is a close epidemiological relationship between drug abuse and HIV infection. There are therefore sound reasons why HIV prevention and drug abuse prevention treatment should be integrated. This need is even more evident when planning care for HIV infected persons.

Low threshold services, outreach programmes and community-based services may prove more efficient when simultaneously dealing with drug abuse and HIV infection issues. Comprehensive approaches, integrating health and social services, psychological support, drug abuse treatment, may in fact offer the best opportunities to create a much needed trustful and long-lasting relationship among care providers and persons with HIV infection (Selwyn 1996, Laraque et al. 1996).

To discuss issues related to the management of HIV infected drug users, it is first necessary to mention a few recent developments in our knowledge of the HIV disease.

Recent developments in biomedical research and new insights into the pathogenesis of the HIV disease

In the 1980s, most researchers thought that HIV may lie latent inside the infected cells during the years-long asymptomatic stage, until some unknown trigger activated viral replication: this led to immune system failure and the resulting clinical progression to AIDS.

More recently, evidence has emerged that viral replication is continuous throughout HIV disease, with high levels of circulating virus in plasma. The dynamic of viral replication has been elucidated by a series of experiments, which have been conducted measuring virus levels in the blood with the new HIV–RNA tests. This has led to very detailed models of the viral kinetic, and to the new concept of viral steady state as the result of highly dynamic viral replication and immune response, taking place in a number of body compartments (Ho et al. 1995, Wei et al. 1995, Coffin 1996). The development of viral load testing has given, for the first time, a direct measure of the activity of infection and the response to therapy. These advances in the knowledge of the pathogenesis of the HIV disease have great clinical relevance. A cautious, wait-and-see approach, could be proposed for what was supposed to be a latent infection caused by a dormant virus, but it does not make sense in a very aggressive and dynamic infection.

Other biological considerations seem to add strength to the early and aggressive treatment approach. Virological studies have shown that, in the course of the infection, the high viral turnover drives the development of extensive genetic diversity, including the accumulation of mutations conferring resistance to antiviral drugs (Coffin 1996); moreover, the immune system, even when retaining CD4+ cell counts close to the normal values, shows signs of progressive functional impairment and late antiretrovirals therapy does not allow complete immune restoration (Connors et al. 1997).

Viral load monitoring

The same tests which allowed the acquisition of new insights on the pathogenesis of HIV disease, are now on the market for routine clinical use. High plasma viral load has been shown to predict the development of immune damage, the subsequent clinical progression, and death. Moreover, changes in viral load while on antiretroviral therapy are highly predictive of immunological and clinical outcomes (Ioannidis et al. 1996, Katzenstein et al. 1996, Mellors et al. 1996, Hogg et al. 1997).

HIV–RNA levels are of proved usefulness in establishing prognosis, in guiding the initiation of antiretroviral therapy, and in assessing the response to antiretrovirals.

Plasma viral load monitoring through HIV–RNA has now to be regarded as an essential part of the clinical follow-up for persons with HIV infection. Viral load assays are expensive, but their use may greatly increase the efficiency of antiretroviral treatment. Viral load monitoring is probably cost-effective if coupled with aggressive antiretroviral therapy (Rose 1997). Where resources are scarce and antiretrovirals poorly available, as it is in most countries with high prevalence of HIV infection, priorities are obviously quite different, and as with previous antiviral agents, the high costs prevent their use.

Controversy still exists on the role of HIV–RNA testing for early diagnosis in the serological window period, and while viral load assays are not yet proposed for routine screening, it seems reasonable to use them for early diagnosis in persons showing symptoms and/or signs of acute HIV infection.

Recent advances in antiretroviral therapy

Antiretroviral therapy is evolving very fast. While guidelines issued in 1993 were deemed obsolete in 1996 (Carpenter et al. 1996), 1996 recommendations have become no longer applicable 11 months after publication (Carpenter et al. 1997).

In 10 years, the number of drugs licensed for antiretroviral therapy has increased from zero to ten. The therapeutic armamentary now include five nucleoside analogues reverse transcriptase inhibitors (didanosine, lamivudine, stavudine, zalcitabine, zidovudine), a non-nucleoside reverse transcriptase inhibitor (nevirapine), and four protease inhibitors (indinavir, nelfinavir, ritonavir, saquinavir). Other drugs may soon be available.

A number of clinical trials have demonstrated the efficacy of the above mentioned drugs and a number of two, three and even four drugs combinations, but long-term studies with clinical endpoints have been completed for only a few possible combinations. Many questions remain to be answered, and much remains to be done to optimize the use of available drugs.

Post-exposure use of antiretrovirals may reduce the risk of infection following sexual intercourse or recreational use of parenteral drugs, but available data are too scarce for any recommendations in this field. If such an approach proved efficacious and feasible, it has been suggested that the availability of post-exposure treatment might result in an increase in hazardous behaviours.

It has been clearly demonstrated that antiretroviral therapy improves the clinical outcome of recently infected persons. For these patients, it remains to be demonstrated if life-long therapy is required, or if antiretrovirals may be safely stopped after an induction period.

One issue which remains unresolved is the possibility of eradicating HIV from an infected person. This point will not be clarified until new data from ongoing studies on recently infected patients are available. Should eradication of HIV infection prove feasible, this would be a very strong point in favour of early and maximal therapy for all the persons with HIV. Patients on intensive combination therapy for a definite period, could more easily accept severe adverse effects, as the price for a possible cure. If eradication proved not feasible, it might be more sensible to identify minimal treatment options for life-long suppressive therapy, aiming at relevant effects (such as long-term suppression of viral replication and prevention of associated immune damage).

Resistance to antiretroviral drugs has emerged as a major problem. Resistant HIV-1 mutants exist in untreated patients. Under drug pressure mutations are likely to be selected in any patient, unless there has been complete suppression of viral replication. This is one main reason for aggressive antiretroviral therapy. Allowing for residual HIV replication will eventually lead to outgrowth of drug resistant viruses and therapy failure. Even very potent antiretrovirals regimens may fail, because of poor compliance, drug interactions and malabsorption. Even a few missed doses of antiretrovirals may favour the emerging of resistance, and nullify the therapeutic effort.

Relevance of recent acquisitions from biomedical research for the management of drug users with HIV infection

Eradication, if at all possible, will probably be much easier in recently infected persons. Eradication is surely going to prove much harder in persons with long-lasting infection.

Should eradication prove possible, it would be a very strong point for early diagnosis of HIV infection and, as mentioned above, it has already been shown that patients receiving antiretrovirals therapy within months since infection , have better clinical outcomes.

The lesson is that healthcare providers should maximize their efforts to identify persons with recent acquisition of HIV infection. Healthcare workers should be able to recognize the symptoms and signs of acute HIV infection and strategy should be implemented to ensure prompt evaluation and testing of patients with suspected recent infection. Moreover, drug users should probably be taught about symptoms of acute HIV infection, and instructed to seek prompt medical advice should the suspicion of acute HIV infection arise.

It is well known that symptoms of acute infection appear only in a few patients, and their prompt recognition may be difficult in drug users, due to coexistence of a number of confounding factors (Dorrucci et al. 1995).

The strategy for early diagnosis should include routine screening for all drug users at risk for parenteral and/or sexual acquisition of HIV infection. The new therapeutic options should induce to more frequent testing than was advised in the past years. Clinical evaluation and HIV testing should probably be offered on at least a 3-monthly basis.

The new assays for HIV antibodies based on saliva samples, offer the possibility of making available on the spot tests and self-testing. The role of this type of testing programmes for drug users requires evaluation (Schopper and Vercauteren 1996).

The current strategy for antiretrovirals therapy is to treat early and hard, with complex drug regimens and strict monitoring. A growing number of specialists are talking about multi-drug chemotherapic treatments in a fashion similar to anti-cancer chemotherapy prescribed by oncology units. Protocols are very frequently updated and changed. Whether it is possible to implement these strategies at the community level remains to be seen. However, compliance and adherence are critical to the efficacy of antiretroviral regimens and the extent to which this can be effective even in hospital-based care is still unknown.

As discussed below, much research is needed in order to identify models of care able to couple state-of-the-art complex therapies with the supportive and personalized approach that is necessary for an effective long-term management of drug users with HIV infection.

Basic things to be done while caring for a person with HIV

Consultation of updated reference literature is necessary in order to be able to provide state-of-the-art care to HIV infected persons (Selwyn and O'Connor 1992, O'Connor et al. 1994, Branson 1995, Wormser 1996, De Vita et al. 1997, Fanning 1997). A few points are summarized here below, stressing issues more relevant for the care of drug users.

Baseline evaluation and follow-up

Baseline evaluation should include a number of things ideally to be done as early as possible, but not necessarily on the very first visit. Practical constraints, patients' preferences, and the need to avoid

Table 7a.1 Baseline evaluation

- Detailed history[1]
- Psychosocial evaluation, including ascertainment of possible risks of transmission of HIV[2]
- Physical examination
- For women: gynaecological examination and Papanicolau smear[3] (testing for *Neisseria gonorrhoeae* and *Chlamydia trachomatis* may also be added)
- Viral load measurement
- CD4+ lymphocytes count
- Tuberculin testing (and chemotherapy for persons who test positive); anergy testing may help in the evaluation of negative tuberculin tests
- Baseline serology for *Cytomegalovirus* infection
- Serological screening for syphilis
- Immunization against *Streptococcus pneumoniae*[4]
- Complete blood and platelets count
- Tests for liver and renal function
- Serology for HBV, HCV, HIV; if indicated for continuing sexual and/or parenteral exposure, HBV vaccination for patients negative for both HBsAg and HBs Ab
- Chest X-ray

Notes:

1. A detailed hisotry should inclde:

    (a) a review of sexual behaviour, contraception, pregnancies, sexually transmitted diseases;
    (b) a review of substance abuse, including alochol and tobacco.
    (c) a review of nutritional habits.
    (d) a review of symptoms possibly related to HIV-infection.

2. A detailed history should include and psychosocial evaluation should lead to:

    (a) identification of persons to be notified and proposed for HIV testing (including sexual partners, persons with whom needles and other injecting equipment were shared, offsprings, and any other persons who could have been exposed to HIV).
    (b) adequate counselling on safe sex and family planning.
    (c) planning of a comprehensive approach to drug abuse; this should include tobacco use and alcohol use (smoke, both of tobacco and of other substances, may concur to the high incidence of respiratory illness in drug users. Alcohol abuse is frequently a major problem, intermingled with the abuse of other substances, unsafe sex and dangerous and illicit behaviour. It may concur to hepatic disease and, because of addictive hepatic and neurological toxicity, may limit the use of anti-retrovirals and other prescribed drugs.

    History and physical examination should provide data for nutritional counselling (and, when indicated, nutritional support), frequently very much needed in HIV-infected drug users.

3. If the result of the initial smear is within normal limits, it has been recommended to obtain a second Papanicolau smear in 6 months, to rule out the possibility of false-negative results. Thereafter, the test should be repeated annually (Centres for Disease Control and Prevention 1993).

4. evidence of clinical efficacy still limited; but HIV-infected drug users may be more prone to develop bacterial pneumonia (Selwyn *et al.* 1988, Hirschtick *et al.* 1995, Mientjes *et al.* 1992, Scheidegger *et al.*, 1996), and may represent a selected target for the use of these vaccines.

Table 7a.2   Follow-up

Every 3 to 4 months:
- Detailed history
- Physical examination
- Counselling and reinforcement to help introduce and maintain safer behaviours
- Discussion of adherence to prescription (both for behavioural changes, and for drug treatment)
- Viral load measurement
- CD4+ cell count
- Tests for liver and renal function
- Serology for *Toxoplasma gondii* (for patients negative on previous examinations)
- Serology for *Cytomegalovirus* infection (for patients negative on previous examinations)

Every year:
- Immunization against influenza[1]
- Tuberculin testing (for patients negative on previous examinations)[2]
- For women: gynaecological examination and Papanicolau testing

Notes:
1. evidence of clinical utility limited.
2. may be omitted for patients with a CD4+ cells count < 100×10^9/L(low negative predictive value of the tuberculin test).

'overloading' of the HIV infected person at his/her first contact with the providers, should encourage the healthcare worker to schedule these measures over more than one consultation.

A number of provisions are required as part of the baseline evaluation and of follow-up, summarized in Tables 7a.1 and 7a.2. Checklists cannot assure quality care and a comprehensive approach should integrate all of these measures. During the first visit, and throughout the course of the disease, the provider of care must assume the responsibility for coordinating care and for arranging access to the resources necessary to meet the medical, psychological and social needs of the the person with HIV infection.

Antiretroviral therapy

Clinicians prescribing antiretrovirals have to refer to recent reference literature for assistance in their decision making (Carpenter *et al.* 1997). Tables 7a.3 and 7a.4 summarize a few critical issues.

Patients should be strongly committed to the antiretroviral treatment. To this end available options have to be extensively discussed with the patient, side effects and adverse reactions have to be frankly exposed. Future perspectives require clarification (monitoring, failure, changing regimen . . .). Time has to be spent discussing how to incorporate pills taking in daily life (timing, interference with eating

Table 7a.3 Antiretroviral therapy: established points

- The goal of therapy is complete viral suppression
- Patients adherence to the drug schedule is critical
- Recommend aggressive therapy to all acutely infected persons
- Start therapy early in the course of HIV infection, when the patient's condition is less complex and the immune system has suffered less immunological deterioration
- Recommend treatment to all symptomatic patients
- Recommend treatment to all patients with rapidly declining CD4+ cells count
- Avoid monotherapy
- Choice the regimen according to: baseline clinical, immunological, and virological status; side effects and drugs interactions profile; prior therapy; potential impact on future treatment options; availability and cost; patient's way of life, preferences, and predicted adherence
- Measure HIV-RNA levels 1 month after initiating or changing therapy, and then every 3–4 months
- Change therapy if viral load monitoring shows persistent viral replication, if CD4+ cells decrease, in case of clinical progression
- Maintain an open dialogue about toxic effects and adherence to the drug regimens: toxicity, intolerance, or non-adherence require an aggressive approach and timely changes of therapy
- When changing a failing regimen, include in the new schedule at least two new drugs

Table 7a.4 Antiretroviral therapy: open points

- Virological and immunological thresholds for initiation of therapy[1]
- Choice of antiretroviral regimens
- Adherence to therapy

Note:
[1]Therapy should be recommended to patients with a viral load above 5000–10 000 RNA copies/mL or a CD4+ cell count below 0.500×10^9/L (or a CD4+ percentage of < 25), but some experts recommend earlier therapy.

habits, privacy). Referral to experienced patients may be precious and this may be attempted on a person-to-person basis, or, in adequate settings, within group discussions. The optimism of patients experiencing clinical improvements with the new drugs is often contagious and may very positively affect the attitude of new patients. The use of written materials is often useful to reinforce the message and the allocation of time for meditation. Developing targeted community specific leaflets and booklets can be helpful, avoiding standard drug companies' materials which are often too optimistic and unfocused.

Follow-up visits should be scheduled according to the specific need of the person (avoid rigid standard follow-ups). Easy access for unplanned visits should be offered (do not leave the patient alone with his/her pills up to the next planned follow-up visit).

Prevention of opportunistic infections

HIV infected persons should be advised on the need to limit exposure to opportunistic pathogens, as detailed in published recommendations. Timely and appropriate initiation and maintenance of prophylaxis of opportunistic infections is critical in delaying progression, increasing survival and improving quality of life. Recent reference literature should be consulted for updated guidelines (Centers for Disease Control and Prevention 1995, De Vita *et al.* 1997).

Effective drug regimens are available for the prevention of *Pneumocystis carinii* pneumonia, toxoplasmic encephalitis, disseminated *Mycobacterium avium* infection, and tuberculosis, while prevention of *Cytomegalovirus* disease is still controversial, with a number of alternative strategies under evaluation.

As for tuberculosis, it has to be noted that intravenous drug use has already been considered a risk factor for tuberculosis before the appearance of the HIV epidemic (Reichman *et al.* 1979) and this has proved even more true in the AIDS era (Selwyn *et al.* 1989, Selwyn *et al.* 1992, Caylà *et al.* 1996). Recommendations for tuberculin screening and preventive therapy are detailed in the literature. The efficiency of preventive therapy remains to be demonstrated in tuberculin-negative, anergic, HIV infected persons from risk groups or geographic areas with a high prevalence (>10%) of *Mycobacterium tuberculosis* infection (Centers for Disease Control and Prevention 1995). In drug users, underlying liver disease and alcohol abuse may interfere with the use of anti-tuberculous drugs.

There is evidence that diagnosis and treatment of tuberculosis can be very effectively integrated into community-based programmes, especially when serving marginalized high-risk HIV infected persons. Counselling, contact tracing, tuberculin testing, sputum collection and examination, are well-established community-based tuberculosis control practices. The feasibility has been shown of directly observed therapy in the community, with professionals and/or volunteers reaching out-patients for daily treatment, at home, in residences, or in the street (Rossi and Reijer 1997, Pascual 1997).

Common mistakes to be avoided

When caring for drug users with HIV infection, prejudices should be avoided.

Symptoms control, and especially pain control, have to be aggressively managed. If indicated, narcotic analgesics can be used. Opiate abusers may require higher total doses of narcotics at more frequent dosing intervals for effective analgesia (this is especially true for patients on methadone). Agonist–antagonist opiates such as bupre-norphine and pentazocine should be used cautiously, because they may precipitate withdrawal.

Implanted long-term intravenous catheters, for maintenance intra-venous therapy, can be implemented in drug users. These patients have a slightly higher rate of infections, but the cumulative incidence of complications is relatively low and does not seem to contraindicate the procedure. Even at home self-administration seems feasible. When adequate training and follow-up are provided, complications occur with a frequency comparable to the one observed when infu-sions are performed by professional carers (Raviglione et al. 1989, Mukau et al. 1992). Whenever contemplating the implantation of an intravenous catheter, a careful balance of risks and benefits should be made. Patients have to be involved in the decision making; counsel-ling and training are mandatory, as well as regular supervision and strict monitoring.

Drug users should not be assumed to have poor adherence to diagnostic and therapeutical prescriptions. In adequate settings, com-pliance may be quite good (Selwyn et al. 1989, 1993).

Drug use and HIV infection: providing universal access to appropriate, effective, affordable care

HIV infected drug users as a marginalized, underserved population

There is evidence that patients often do not take full advantage of available measures of proved efficacy in preventing transmission, delaying progression, increasing survival, improving quality of life (Stein et al. 1991). In this respect, drug users often represent a disadvantaged group, with poor access to health and social services, inadequate referral processes, discrimination, lack of efficacious advocacy, low level of self-esteem and poor awareness of their right to obtain quality care. Joblessness, homelessness, illegal immigrant status, may reinforce marginalization (Solomon et al. 1991, Rosenberg et al. 1991, Moore et al. 1994, Breibart et al. 1996). Drug users often undergo frequent, short-term imprisonments and while drug use and HIV infection may be highly prevalent in many correctional facilities, these institutions often fail to provide good quality care for HIV infection and drug abuse. Moreover, detention disrupts social net-working and discontinues the process of care.

Women may be even more disadvantaged than men when bearing the double burden of HIV infection and drug use (Michell et al. 1992).

Reasons for an early, aggressive, comprehensive approach

Early diagnosis of HIV infection in drug users may reduce the risk of spreading the infection. Moreover, new therapeutic options make early diagnosis and aggressive treatment high priorities. A number of interventions may improve such outcomes as progression to AIDS and survival, and care must be given to implementing state-of the-art treatment for all groups based on economic, social or ethnic or other minority origin. The provision of pyschosocial support, methadone prescribing and detoxification treatment needs to be closely linked with assessment of the antiviral needs of the individual.

Models of care

Treatment for HIV infection has evolved into a very complex, ever changing specialist area. The discussion on models of care has become more and more relevant, and difficult. Mainstreaming and decentralization of services or central HIV dedicated services may be seen by many as a fundamental issue in designing services.

The pros and cons of AIDS-dedicated hospitals have been discussed for years. The same has been for AIDS-dedicated units within general hospitals (Pinching 1989, Rothman and Tynan 1990, Emanuel and Weinberg 1991, Turner and Ball 1992, Fahs et al. 1992). In fact, hospital AIDS units and centres for excellence in HIV/AIDS care have been very important in a few countries, as places for research, care and policy making.

Outside the hospitals, at the community level, a similar issue has been debated; are specialist AIDS units required or can generic services be developed as the agency to deliver care to this group? Models have been developed with dedicated generalists and dedicated community teams (Smits et al. 1990, Butters et al. 1991). This resembles a long-lasting debate in the field of drug abuse: is this to be treated by generalists, dedicated drug units, or even hospital-based services?

For HIV infected drug users, the problem has two elements: how to integrate care for HIV infection and for drug abuse and how to provide a continuum of care, integrating social and health service, and primary and secondary care? Experiences are very diversified.

At one extreme of the spectrum, care for HIV infected drug users has been regarded as 'a primary care disease' (Northfelt et al. 1988, Paauw and O'Neill 1990) cared for by generalists, with no special qualification or expertise. In other instances, during the course of the HIV epidemic, a process of selection (often self-selection) of providers has taken place: a few General Practitioners, and other providers of generalist services, have developed a special interest and a greater experience in the field of care for HIV infection and drug abuse. These providers have often become well known both among patients and providers, and beside providing primary care, often play a pivotal role within the community, acting as role models, consultants for healthcare and social workers, counsellors for local policy makers, advocates for patients and other persons involved in the epidemic. Relevant contribution to research may also be offered.

One more step ahead in the direction of specialization, is the institution of dedicated services, providing primary care for HIV infection and drug abuse. This has been a natural evolution in countries where drug abuse units had been well established before the HIV epidemic. These units had often expanded their activities beyond the limited scope of drug abuse, and, in an effort to provide comprehensive services, had been caring for viral hepatitis and other medical complications of drug abuse, family planning, psychiatric help, and so on. HIV was one more thing to look after, and in a few drug abuse units with a higher load of HIV infected users, the new disease became very relevant. In some instances, as in Italy, extra resources have been allocated, so as to allow drug abuse units to provide the extra services required by the HIV epidemic. In this way, HIV infected drug users may often find at the drug abuse units quality and comprehensive care. It may be noted however that this 'parallel track' for drug users within the health system sustains a sort of marginalization, and may reinforce stigma and prejudice (O'Connor *et al.* 1992).

Even more specialized, a few hospital units have evolved AIDS dedicated services, providing comprehensive care for HIV infected drug users, offering a wide array of health and social interventions, on an out- and in-patient basis (Brettle 1990).

Networking

No magic model may fit a very diversified reality. To provide care for HIV infected drug users flexibility is mandatory. A careful assessment of the needs and resources of the involved community is necessary, as well as the keenest attention to feedback inputs from patients and other community members.

A few points usually require careful evaluation. Only under very exceptional circumstances may a single provider care for an HIV infected drug user, through the entire course of the disease. Most models of care involve a number of providers, operating within a network which is articulated in two or more levels of care: patients/ relevant others/volunteers/generalist providers/generalist providers with a special interest/community-based dedicated units/hospital-based units/dedicated hospital-based units: these providers have to cooperate (to share care) in order to assure comprehensiveness and continuity of care.

- Networking requires a common base of knowledge: education and training programmes for care workers are mandatory.
- Networking requires a common language and some degree of agreement on the global vision (for instance, bias and prejudice against drug users still exist within the caring system and may render cooperation very difficult; community-based and hospital workers often have very different points of view and priorities and even language may be a barrier; health and social workers too often fail to communicate). Open and frank discussion among providers should be promoted and encouraged.
- Shared care requires agreement on a number of procedures: written protocols regularly discussed and updated, should define guidelines (for baseline evaluation and follow-up, detoxification, antiretrovirals therapy, prevention of opportunistic infections, symptoms management and palliative care, crisis interventions, death-related issues, professional exposures to HIV . . .).
- Whatever the model of care, referral procedures are crucial – they should be openly discussed and written policies should clarify the role of each provider.
- The transfer of information is critical. There is evidence that concern about disclosure of their diagnosis by general practitioners or other primary care providers may be a main reason for patients referring to centralized hospital services (Singh *et al.* 1997, Tomlinson *et al.* 1997). A written policy should be developed and confidentiality should be ensured.
- A wide network, with a very diversified number of providers and offered services, may in fact fail because of lack of coordination. Case management should be provided. A case manager could be one of a variety of health professionals, including doctors, nurses, social workers. Case managers have been playing a pivotal role for organizing the delivery of day-to-day care in the United States of America due to the lack of national health system and the many gaps that the system of care presents for marginalized patients. In other countries, with a well-developed primary care network, case managers may often act more as promoters and facilitators.

Quality assurance

A comprehensive network, with an expanded role for community-based services, requires very complex management procedures. It cannot be the result of spontaneous efforts by isolated workers and volunteers and it requires careful monitoring (Rizzi and Arici 1995). This is of special importance when caring for drug users, who often are marginalized and unable to negotiate with the health system.

We have no conclusive evidence of the superiority (or inferiority) of community-based models of care, both in terms of efficacy and effectiveness. Few published reports present discordant data (Markson *et al.* 1994, Mauskpof *et al.* 1994, Turner *et al.* 1994, Curtis *et al.* 1995, Paauw *et al.* 1995, Smith *et al.* 1996, Kitahata *et al.* 1996, Fleerackers *et al.* 1997).

Traditional clinical outcomes (such as survival, performance status, symptoms control) seem poorly influenced by the model of care. This may change with the introduction of the new, more effective therapies.

The limited available experience with quality of life and health-related quality of life measurements does not yet allow models evaluations and comparisons. Standard tools have to be adapted and validated for employment in drug users with HIV infection (Gill and Feinstein 1994, Rizzi *et al.* 1994, Cohen *et al.* 1996, Carretero *et al.* 1996).

It would also be desirable to include in the evaluation process a measure of the degree of the patient's satisfaction. Again, it seems difficult to define easy and reliable indices and standards (Kassirer 1993).

Most studies in fact fail to analyse the domains which are more peculiar to community-based services: comprehensiveness, continuity, coordination, and attention to psychosocial issues, are not easily accounted for.

Much more research is needed in order to improve our ability to deliver quality care to HIV infected drug users. Meanwhile, an open and flexible approach has to be adopted, and quality assessment programmes should be incorporated in any system providing care for HIV infection.

References

Branson, B.M. 1995: Early intervention for persons infected with human immunodeficiency virus. *Clinical Infectious Diseases* **20** (suppl. 1), S3–22.

Breibart, W., Rosenfeld, B.D., Passik, S.D., McDonald, M.V., Thaler, H., Portenoy, R.K. 1996: The undertreatment of pain in ambulatory AIDS patients. *Pain* **65**, 243–9.

Brettle, R.P. 1990: Hospital health care for HIV infection with particular reference to injecting drug users. *AIDS Care* **2**, 171–81.

Butters, E., Higginson, I., Wade, A., McCarthy, M., George, R., Smits, A. 1991: Community HIV/AIDS teams. *Health Trends* **23**, 59–62.

Carpenter, C.C.J., Fischl, M.A., Hammer, S.M., Hirsch, M.S., Jacobsen, D.M., Katzenstein, D.A., Montaner, J.S., Richman, D.D., Saag, M.S., Schooley, R.T., Thompson, M.A., Vella, S., Yeni, R.G., Volberding, P.A. 1996: Antiretroviral therapy for HIV infection in 1996. *Journal of the American Medical Association* **276**, 146–54.

Carpenter, C.C.J., Fischl, M.A., Hammer, S.M., Hirsch, M.S., Jacobsen, D.M., Katzeustein, D.A., Montaner, J.S., Richman, D.D., Saag, M.S., Schooley, R.T., Thompson, M.A., Vella, S., Yeni, P.G., Volberding, P.A. 1997: Antiretroviral therapy for HIV infection in 1997. Updated recommendations of the International AIDS Society–USA panel. *Journal of the American Medical Association* **277**, 1962–9.

Carretero, M.D., Burgess, A.P., Soler, P., Soler, M., Catalàn, J. 1996: Reliability and validity of an HIV-specific health-related quality-of-life measure for use with injecting drug users. *AIDS* **10**, 1699–705.

Caylà, J.A., de Olalla, P.G., Galdòs-Tanguis, H., Vidal, R., Lopez-Colemes, J.L., Gatell, J.M., Jans'a, J.M. 1996: The influence of intravenous drug use and HIV infection in the transmission of tuberculosis. *AIDS* **10**, 95–100.

Centers for Disease Control and Prevention, 1993: Sexually transmitted diseases treatment guidelines. *Morbidity and Mortality Weekly Report* **42** (RR-14), 1–102.

Centers for Disease Control and Prevention, 1995: USPHS/IDSA guidelines for the prevention of opportunistic infections in persons infected with Human Immunodeficiency Virus: a summary. *Morbidity Mortality Weekly Report* (RR-8), 1–36.

Coffin, J.M. 1996: HIV viral dynamics. *AIDS* **10**, S75–84.

Cohen, S.R., Hassan, S.A., Lapointe, B.J., Mount, B.M. 1996: Quality of life in HIV disease as measured by the McGill quality of life questionnaire. *AIDS* **10**, 1421–7.

Connors, M., Kovacs, J.A., Krevat, S., Gea-Banaeloche, J.C., Sneller, M.C., Flanigan, M., Metcalf, J.A., Walker, R.E., Falloon, J., Baseler, M., Feuerstein, I., Masur, H., Lane, H.C. 1997: HIV infection induces changes in CD4+ T cell phenotype and depletions within the CD4+ T cell repertoire that are not immediately restored by antiviral or immune-based therapies. *Nature Medicine* **3**, 533–40.

Curtis, J.R., Paauw, D.S., Wenrich, M.D., Carline, J.D., Ramsey, P.G. 1995: Physicians' ability to provide initial primary care to an HIV-infected patient. *Archives of Internal Medicine* **155**, 1613–18.

DeVita, V.T., Hellman, S., Rosenberg, S.A., Curran, J., Essex, M., Fauci, A.S. (eds). 1997: *AIDS. Etiology, diagnosis, treatment and prevention.* Lippincott-Raven, Philadelphia.

Dorrucci, M., Rezza, G., Vlahov, D., Pezzotti, P., Sinicco, A., Nicolosi, A., Lazzarin, A., Galai, N., Gafa, S., Pristera, R. for the Italian Seroconversion Study. 1995: Clinical characteristics and prognostic value of acute retroviral syndrome among injecting drug users. *AIDS* **9**, 597–604.

Emanuel, E.J., Weinberg, D.S. 1991: Is it time for a comprehensive AIDS medical center? *American Journal of Medicine* **91**, 74–9.

Fahs, M.C., Fulop, G., Strain, J., Sacks, H.S., Muller, C., Cleary, P.D., Schmeidler, J., Turner, B. 1992: The inpatient AIDS unit: a preliminary empirical investigation of access, economic, and outcome issues. *American Journal of Public Health* **82**, 576–80.

Fanning, M.M. (ed.) 1997: *HIV infection. A clinical approach.* W.B. Saunders, Philadelphia.

Fleerackers, Y., Haegenborgh, T., De Cock, R., Colebunders, R. 1997: *Is general practitioner care cheaper for the Belgian patient?* Proceedings of the Third International Conference on Home and Community Care for Persons Living with HIV/AIDS, Amsterdam, 0149.

Gill, T.M., Feinstein, A.R. 1994: A critical appraisal of the quality of quality-of-life measurements. *Journal of the American Medical Association* **272**, 619–26.

Hirschtick, R.E., Glassroth, J., Jordan, M.C., Wilcosky, T.C., Wallace, J.M., Kvake, P.A., Markowitz, N., Rosen, M.J., Mangura, B.T., Hopewell, P.C. and the Pulmonary Complications of HIV Infection Study Group. 1995: Bacterial pneumonia in persons infected with the human immunodeficiency virus. *New England Journal of Medicine* **333**, 845–51.

Ho, D.D., Neuman, A.U., Perelson, A.S., Chen, W., Leonard, J.M., Markowitz, M. 1995: Rapid turnover of plasma virions and CD4 lymphocytes in HIV-1 infection. *Nature* **373**, 123–6.

Hogg, R.S., Sherlock, C.H., Yip, B., Craib, K.J.P., Schechter, M., Montaner, J.S.G., O'Shaughnessy, M.V. 1997: *Evaluation of plasma HIV-1 RNA copy number in 2327 HIV-infected individuals.* Proceedings of the Fourth Conference on Retroviruses and Opportunistic Infections, Washington, DC, 153.

Ioannidis, J.P.A., Cappelleri, J.C., Lau, J., Sacks, H.S., Skolnik, P.R. 1996: Predictive value of viral load measurements in asymptomatic untreated HIV-1 infection: a mathematical model. *AIDS* **10**, 255–62.

Kassirer, J.P. 1993: The quality of care and the quality of measuring it. *New England Journal Medicine* **329**, 1263–5.

Katzenstein, T.L., Pedersen, C., Nielsen, C., Lundgren, J.D., Jakobsen, P.H., Gerstoft, J. 1996: Longitudinal serum HIV RNA quantification: correlation to viral phenotype at seroconversion and clinical outcome. *AIDS* **10**, 167–73.

Kitahata, M.M., Koepsell, T.D., Deyo, R.A., Maxwell, C.L., Dodge, W.T., Wagner, E.H. 1996: Physicians' experience with the Acquired Immunodeficiency Syndrome as a factor in patients' survival. *New England Journal of Medicine* **334**, 701–6.

Laraque, F., Greene, A., Triano-Davis, J.W., Altman, R., Lin-Greenberg, A. 1996: Effect of comprehensive intervention program on survival of patients with human immunodeficiency virus infection. *Archives of Internal Medicine* **156**, 169–76.

Markson, L.E., Cosler, L.E., Turner, B.J. 1994: Implications of generalists' slow adoption of zidovudine in clinical practice. *Archives of Internal Medicine* **154**, 1497–504.

Mauskopf, J., Turner, B.J., Markson, L.E., Houchens, R.L., Fanning, T.R., McKee, L. 1994: Patterns of ambulatory care for AIDS patients, and association with emergency room use. *Health Services Research* **29**, 489–510.

Mellors, J.W., Rinaldo, C.R., Gupta, P., White, R.M., Todd, J.A., Kingsley, L.A. 1996: Prognosis in HIV-1 infection predicted by the quantity of virus in plasma. *Science* **272**, 1167–70.

Mientjes, G.H., van Ameijden, E.J., van den Hoek, A.J.A.R., Coutinho, R.A. 1992: Increasing morbidity without rise in non-AIDS mortality among HIV-infected intravenous drug users in Amsterdam. *AIDS* **6**, 207–12.

Mitchell, J.L., Tucker, J., Loftman, P.O., Williams, S.B. 1992: HIV and women: current controversies and clinical relevance. *Journal of Women's Health* **1**, 35–9.

Moore, R.D., Hidalgo, J., Bareta, J.C., Chaisson, R.E. 1994: Zidovudine therapy and health resource utilization in AIDS. *Journal of Acquired Immune Deficiency Syndrome* **7**, 349–54.

Mukau, L., Talamini, M.A., Sitzmann, J.V., Cartland Burns, R., McGuire, M.E. 1992: Long-term central venous access vs other home therapies: complications in patients with Acquired Immunodeficiency Syndrome. *Journal of Parenteral and Enteral Nutrition* **5**, 455–9.

Northfelt, D.W., Hayward, R.A., Shapiro, M.F. 1988: The acquired immunodeficiency syndrome is a primary care disease. *Annals of Internal Medicine* **109**, 773–5.

O'Connor, P.G., Molde, S., Henry, S., Shockcor, W.T., Schottenfeld, R.S. 1992: Human immunodeficiency virus infection in intravenous drug users: a model for primary care. *American Journal of Medicine* **93**, 382–6.

O'Connor, P.G., Selwyn, P.A., Schottenfeld, R.S. 1994: Medical care for injection-drug users with human immunodeficiency virus infection. *New England Journal of Medicine* **331**, 450–59.

Paauw, D.S., O'Neill, J.F. 1990: Human immunodeficiency virus and the primary care physician. *Journal of Family Practice* **31**, 646–50.

Paauw, D.S., Wenrich, M.D., Curtis, J.R., Carline, J.D., Ramsey, P.G. 1995: Ability of primary care physicians to recognize physical findings associated with HIV infection. *Journal of the American Medical Association* **274**, 1380–82.

Pascual, J. 1997: *Directly observed treatment (DOT) at home for tubercolosis patients with AIDS in Catalonia*. Proceedings of the Third International Conference on Home and Community Care for Persons Living with HIV/AIDS, Amsterdam, 017.

Pinching, J.A. 1989: Models of clinical care. *AIDS* **3**, S209–13.

Raviglione, M.C., Battan, R., Pablos-Mendez, A., Aceves-Casillas, P., Mullen, M.P., Taranta, A. 1989: Infections associated with Hickman catheters in patients with acquired immunodeficiency syndrome. *American Journal of Medicine* **86**, 780–86.

Reichman, L.B., Felton, C.P., Edsall, J.R. 1979: Drug dependence, a possible new risk factor for tuberculosis disease. *Archives of Internal Medicine* **139**, 337–9.

Rizzi, M., Marchesi, S., Morelli, E., Avogadri, M. 1994: Quality of life in persons with AIDS: evaluation by the 'Medical Outcomes Study' instrument. *AIDS Patient Care* **8**, 265–8.

Rizzi, M., Arici, C. 1995: A quality assurance programme for the care of persons living with HIV infection. *AIDS Patient Care* **9**, 182–8.

Rose, D.N. 1997: *Cost-effectiveness of viral load testing in the management of HIV disease.* Proceedings of the Fourth Conference on Retroviruses and Opportunistic Infections, Washington, DC, p. 180.

Rosenberg, P.S., Gail, M.H., Schrager, L.K., Vermund, S.H., Creagh-Kirk, T., Andrews, E.B., Winkelstein, W. Jr., Marmor, M., Des Jarlais, D.C., Biggar, R.J.. 1991: National AIDS incidence trends and the extent of zidovudine therapy in selected demographic and transmission groups. *Journal of Acquired Immune Deficiency Syndrome* **4**, 392–401.

Rossi, M.M., Reijer, P.T. 1997: *Decentralized model of tuberculosis treatment (D.O.T.S.) in community based home care programmes for people living with HIV/AIDS.* Proceedings of the Third International Conference on Home and Community Care for Persons Living with HIV/AIDS, Amsterdam, 015.

Rothman, D.J., Tynan, E.A. 1990: Advantages and disadvantages of special hospitals for patients with HIV infection. *New England Journal of Medicine* **323**, 764–8.

Scheidegger, C., Zimmerli, W. 1996: Incidence and spectrum of severe medical complications among hospitalized HIV-seronegative and HIV-seropositive narcotic drug users. *AIDS* **10**, 1407–14.

Schopper, D., Vercauteren, G. 1996: Testing for HIV at home: what are the issues? *AIDS* **10**, 1455–65.

Selwyn, P.A., Feingold, A.R., Hartel, D., Schoenbaum, E.E., Alderman, M.H., Klein, R.S., Friedland, G.H. 1988: Increased risk of bacterial pneumonia in HIV-infected intravenous drug users without AIDS. *AIDS*, **2**, 267–72.

Selwyn, P.A., Feingold, A.R., Iezza, A., Feingold, A.R., Iezza, A., Satyadeo, M., Colley, J., Torres, R., Shaw, J.F.M. 1989: Primary care for patients with human immunodeficiency virus (HIV) infection in a methadone maintenance program. *Annals of Internal Medicine* **110**, 761–3.

Selwyn, P.A., Hartel, D., Lewis, V.A., Schoenbaum, E.E., Vermund, S.H., Klein, R.S., Walker, A.T., Friedland, G.H. 1989: A prospective study of tubercolosis among intravenous drug users with human immunodeficiency virus infection. *New England Journal of Medicine* **320**, 545–50.

Selwyn, P.A., O'Connor, P.G. 1992: Diagnosis and treatment of substance users with HIV infection. *Primary Care* **19**, 119–56.

Selwyn, P.A., Sckell, B.M., Alcabes, P., Friedland, G.H., Klein, R.S., Schoenbaum, E.E. 1992: High risk of active tuberculosis in HIV-infected drug users with cutaneous anergy. *Journal of the American Medical Association* **268**, 504–509.

Selwyn, P.A., Budner, N.S., Wasserman, W.C., Arno, P.S. 1993: Utilization of on-site primary care services by HIV-seropositive and -seronegative drug users in a methadone maintenance program. *Public Health Reports* **108**, 492–500.

Selwyn, P.A. 1996: Can we reduce the burden of morbidity in HIV-infected injecting drug users? *AIDS* **10**, 1429–30.

Singh, S., Raab, J., Wright, L., King, M. 1997: *General practice and HIV/ AIDS in London, UK: a quantitative and qualitative analysis.* Proceedings of the Third International conference on Home and Community Care for Persons Living with HIV/AIDS, Amsterdam, 0146.

Smith, S., Robinson, J., Hollyer, J., Bhatt, R., Ash, S., Shaunak, S. 1996: Combining specialist and primary health care teams for HIV positive patients: retrospective and prospective studies. *British Medical Journal* **312**, 416–20.

Smits, A., Mansfield, S., Singh, S. 1990: Facilitating care of patients with HIV infection by hospital and primary care teams. *British Medical Journal* **300**, 241–3.

Solomon, L., Frank, R., Vlahov, D., Astemborski, J. 1991: Utilization of health services in a cohort of intravenous drug users with known HIV-1 serostatus. *American Journal of Public Health* **81**, 1285–9.

Stein, M.D., Piette, J., Mor, V. 1991: Differences in access to zidovudine (AZT) among symptomatic HIV-infected persons. *Journal of Internal Medicine* **6**, 35–40.

Tomlinson, D.R., Farnham, C, Higginson, I., Shaw, M. 1997: *Utilization of GP services by HIV positive patients. Factors affecting registration and disclosure.* Proceedings of the Third International Conference on Home and Community Care for Persons Living with HIV/AIDS, Amsterdam, 0148.

Turner, B.J., Ball, J.K. 1992: Variations in inpatient mortality for AIDS in a national sample of hospitals. *Journal of Acquired Immune Deficiency Syndrome* **5**, 978–87.

Turner, B.J., McKee, L., Fanning, T., Markson, L.E. 1994: AIDS specialist versus generalist ambulatory care for advanced HIV infection and impact on hospital use. *Medical Care* **32**, 902–16.

Wei, X., Ghosh, S.K., Taylor, M.E., Johson, V.A., Emini, E.A., Deutsch, P., Lifson, J.D., Bonhoeffer, S., Nowak, M.A., Hahn, B.A.. 1995: Viral dynamics in human immunodeficiency virus type 1 infection. *Nature* **373**, 117–22.

Wormser, G.P. (ed.) 1996: *A clinical guide to AIDS and HIV.* Lippincott-Raven, Philadelphia.

7b HIV/AIDS – care and management

Fergus D. O'Kelly

Introduction

Illegal drug use, especially injecting drug use, has caused economic, social and medical problems for industrialized societies, increasingly in the last 30 years. Societies through their government agencies and health services have adopted various strategies to address these issues, with little success. The problem posed by injecting drug users is now greater than at any time in recent history.

The advent of the HIV/AIDS epidemic in the early 1980s also caused major difficulties for societies around the globe. It has caused economic devastation in some nations and challenged others to recognize sexual and drug using behaviour previously ignored or inadequately understood, and in doing so to put into place services that were acceptable and accessible to persons who acquired infection through such behaviours.

Those countries affected early in the epidemic currently carry the most serious economic impacts. In many countries, particularly Eastern Europe, South America and Asia the full impact has yet to be felt, but will be, as the incubation period expires and spread remains high.

Thus the combination of HIV infection and problem drug use in a sizeable proportion of its population has posed particular public health problems for many communities. In addressing these important health problems not only have the health services been forced to change and embrace new strategies, but also welfare services and society in general have also had to adapt. This process of adaptation can be likened to the stages in a grief reaction. The first reaction is denial that this could happen in our own communities, followed by anger at certain minority groups, especially when their behaviours were outside of the 'accepted' norm, and blame levelled at the health and other governmental services for not anticipating the problem, or for not supplying services quickly enough. Finally acceptance occurs and recognition that this problem must be addressed in a comprehensive, professional and humane way, which allows us to treat the individual and minimize spread of HIV infection.

HIV spread began in the late 1970s and early 1980s in East and Central Africa among heterosexual men and women with multiple sexual partners. Within a few years spread began among homosexual and bisexual men in some urban areas of the Americas, Western Europe, Australia and New Zealand. Today the virus is being transmitted in all countries. It is estimated that 22.6 million people worldwide are living with HIV infection or AIDS. Of these 830 000 are children and about 42% of the adults are women. This proportion is growing. The majority of newly infected adults are under 25 years old.

Between 5% and 10% per cent of all adult infection results from sharing HIV infected injection equipment by drug users. This proportion is also growing, and in many areas of the world injecting drug use is the dominant mode of transmission of HIV (United Nations 1996).

Within Europe, the pattern of spread of HIV/AIDS has changed with time. In the early 1980s the epidemic was characterized by male homosexual and bisexual cases forming the majority of those infected. This changed through the early 1990s to a situation where injecting drug users accounted for the highest proportion of newly

Table 7b.1 Regional HIV/AIDS statistics and features, December 1997

Region	Epidemic started	Adults and children living with HIV/AIDS	Adult prevalence rate	Cumulative no. of orphans	Percent women	Main mode of transmission for those living with HIV/AIDS
Sub-Saharan Africa	late '70s–early '80s	20.8 million	7.4%	7.8 million	50%	Hetero
North Africa, Middle East	late '80s	210 000	0.13%	14 200	20%	IDU, Hetero
South and South-East Asia	late '80s	6.0 million	0.6%	220 000	25%	Hetero
East Asia, Pacific	late '80s	440 000	0.05%	1 900	11%	IDU, Hetero MSM
Latin America	late '70s–early '80s	1.3 million	0.5%	91 000	19%	MSM, IDU, Hetero
Carribean	late '70s–early '80s	310 000	1.9%	48 000	33%	Hetero, MSM
Eastern Europe and Central Asia	early '90s	150 000	0.07%	30	25%	IDU, MSM
Western Europe	late '70s–early '80s	530 000	0.3%	8 700	20%	IDU, MSM
North America	late '70s–early '80s	860 000	0.6%	70 000	20%	MSM, IDU, Hetero
Australia and New Zealand	late '70s–early '80s	12 000	0.1	300	5%	MSM, IDU
Total		30.6 million	1.0%	8.2 million	41%	

Hetero: heterosexual transmission; IDU: injecting drug use; MSM: men who have sex with men

Source: UN AIDS 1996.

diagnosed cases; 43% of adult/adolescent cases; in 1996. At the end of the first quarter of 1997 the WHO (European Region) reported 19 625 AIDS cases of which 3.7% were paediatric cases, that is under 13 years old (WHO 1997).

Recently, however, the annual incidence of AIDS cases in Europe appears to have decreased. It reached a plateau in 1994–95 and decreased by 10% in 1996. The largest decrease is amongst homo-sexual men, down 20% with a decrease of 7% for injecting drug users and a decrease of 0.4% for heterosexually infected persons. Whilst this is welcome news, only time will tell if this is to be sustained. It is noteworthy that the greatest fall is among homosexual men who as a group have been targeted for specific health promotion and education and that the smallest reduction is in heterosexual infected persons who would have only been exposed to general health promotion information, and who would feel less at risk of HIV.

There is a significant public health problem associated with HIV infection in the drug using population. There are approximately 68 000 AIDS cases in Europe whose principal mode of infection is injecting drug use.

HIV/AIDS in the injecting drug using population could be said to be a disease of relative affluence in that it has been a feature of the wealthier industrialized nations. However the infected injecting drug users are found amongst the poorest within those societies. It is said therefore to be a disease of poverty within an affluent society. Recent reports of spread of HIV by injecting drug users in Russia, India and other Asian countries are likely to have a major impact on this picture (UN AIDS 1996). This poses many challenges for these societies. Medicine and the wider health and welfare services cannot be expected to meet all these challenges, but we must address the problems brought to us by the individual to his/her maximal benefit whilst attempting to minimize the spread of infection by reasonable measures such as harm minimization strategies. These challenges include adopting public health policies targeted at, and acceptable to minority groups with high risk sexual and drug use practices.

HIV infection

It is now accepted by the medical and scientific community that infection with the HIV viruses leads to AIDS. It is thought that there may be cofactors such as coexisting infection, which speed up the progress from initial infection to severe depression of the immune system with its consequent clinical presentation.

HIV exists in two main forms, HIV-1 and HIV-2. HIV-1 causes most HIV diseases world-wide and HIV-2 appears to be confined mainly to West Africa, but cases have been reported from East Africa, Europe, Asia and Latin America. Ten different genetic sub-types of HIV-1 have been found, but their biological and epidemiological significance is as yet unclear. Both HIV-1 and HIV-2 are transmitted in the same way, that is the virus enters the body through three main routes:

- Sexual spread – through unprotected sexual intercourse between man and woman (heterosexual) or between men (homosexual). There are no documented cases of sexual spread between women.
- Blood-borne – through blood, blood products and sharing infected injecting equipment.
- Materno-foetal – from infected mother to her foetus or infant during pregnancy, delivery or when breast-feeding.

HIV-2 appears to be less easily transmitted than HIV-1 and progression from HIV-2 infection to AIDS is slower. However AIDS appears to be identical whether from HIV-1 or HIV-2 infection (Wright 1996).

After entering the body, the virus infects the CD4 positive T-lymphocytes, impairs the cells, invades, multiplies and then destroys the cells with resultant immunodeficiencies. This renders the infected person open to opportunistic infection and malignancies which characterize the acquired immunodeficiency syndrome. The average time between infection and death from AIDS, if untreated, is about 10–12 years. It would seem that there is no difference in the incubation period despite the source of infection, socioeconomic indicators and gender, but that mortality within the injecting drug use group from causes other than HIV infection is much higher (Prins and Veugelers 1997, Selwyn et al. 1992). There is a well-established connection between older age at time of infection and more rapid progressive disease.

Clinical presentation of HIV disease

There are no signs or symptoms which are unique to HIV/AIDS as it is a multisystem disorder with a high variety of manifestations. HIV disease should be part of a differential diagnosis in any unexplained clinical presentation. It has been likened to tuberculosis in its protean manifestations and physicians hold that to know and understand HIV diseases is to 'know' medicine.

A full history including sexual and drug details may reveal the possibility of HIV infection. This possibility may be confirmed by testing for the presence of antibodies to the HIV virus. It should be remembered that not all laboratories routinely test for antibodies to HIV-2 and it should be borne in mind if HIV-2 infection is suspected in somebody recently arrived from West Africa, or who has a partner from West Africa.

The enzyme immunoassay EIA, also known as ELISA, is the standard test used for screening for antibodies to HIV. EIAs using both HIV-1 and HIV-2 antigens are commonly used in Europe, USA, Australia and New Zealand. The sensitivity and specificity of the EIA test is very high (greater than 99%) so false positive or negative results are uncommon. However it is common practice to confirm a reactive test with a supplemental test either a second separate type of ELISA or the Western Blot assay (Wright 1996).

Ninety-five per cent of individuals infected with HIV will sero-convert, that is they will give a positive test for HIV antibodies, within 3 months of exposure. It is therefore important to find out from the individual requiring the test when they were exposed to risk. A baseline test can be performed at the time of consultation with further tests at 3 months and 6 months. If all these tests are negative and no further possible exposure has taken place, the individual can be reassured that they are negative for HIV infection.

Pre- and post-test counselling

A diagnosis of HIV infection in an individual is an emotionally overpowering event, often causing an acute grief reaction. The psychological impact is profound in most individuals. In addition to the possible serious medical implication there are also social implications, such as strain on their immediate family supports, employment prospects, insurance and housing eligibility.

Therefore, pre-test counselling and confidentiality are essential in the care of all people thought to be at risk of HIV infection. The World Health Organization (WHO 1988) and the General Medical Council (London) (GMC 1995) both insist on the importance of pre-test counselling and stress the need for confidentiality, as do most health-care services in developed countries. This counselling should be carried out by the clinician managing the individual case, or by a trained counsellor. Sometimes the individual may need time to think over the implications of possible infection and may need to return on another occasion for testing. If an individual declines to be tested on the first occasion he/she should be counselled as to their risk behaviour and the need to prevent or at least limit possible exposure, to themselves and others.

Pre-test counselling

This should (a) assess the individual's risk of HIV infection; (b) educate them about risk prevention or risk reduction; (c) ensure that they understand the test and its implications. Table 7b.2 provides a list of issues and topics which should be included in such a session.

Table 7b.2   HIV testing and pre-test counselling

- Must be voluntary, and with informed consent
- Information provided must include:
  - What a positive result means
  - How the virus can be passed on
  - That it does not necessarily mean that the person will develop AIDS
  - That the person being tested has a duty to avoid transmission
  - Safer sex practices and condom use should be explained
  - Implications regarding infringements of rights in housing, employment, or other areas arising from potential breach of confidentiality
- Implications of a positive or negative result in insurance applications.

  - Information obtained must include:
    - Why the person wants to take the test
    - Risk behaviour including sexual practice, needle sharing etc.
    - Psychosocial history including
    - Psychiatric history if any
    - Social supports
    - Methods of coping with stress
    - Reaction to a positive test result

Adapted from WHO Guidelines on Counselling for HIV Testing.

Post-test counselling

This should (a) help the person understand the test results; (b) provide appropriate emotional support and follow-up; (c) modify behaviour in the individual by negotiating a risk reduction strategy. Table 7b.3 is a list of areas which need to be addressed.

Table 7b.3   Post-test counselling

- Test results should be given in face to face consultation, with appropriate emotional support
- Individuals should be given access to written information on AIDS and the meaning of the test and other appropriate support literature.
- Follow-up counselling and access to appropriate care for the HIV positive individual.
- Risk reduction plans should be negotiated for the individual whether positive or negative. (This will have limited impact on the individual who has just received a positive result and therefore must be followed up at subsequent meeting.)

Adapted from WHO Guidelines for Counselling HIV Testing.

Clinical course and classification

The natural history of a person infected with the HIV virus is that they will progress more or less step-wise though a series of character-istic clinical stages in line with progressive depletion of CD4 lympho-cyte levels. This clinical picture may be radically altered with the new anti-viral triple therapies outlined at the Vancouver AIDS Conference 1996. However it should be remembered that up to 90% of people with HIV disease do not have access to these newer therapies and in many areas, especially Sub-Saharan Africa, they may not have access to what many would see as basic medications for palliative care such as appropriate analgesics, antifungal treatments and other antibiotics (Odongo-Aginya *et al*. 1997).

As the clinical course of the disease progresses, many symptoms and signs may be present. Table 7b.4 includes a list of some of the important features of the earlier part of the illness often present prior to the diagnosis of the full AIDS syndrome.

The American Centre for Disease Control (CDC) revised its classifi-cation for HIV disease in 1993 (CDC 1993). This classification attempts to combine clinical manifestation with laboratory mar-kers, that is CD4 cell counts. This new definition was adopted by European authorities with the exception of the use of CD4 count level as a diagnostic feature of progression or advanced disease.

Table 7b.4 Checklist of clinical features in early to mid-course of HIV infec-tion

General:	Mouth:
Risk behaviour	Gingivitis
Sweats and rigours	Oral candidiasis
Weight loss	Hairy oral leukoplakia
Lymphadenopathy	Kaposi's sarcoma
General well-being	**Gastrointestinal tract:**
Skin:	Diarrhoea
Dry skin	Dysphagia
Seborrhoeic dermatitis	Pain
Psoriasis	Peri-anal disease
Folliculitis	**Central nervous system:**
Herpes simplex	Mood
Herpes zoster	Concentration
Kaposi's sarcoma	Memory
Respiratory system:	Peripheral neuropathy
Cough	Motor weakness
Dyspnoea	Retinopathy

Clinical categories

Table 7b.5 gives the CDC clinical submissions used in North America.

Table 7b.5 Clinical categories

CD4 categories	Asymptomatic HIV, or persistent generalized lymphadenopathy	Symptomatic, not A or C conditions	AIDS– indicator conditions
1. > 500 cells/mm	A1	B1	*C1
2. 200–499 cells/mm	A2	B2	*C2
3. < 200 cells/mm	*A3	*B3	*C3

*Denotes AIDS cases by surveillance definition.

Category A

Acute HIV seroconversion illness

Between 50 and 90% of people with HIV will go through a sero-conversion illness within 2–4 weeks of exposure. The illness starts usually between 3 and 14 days, and has features similar to a 'flu-like syndrome. In some cases a more severe reaction causes the appearance of an infectious mononucleosis infection. The patient will have fever, sore throat, enlarged lymph glands and a discreet rash over the body. Occasionally the illness can be more profound and include severe systematic disturbance, confusion and neurological involvement.

Asymptomatic stage of HIV

Most HIV infected individuals remain symptom-free for many years following infection. There are no abnormal physical findings, but laboratories' examinations of CD4 counts may show a decline towards the end of the period.

Persistent generalized lymphadenopathy

This is common feature of chronic HIV infection and is defined as enlarged lymph nodes one centimetre in diameter in two or more extra inguinal sites persisting for at least 3 months, without any current illness or medication known to cause enlarged nodes. Patients are usually well.

Category B

Early symptomatic illness, not A or C conditions

Category B consists of symptomatic conditions in an HIV infected adolescent or adult that are not included among conditions listed in clinical Category C and that meet at least one of the following criteria: (a) the conditions are attributed to HIV infection or are indicative of a defect in cell mediated immunity; or (b) the conditions are considered by physicians to have a clinical course or to require management that is complicated by HIV infection. Examples of conditions in clinical Category B include, but are not limited to:

- Bacillary angiomatosis
- Candidiasis, oropharyngeal (thrush)
- Candidiasis, vulvovaginal, persistent, frequent, or poorly responsive to therapy
- Cervical dysplasia (moderate or severe)/cervical carcinoma *in situ*
- Constitutional symptoms, such as fever (38.5°C) or diarrhoea lasting >1 month
- Hairy leukoplakia, oral
- Herpes zoster (shingles), involving at least two distinct episodes or more than one dermatome
- Idiopathic thrombocytopenic purpura
- Listeriosis
- Pelvic inflammatory disease, particularly if complicated by tubo-ovarian abscess
- Peripheral neuropathy.

For classification purposes, Category B conditions take precedence over those in Category A. For example, someone previously treated for oral or persistent vaginal candidiasis (and who has not developed a Category C disease) but who is now asymptotic should be classified in clinical Category B.

Category C

Symptomatic illness – AIDS indicator illness

This long list of illnesses which indicate the presence of severe immunodeficiency and once diagnosed qualify the patient as having AIDS.

Table 7b.6   Conditions included in the 1993 AIDS surveillance case definition

- Candidiasis of bronchi, trachea, or lungs
- Candidiasis, esophageal
- Cervical cancer, invasive*
- Coccidiodomycosis, disseminated or extrapulmonary
- Cryptosporidiosis, chronic intenstinal (> 1 month's duration)
- Cytomegalovirus disease (other than liver, spleen, or nodes)
- Cytomegalovirus retinitis (with loss of vision)
- Encephalopathy, HIV-related
- Herpes simplex: chronic ulcer(s) (> 1 month's duration); or bronchitis, pneumonitis, or esophagitis
- Histoplasmosis, disseminated or extrapulmonary
- Isosporiasis, chronic intestinal (> 1 month's duration)
- Kaposi's sarcoma
- Lymphoma, Burkitt's (or equivalent term)
- Lymphoma, primary, or brain
- *Mycobacterium avium* complex or *M. kansasii*, disseminated or extrapulmonary
- *Mycobacterium tuberculosis*, any site (pulmonary* or extrapulmonary)
- *Mycobacterium*, other species or unidentified species, disseminated or extrapulmonary
- *Pneumocystis carinii* pneumonia
- Pneumonia, recurrent*
- Progressive multifocal leukoencephalopathy
- *Salmonella* septicaemia, recurrent
- Toxoplasmosis of brain
- Wasting syndrome due to HIV

*Added in the 1993 expansion of the AIDS surveillance case definition.

HIV in drug users

There is little clinical difference in the presentation of HIV disease in drug users and others with HIV infection. There are however additional medical problems which may arise such as abscesses, endocarditis and pneumonia. Other problems would include concurrent infection such as hepatitis A, B, C, and D, sexually transmitted diseases and overdoses. More discussion and descriptions of these and other illnesses experienced by drug users are included in Chapter 6.

Many symptoms which arise in drug users may mimic symptoms common to HIV diseases such as respiratory problems, gastrointestinal and non-specific problems such as weight loss. Table 7b.7 illustrates this sometimes confusing overlap.

However, clinical differences do occur, for instance Kaposi's sarcoma appears to be more common among homosexual and bisexual men than amongst drug users. The incidence of tuberculosis and pneumonia other than *Pneumocystis carinii* pneumonias is higher

Table 7b.7   Comparison of drug-related and HIV-related problems

Symptom complex	Drug-related	HIV-related
Respiratory syndrome (Cough, SOB, etc)	Bacterial pneumonia Bronchitis Endocarditis Heroin asthma	P. carinii pneumonia Tuberculosis
Neurological syndrome (Fits, LOC, confusion, etc)	Any infection Drug excess Drug withdrawals	Toxoplasmosis Meningitis Lymphoma
Weakness	Nerve injury after drug injection	Myopathy Neuropathy AZT myopathy
Visual loss	Candida Ophthalmitis	Crytomegalovirus (CMV)
Gastrointestinal syndrome (Diarrhoea, vomiting)	Drug withdrawal	Cryptosporidiosis Isoporiasis CMV colitis
Abdominal pain	Opiate withdrawal	Oesophagitis ddl-associated pancreatitis
Skin (Rashes)	Drug injury Abscess Poor diet	Seborrhoeic dermatitis Kaposi's sarcoma Scabies Thrombocytopenia Herpes zoster
Constitutional; syndrome (fever, sweats, weight loss)	Drug withdrawals Stimulants Excessive opiates	CDC IVA Tuberculosis or M. avium intracellulare P. carinii pneumonia or other opportunistic infection

Note: Neuropathic symptoms are associated with the newer antiviral drugs such as didanosine, zalcitabine and stavudine. Pancreatitis is associated with didanosine, zalcitabine, lamivudine and rashes and gastro-intestinal infection infection occur with the use of many of these drugs.
Modified from Brettle (1993).

amongst drug users, as is infective endocarditis. These conditions are probably secondary to repeated use of injecting equipment, poor personal care and social circumstances. Drug users, especially those outside treatment, have a higher mortality than is found in their non-drug using peers. There is an excess mortality of about 15 times the expected rate, much of which is due to drug overdose (Carnwath 1997).

Special issues for women

'By the year 2000, women will comprise half of 30–40 million people infected with HIV and approximately one-third of their children will also carry the virus. Women are biologically more vulnerable to HIV infection and their low social and economic status increases the risk of infection' (WHO 1995).

Female drug users are at an increased risk of medical problems than their male counterparts. They are more likely to suffer from sexually transmitted disease, HIV, hepatitis and anaemia. In addition there are problems around pregnancy, contraception and gynaecology. They have higher stress levels and are likely to suffer from anxiety and depression – much of this may derive from low-esteem.

Many have a background of abuse of all types in childhood which may predispose to self-neglect and abuse, including drug use. As well as caring for themselves they often have the added responsibility of children, a partner and keeping a home. All these factors make them more vulnerable and in need of appropriate supportive care. Some centres now recognize the particular problem of women IDUs, and have dedicated services for these women (Bourke 1997).

Drug users in prison

Many large urban centres report a close relationship between heroin use and crime, and drug misuse in prisons is widespread (Task Force Report 1997). Recent studies reporting on the British Prison System show the underestimation and therefore under-reporting on the extent of drug use and HIV infection in the prisons. One study showed that over half the male remand prisoners in one prison had a history of drug use prior to their detention and that this was underestimated on initial screening. Only 5% of those needing detoxification received it (Mason et al. 1997). A further study showed that 16% of injecting drug users had shared needles in prison and some had started injecting in prison (Bellis et al. 1997).

In Scotland Yirrel (Yirrell et al.1997) found using molecular linkage techniques on viral samples taken from HIV positive prisoners that 13 of 14 infected men had 'viral sequences similar enough to indicate that one source of infection was common to all'. This gives strong evidence to show that these prisoners were likely to have acquired HIV infection within the prison through the sharing of injection equipment. The authors summed up their findings with the ominous statement: 'Injecting drug use is a potentially explosive health care problem in prison'. Health services in some prison systems are now being shared between the criminal justice system and the healthcare system.

In the Irish prison system it is estimated that 70% of inmates in the state's largest prison have a history of drug misuse, prisoners have a well developed drug habit prior to entering prison and that approximately 50% of them have no desire to receive treatment for their addiction. Further there is evidence of extensive smuggling of drugs into the prison despite controls and screening. As in other countries the vast majority of prisoners who use drugs come from economically and socially deprived backgrounds (Task Force Report 1997).

As in other countries, it is now being considered whether or not it is necessary to imprison drug users for offences connected with their addiction, such as possession or larceny. It might be more appropriate to intercept offenders at their earliest experience with the criminal justice system and divert them to properly supervised treatment and rehabilitation services – that is non-custodial sanctions linked to treatment option. In the US a system of Drug Courts operate in some States. The Drug Court is a court-operated rehabilitation programme whose ethos is that defendants arrested for non-violent drug-related offences are retained in the programme until they achieve set goals. If they re-offend they are diverted back into the criminal justice system (Task Force Report 1997).

Other countries have less formal programmes which have broadly the same goals as the US Drugs Court System. This system depends upon the presence of adequate alternative treatment facilities which have the confidence of the courts. Drug users sentenced to prison need to be offered detoxification, or maintenance programmes if the problem of HIV infection in our prisons is not to get worse. Those prisoners who have not used drugs or who have stopped need to be housed in a 'drug-free' section of the prison.

Provision of services for drug users with HIV

Good management is based on optimal care for the individual to prevent or limit further progression of the disease, and to prevent further spread from the infected individual to others. That is, care for the individual, his or her family and for the wider public. This will involve a variety of treatment services both voluntary and statutory with psychosocial and educational supports. Many drug users and their families fail to access appropriate services for a variety of reasons, including indifference and hostility from healthcare services and previous negative experiences with healthcare workers. Important advances in the clinical management of HIV make it difficult for clinical workers to keep up to date even in specialist services; clinicians often need to inform themselves through current medical journals. Chapter 7a deals in some detail with the new antiviral chemotherapy which has made such a dramatic impact since 1996.

As yet there is no vaccine available to protect against HIV infection and so preventative strategies still rest with education. This includes information leading to behaviour modification. This needs to be addressed at the public at large and to have targeted approaches to certain sub-groups such as homosexual or bisexual men and injecting drug users in order to alter their sexual and drug using behaviour.

The management of HIV/AIDS amongst homosexual and bisexual men has been aided, and in fact driven, by self-help groups who have insisted on being recognized as partners in care. By their actions they have challenged the paternalistic model of medical care and have been influential in changing this model of care to one of partnership between the clinician and the patient. This is beginning to have a beneficial effect on all aspects of clinical care.

These changes have been achieved because the gay community have been organized, active, articulate and health conscious. The picture is very different from that in the drug using group, whose activities in most countries are illegal. The illegal use of drugs and the expense of maintaining a constant supply of drugs means that theft and prostitution are often used to finance a habit. This brings drug users constantly into contact with the criminal justice system and as a group they often have little trust in state agencies and services. There are, however, examples of organizations representing drug users and acting as advocates for their needs. In Amsterdam drug users through their group Junky Union have engaged the city medical authority in dialogue and have been influential in fashioning Amsterdam's pragmatic drug policy (Buning *et al.* 1991).

Even when they use services, the attendance of drug users tends to be poor especially if drug services and HIV services are separate. By its nature drug addiction tends to be a chronic relapsing condition. The best care for drug users should involve treating their drug problem and HIV at the same time. Indeed, treating their drug problem is the key to engaging this group so that their HIV disease is effectively managed, for their own sake and so that the potential for infecting a wider population is reduced.

The role of the General Practitioner

The care of drug users is best achieved by treating them as close to their community as possible with secondary support for specialist drug treatment centres and HIV services. This is further expanded in Chapters 13 and 14. The General Practitioner or family doctor, as present in many national healthcare systems, is ideally placed in the community to be able to offer this care. He or she works in a defined small area, serving individual and family medical needs, with a knowledge of local conditions and support networks. In reality however the role of the General Practitioner in the care of injecting drug users has depended largely on the outlook and enthusiasm of the individual. Such care has been described as – 'reactive and pragmatic rather than planned and strategic' (Glanz 1994). General Practitioners have largely been reluctant to work with drug users, and drug problems in patients with HIV have been seen as the greatest deterrent for caring for these patients (Sibald and Freeling 1988). However many studies into doctors' attitudes were conducted early in the epidemic and as time has gone on more and more GPs have been prepared to take on the management of drug users with or without HIV infection when properly supported and resourced (Bury *et al.* 1997, Waller 1997). The doctor's greatest fear is one of personal safety and this can be largely overcome by GPs treating individuals with the support of dedicated drug workers, working in close co-operation with the drug services and supported by appropriate specialist HIV services.

The General Practitioner or family doctor is also ideally placed to provide continuing care to the individual, but also and just as importantly, to the individual's family. Here the doctor can advise, counsel, treat and generally support the whole family in this difficult clinical area.

Harm reduction

Up until the mid 1980s, drug treatment services around the world were mainly directed towards 'curing' addiction, that is moving the drug user to a drug-free state and supporting them in this abstinent state to engage in 'normal' social behaviour. Initial help was provided by medical drug treatment services supported by drug-free 'therapeutic' communities, examples of which include Day Top in the USA, Phoenix House in the UK, and Coolmine in Ireland. It quickly became apparent that there was a large reservoir of HIV infection amongst injecting drug users when HIV antibody testing became widely available in 1985. This posed a public health threat, not only within in drug using community but by sexual spread and vertical (materno-foetal) spread from drug users to a much wider community. This alarmed and prompted the drug services to review their approach. To varying degrees over the next decade, drug services in most western countries adopted a more pragmatic approach and whilst many services retain the goal of abstinence from drugs for the individual, they accept that many drug users, especially opiates users, cannot or will not stop using drugs. The reasons for not being able to stop include physical addiction and complex psychosocial problems. This pragmatic approach is one of harm reduction – that is to reduce the harm that drug users can do to themselves and to other by their continuing drug use and sexual activities.

In 1985 the Advisory Council, on The Misuse of Drugs (ACMD 1988) stated: 'The spread of HIV is a greater danger to individual and public health than drug misuse. Accordingly, we believe that services which aim to minimize HIV risk behaviour by all available means should take precedence in development plans.' The report goes on to say that 'There need to be changes in professional and public attitudes to drug misuse' and that 'we must be prepared to work with these who continue to misuse drugs' not to do so would 'have a major effect on ability to contain the spread of HIV'. This report has had a major effect on the drug services in the UK and beyond.

The services which aim to minimize HIV risk behaviour in injecting drug users are needle and syringe exchange, oral methadone substitution of opiates, provision of 'safer' sex education and easy access to condoms, at no cost to the individual. These services need to relate to the drug users, that is they need to be easily accessible and available, if they are to make any impact.

The experiences in Amsterdam (Buning *et al*. 1991) and Glasgow (Bloor *et al*. 1994) appear to show that harm minimization/reduction programmes help to keep the seroprevalence of HIV amongst drug users in these cities at a low level. Multicentre studies in London (Stimson *et al*. 1996) and Australia (Hurley *et al*. 1997) show HIV incidence amongst injecting drug users can be reduced by harm minimization programmes. However the implementation of these services in affected communities and cities has often been resisted by local communities, and local businesses. They fear that setting such services in their communities will have an adverse effect on their business and that such areas will be labelled as 'drug areas' (Barry 1996).

So whilst the health authorities and their drug services have tried to implement these harm reduction services with varying enthusiasm, they have met strong, sometimes unexpected, resistance from communities. The lesson which has been learnt is that the drug services need to enter into dialogue with affected communities in which they hope to introduce services, so as to listen to legitimate grievances and fears and introduce a service that all can support.

The Dublin experience

Dublin's experience with injecting drug users has been a relevantly recent one. There was little injecting opiate drug use in Dublin prior to the early 1980s (Butler 1991). At that time it became apparent that there was a growing problem with injecting opiate use in the large more deprived, public authority housing units around the city. HIV infection was probably introduced into this group in 1982 (Hillery 1990). Drug users form the largest group of HIV positive individuals in Ireland accounting for over 40% of those who are HIV positive (Virus Alert 1997).

In the mid 1980s there was only one drug treatment centre (Trinity Court) with ten in-patient beds for detoxification. This service struggled to cope with a large and growing problem through the 1980s. Trinity Court at this time only offered drug detoxification. It became evident that more comprehensive services were needed and it is now only in 1997 after an injection of £IRL14 million that such an adequate service has been achieved. In the interim period many bodies were engaged in dialogue, some of it 'heated' dialogue, to initiate appropriate services. This process has involved the Department of Health, the Eastern Health Board, Trinity Court, the Irish College of General Practitioners, Pharmacists and voluntary drug organizations. This took place against a background of resistance by organized community groups. It is known anecdotally that criminal elements who were profiting from illicit drug supply were 'supportive' of community resistance to locally placed drug services.

The service now consists of six medical drug treatment centres under the supervision of three psychiatrists who are specialists in addiction problems. These six centres have in turn responsibility for a number of satellite clinics, 12 in total. The satellite clinics are based in the heart of local communities and are run by local voluntary drug agencies, and are supported by local General Practitioners who work on a sessional basis in these clinics. They provide methadone maintenance and detoxification programmes and whilst they provide limited medical support they encourage drug users to go to their own GPs for ongoing medical care. When drug users are stabilized, the intention is that their GPs would also take over care for their methadone maintenance along the lines of a national protocol.

There is now a centrally held treatment list of all drug users receiving methadone maintenance and protocol for implementation of this programme. The protocol was agreed between the Department of Health, the Irish College of General Practitioners and the representatives of the Pharmacists Associations.

In addition to the services already mentioned, there are now 34 in-patient beds for detoxification in three units. All the services are supported by community drug counsellors and education officers, and are under the direction of three area administrators, all answerable to one programme manager. In addition to the service listed there is a Gay Men's Health Project and Women's Health Project for Street Women.

Outside these services, there are a further 75 General Practitioners (family doctors) who treat and prescribe methadone linctus in their own practice. These doctors prescribe for 1100 drug users whilst the services treat a further 1400 people (Trinity Court June 1997).

These services are provided in conjunction with community pharmacists who dispense either daily or weekly to individuals. The total number of drug users is estimated as 3600 persons (Task Force Report 1996) and is made up of those known to be in treatment and those on the waiting list. The services are to expand further and the stated aim of the services is to reduce the waiting lists to zero, so that drug users would have easy and early access to full treatment services. It is expected that this will be achieved before the end of 1997.

However, many countries from the developing world, such as Malaysia, cannot afford to develop such services. Yoong in a recent paper (Yoong and Cheong 1997) stated that 'These patients (i.e. drug users) use up a disproportionate share of health resources, something that developing countries cannot afford'. The paper goes on to note, however, that if services are not developed, the number of drug users will increase and with it HIV infection. Therefore it is important for all nations, all communities with a drug use problem, to develop harm reduction strategies in line with available resources.

References

ACMD 1988: *AIDS and drug misuse, Part 1*. Report by Advisory Council on the Misuse of Drugs. HMSO, London.

Barry, J. 1996: *Personal communication* from Dr Joe Barry, HIV/AIDS and Drugs Medical Co-ordinator, Eastern Health Board, Ireland.

Bellis, M.A., Weild, A.R., Beeching, N.J., Mutton, K.J., Quttub, S. 1997: Prevalence of HIV and injecting drug use in men entering Liverpool Prison. *British Medical Journal*, **315**, 30–31.

Bloor, M. Frischer, M., Taylor, A., Covell, R., Goldberg, D., Green, S., McKeganey, N., Platt, S. 1994. *Tideline and turn: Possible reasons for continuing low HIV prevalence among Glasgow's injecting drug users*. Sociological Review, Blackwell, Oxford.

Bourke, M. 1997: *Working with drug users in general practice*. Irish College of General Practitioners.

Brettle, R.P. 1993. HIV Infection related to injection drug use. In: Adler, M.W. (ed.) *ABC of AIDS*, 3rd Edn. BMJ Publication, London.

Buning, E., van Brussel, V., van Santen, G. 1991. The impact of harm reduction drug policy on AIDS prevention in Amsterdam. In: *The reduction of drug related harm.* Routledge, London, pp. 30–38.

Bury, J., Simmonte, M., Jacquet, E. 1997: *Training primary care staff about HIV prevention.* Paper read at Third International Conference on Home and Community Care for Persons Living with HIV/AIDS, Amsterdam.

Butler, S. 1991: Drug problems and drug policies in Ireland: a quarter of a century reviewed. *Administration (Journal of Institute of Public Administration)* **39**, 210–33.

Carnwath, T. 1997: Fatal methadone overdose. Letter. *British Medical Journal* **315**, 55.

CDC 1993: Center of Disease Control 1993. Revised classification system for HIV infection and expanded surveillance case definition for AIDS among adolescents and adults. *Morbidity and Mortality Weekly Report* **41**, 17.

GMC 1995: *HIV and AIDS: the ethical considerations.* Guidelines from the General Medical Council, London.

Glanz, A. 1994: The fall and rise of the general practitioner. In: Strang, J. and Gossop, M. (eds). *Heroin addiction and drug policy, the British System.* Oxford Medical Publications.

Hillery, I. 1990: *Personal communication* from Professor Irene Hillery, Virus Reference Laboratory, University College Dublin, Dublin 4.

Hurley, S., Jolley, D.J., Kaldor, J.M. 1997: Effectiveness of needle exchange programmes for prevention of HIV infection. *Lancet* 1997, **349**, 1797–800.

Mason, D., Birmingham, L., Grubin, D. 1997: Substance use in remand prisoners: a consecutive case study. *British Medical Journal,* **315**, 18–21.

Odongo-Aginya, A.D., Madrae, E., Muva, E. 1997: *A need assessment for community based home care for persons living in HIV/AIDS in Uganda.* Paper read at Third International Conference on Home and Community Care for Persons Living with HIV/AIDS, Amsterdam.

Prins, M., Veugelers, P.J. 1997: Comparison of progression and non-progression in injecting drug users and homosexual men with documented dates of HIV-1 seroconversion. *AIDS,* **11**, 621–31.

Selwyn, P.A., Alcabes, P., Hartel, D., Buono, D., Schoenbaum, E.E., Klein, R.S., Davenny, K., Friedland, G.H. 1992: Clinical manifestations and predictors of disease progression in drug users with human immunodeficency virus infection. *New England Journal of Medicine,* **327**, 1697–703.

Sibald, B., Freeling, P. 1988: AIDS and the future general practitioner. *Journal of the Royal College of General Practitioners,* **38**, 500–502.

Stimson, G.V., Hunter, G.M., Donoghoe, M.C., Rhodes, T. Darry, J.V., Chalmers, C.P. 1996: HIV-1 Prevalence in community wide samples of injecting drug users in London, 1990–1993. *AIDS,* **10**, 657–66.

Task Force Report 1996. *First report of the ministerial task force on measures to reduce the demand for drugs.* Government Information Office, Dublin.

Task Force Report 1997: *Second report. Government Information Office, Dublin.*

Trinity Court 1997: *Internal report to the board of Trinity Court.* Trinity Court, Pearse Street, Dublin.

UN AIDS 1996: *HIV/AIDS: The Global Epidemic December 1996.* UNAIDS/SC/96039–4.

Virus Alert 1997. *Bulletin of the Virus Reference Laboratory* No. 2. University College, Dublin.

Waller, T. 1997: A general practitioner's role: past, present and future. In: Beaumont, B. (ed.) *Care of drug users in general practice.* Radcliffe, Oxford.

WHO/SPA/IMF 1988: *Counselling in HIV infection and disease.* WHO, Geneva.

WHO 1995: *Effective approaches for the prevention of HIV/AIDS in women.* WHO, Geneva.

WHO-EC 1997: *HIV/AIDS surveillance in Europe.* Second Quarterly Report. WHO EC collaborating centre on AIDS, Saint Maurice, France.

Wright, E. 1996: Natural history and laboratory markers of HIV infection. In: *Management of the HIV-infected patient.* Cambridge University Press.

Yirrell, D.L., Robertson, P., Goldberg, D.J., McMenamin, J., Cameron, S., Leigh Brown, A.J. 1997: Molecular investigation into and outbreak of HIV in a Scottish Prison. *British Medical Journal*, **314**, 1446–50.

Yoong, K., Cheong, I. 1997: A study of Malaysian drug addicts with human immunodeficency virus infections. *International Journal of STD and AIDS*, **8**, 118–23.

Patient assessment

Marc N Gourevitch, Peter A Selwyn and
Patrick G O'Connor

Introduction

Despite the high lifetime prevalence of substance abuse found in many studies, it is consistently under-recognized in practice (Kamerow *et al.* 1986, Coulehan *et al.* 1987). Even when identified, it is commonly ignored, frequently because of a lack of comfort and skill on the part of the clinician. In this chapter, we attempt to present a cohesive approach to the drug using patient, focused on assessing and engaging the patient in a constructive relationship.

Overall approach

To succeed in eliciting from the patient the information needed to address his/her drug use effectively, the relationship between patient and clinician must be based in trust. This may take time to establish, as it relies upon the patient coming to appreciate that the physician is genuinely interested in helping. The clinician may move this process along considerably by adopting a non-judgmental and accepting attitude towards the information and behaviours related by the patient. Shame and diminished self-esteem are prevalent traits among drug users. The physician must take care to avoid disapproving or critical remarks, as patients will often respond by withholding information they fear might provoke such reactions in the future. Such damage to the therapeutic alliance can severely restrict the work that can be accomplished on the patient's behalf.

The issue of confidentiality frequently arises when caring for the drug using patient. A direct approach is most effective here as well. When the physician is part of a larger treatment team in which the expectation is that patient data will be shared among members of the team, this arrangement is best made clear to the patient at the beginning of the relationship. Splitting and perceived betrayal can thus be avoided. The physician must educate himself or herself regarding the laws governing confidentiality of information about patients' substance abuse behaviour and treatment. Sensitivity to this issue by the treating clinician will enhance the development of trust in the clinician by the patient.

To engage the patient most effectively, the provider must determine and attend to the patient's agenda. Particularly at the outset, the drug user may or may not perceive or acknowledge his/her drug use as a problem in need of attention. By enquiring about and addressing the primary concerns of the patient, the clinician will make evident his/her interest in helping the patient. This will likely result in greater receptiveness later, on the part of the patient, to the clinician's concern regarding the patient's drug use.

History

Substance abuse is notoriously under-recognized by providers of medical care. Many physicians (primary care doctors and specialists) are inadequately trained to recognize drug use. This deficiency is compounded by the stigma associated with drug use and the consequent reluctance of many patients to acknowledge these behaviours. As a result, many opportunities to aid patients, whether by reducing the riskiness of behaviours or helping achieve abstinence altogether, are missed. For this reason, and because of the often grave health risks that drug use poses to the patient and his/her contacts, it is critical that clinicians incorporate the drug use history into their routine evaluation of all patients.

An understanding of the terminology and diagnosis of drug misuse is necessary to be able to interpret the results of the patient's history. The *Diagnostic and Statistical Manual IV* specifies two categories of drug use: dependence and abuse. *Dependence* refers to drug use that becomes associated with physiologic tolerance and the presence of an abstinence syndrome. Tolerance signifies that progressively higher doses of a drug are required by a chronic user to achieve a desired effect such as euphoria. Abstinence syndromes are drug specific and occur following withdrawal of the drug. The severity of an abstinence syndrome may be lessened medically by using one of several detoxification techniques. Along with these important physiologic characteristics, dependence connotes a habitual and compulsive or consuming involvement with using the drug or drugs in question. *Abuse* implies a pattern of persistent drug use associated with recurrent intoxication and loss of control, despite significant medical and social consequences. Abuse is more likely to characterize intermittent drug use, in which tolerance and withdrawal do not develop, but some physical or social harm befalls the user. The distinction between dependence and abuse is useful to the clinician trying to assess the extent and severity of a patient's drug use, and the options for intervention.

The concept of substance use as a 'disease' has engendered much controversy, although it has gained significant acceptance. It is often helpful for primary care providers to think of substance use as a 'chronic disease,' with features common to other chronic diseases with which they are more familiar, such as diabetes, chronic lung disease, arthritis and HIV infection. Like these illnesses, substance use is a persistent condition typically characterized by exacerbations and remissions. Primary care providers have little difficulty managing exacerbations of other chronic diseases and are familiar with strategies to induce remission or to slow progression of diseases they cannot cure. When a 'sober' intravenous drug user relapses to active use, however, the clinician often gives in to frustration, assuming despite evidence to the contrary (Daley and Marlatt 1992) that further attempts at treatment will be fruitless. Care givers who accept relapse as a common clinical presentation of drug use, and who are aware of available treatment options, may remain more successfully engaged with the drug using patient, thus enhancing the quality and continuity of care provided.

Conceptually, there are two principal phases to the initial assessment of an individual's drug use behaviour: a screening history and, if positive, a more detailed history. Screening, of patients not known to be current or former drug users, refers to the determination of whether drug use/misuse is or has been present. If screening elicits a history of drug use, or if a patient volunteers such information without probing by the practitioner, then a more detailed drug use history is indicated. Although in practice, screening and (if positive) more detailed history questions are often woven together, we will discuss them here separately for the sake of clarity.

Screening history

Depending on the context, it may be useful for the clinician to preface questions about drug use with a statement that these important questions are a standard component of history taking. Drug use questions may be most comfortably situated following questions about smoking cigarettes. Whatever the sequence, physicians should become familiar with a set of drug use questions and apply them consistently.

In keeping with the meanings of addiction and dependence, the clinician must search not only for acknowledgment of drug use, but also for indications of the impact of such use on the patient's life. Loss of control, interference with social and physical functioning, guilt, and physical withdrawal are all signs of problem drug use. Instruments to screen for such signs in alcohol users, such as the four CAGE questions, have not been formally validated among other drug users. However, they may serve as a template for asking about all forms of drug use. The CAGE questions are:

1 Have you ever felt you ought to Cut down on your drinking?
2 Have people Annoyed you by criticizing your drinking?
3 Have you ever felt Guilty about your drinking?
4 Have you ever had a drink first thing in the morning to steady your nerves (an Eye opener)? (Mayfield et al. 1974).

Used together, these questions have been reported to be 85% sensitive and 89% specific in detecting alcohol abuse. The principles upon which the CAGE questions are based form an excellent basis from which to explore a patient's use of any addictive drug. Although other instruments have been developed to screen patients for use of drugs other than alcohol, none has been extensively evaluated in the general medical setting (Schorling and Buchsbaum 1997).

Denial may complicate the process of screening for drug use. Denial can be both unconscious and conscious. Patients often work hard to rationalize their substance abuse problems to themselves, to the point that they are convinced no problem exists despite evidence to the contrary. Denial occurs on a conscious level when patients, fearful of rejection or feeling shame, deny drug use despite the presence of obvious complications. Clinicians often participate in such denial. Because of their own discomfort regarding substance use, providers may reinforce patients' denial by not inquiring about substance use or by accepting the denial of drug use too readily.

When screening for a history of substance abuse is negative, other elements of the history may still serve as important clues or 'red flags' regarding drug use. These include common medical, behavioural, or social symptoms and signs that, although sometimes non-specific, may give a clue to underlying substance abuse. Trauma resulting from physical abuse, altercations, or motor vehicle accidents also often suggests hidden drug use (Schorling and Buchsbaum 1997).

Detailed history

Regardless of the type of substance used, the history should include information on five major points: drug(s) used, route(s) of administration, patterns of use, complications, and history of treatment.

The identity of the drug or drugs used must be explored. Terminology may be an issue, and must be clarified at the outset. Clinicians unfamiliar with a drug cited by a patient should not be embarrassed to ask the patient if it might go by another name. Most patients will take such inquiries as a sign of genuine interest, rather than of naïvete. Alternatively, the physician may consult a published list of common 'street' names of drugs of abuse (Cherubin and Sapira 1993) ideally one tailored to the geographic area of their practice. Polysubstance abuse is common, particularly among drug injectors. The clinician must not conclude the history after characterizing the patient's use of a single drug, but rather should follow with questions like 'what other drugs do you use?' until the inventory has been completed.

The route of administration is particularly important, as it is directly related to the drug's harmful effects. Many drugs may be taken by more than one route. Heroin, cocaine and amphetamine can be injected, snorted intranasally, or smoked alone or together with tobacco or marijuana. Drug injection is the most dangerous form of administration, because of the high blood levels attained and because of the many infectious and other complications of needle use, discussed further below. No form of administration is benign, however. Intranasal use may be complicated by erosion of the intranasal septum and sinusitis (Warner 1993), and smoking with acute and chronic respiratory symptoms and pneumonia (Tashkin *et al.* 1990, 1993, Caiaffa *et al.* 1994). Knowledge of the route of use is thus essential in assessing the patient's risk for complications and in developing a strategy to minimize drug use-related harm. This section of the patient interview often presents the greatest opportunity for introducing education about strategies for preventing complications of drug abuse (see below).

Patterns of drug use give an indication of the extent of the patient's involvement with drug taking. The duration of use, frequency of use, most recent use, and amount used are useful data in this regard. Intermittent use does not necessarily reflect a lesser problem than daily use. Binge drinking or 'runs' of cocaine use can be acutely dangerous and associated with particularly risk-prone behaviour. The use of several drugs concurrently, often with opposing effects, should also be explored. The mixture of heroin and cocaine (speedball) is perhaps the best known combination. Assessing patterns of use provides a window onto the intensity of the patient's drug using behaviour.

Addressing and reducing the medical and social complications of drug use are the principal reasons for assessing patients' drug using behaviours. The medical complications of drug use are legion (Cherubin and Sapira 1993, Warner 1993, Leiber 1995), and include direct drug effects (narcotic overdose, heroin pulmonary edema, cocaine-induced myocardial infarction and rhabdomyolysis, alcoholic hepatitis, etc.) and indirect effects (e.g. injection-related infections). When taking the history, it may be most practical simply to ask the patient whether he/she has had any of the medical complications most commonly associated with the drug(s) in question. Later, during the physical and laboratory examinations, evidence for other sequelae of drug use may be sought.

The social complications of drug abuse are frequently more difficult for patients to discuss than the physical complications. Damaged family ties and friendships, unemployment or difficulty at work, dependence on others or on the state, unstable housing, and time in prison are but a few of the direct or indirect consequences of chronic drug use for many patients. Not infrequently, these complications may be the patient's principal concern, as opposed to the medical conditions with which many clinicians are more comfortable. It is critical to pay close attention to the needs felt most acutely by the patient. As with the rest of the history, the object of enquiring into these issues is not simply to take exhaustive inventory. Rather, it is to develop an understanding of the specific impact of drug use on the patient's life, with a view towards assessing, focusing and ultimately harnessing the patient's motivation to alter his or her behaviour.

An understanding of the patient's history of treatment for drug use is valuable. Therapies that proved ineffective in the past should not be chosen again without careful consideration. If a method of treatment has failed, it is important to enquire why. The definition of 'successful' treatment must be formulated thoughtfully. If a cocaine injector's first residential treatment was followed by 2 years of abstinence and then gradual resumption of intranasal use, the treatment might well be considered a success. Similarly, other correlates of reduced drug use or abstinence, while not meeting the definition of treatment, must be explored. If employment is consistently associated with abstinence and loss of work with drug use, then the primary objective might be to assist the patient in obtaining work, not drug treatment in the traditional sense. Instruments developed specifically to take inventory of patients' treatment histories (McLellan *et al.* 1992) may have only limited applicability in the general primary care setting.

Obtaining a thorough drug use history may require multiple visits. Once a trustful relationship is developed, patients will likely feel more comfortable discussing their substance use and a more complete picture may emerge. Multiple sources of information may be required, especially family members and friends. Medical records, when available, may also be helpful in revealing a history of and medical complications related to drug use.

Physical examination

When examining the drug using patient, attention should be focused on the systems directly affected by the substances the patient is known to use, while not neglecting evidence of use of other drugs. Special attention should be paid to the presence of a variety of signs. Injection ('track') marks may be recent (appearing as fresh punctate marks, often with mild surrounding erythema) or old (linear, hyper-pigmented scars representing the confluence of multiple past injection sites). They are found wherever veins are accessible, most often in the antecubital fossae, on the forearms, hands and legs, and less commonly in the neck and groin. Lymphedema of the hands is not uncommon among patients with an extensive injection history. Fresh or old healed abscesses, and cellulitis, are common among injectors, typically reflecting poor hygiene in injecting technique. A cardiac murmur consistent with mitral or tricuspid regurgitation may suggest a past or current history of endocarditis. The nasal septum should always be examined for erosion or infection, signifying intra-nasal drug use. Tachycardia and tremulousness may signify withdrawal from alcohol or other drugs. The stigmata of chronic alcohol abuse and cirrhosis must be looked for as well.

Laboratory examination

There are two principal components to the laboratory examination of the drug using patient in the primary care setting: screening for drugs used, and screening for the sequelae of their use. Testing of the urine for drugs or their metabolites is commonly performed, though its sensitivity may be significantly affected by such factors as the nature of the assay employed, the interval between drug use and urine sampling, and the quantity of drug used by the patient. False positive results are not uncommon. Unless used to corroborate patient self-report, it is rarely advisable to treat a single urine toxicology result as definitive evidence of drug misuse. In addition, in the primary care setting, it is not generally appropriate to obtain urine for toxicologic screening without making clear to the patient the nature of the test being ordered. Urine toxicologic screening is particularly insensitive in detecting alcohol use. While a blood alcohol determination may be used for this purpose, an elevated level may often be already apparent as 'alcohol on the breath', and thus of limited use as a screening test.

Results of several routinely conducted laboratory tests may also suggest the presence or severity of drug use. Elevation of hepatic enzymes is a common finding in drug users (Stimmel *et al.* 1975), usually reflecting viral or alcoholic hepatitis. Serologic evidence of hepatitis B and C should alert the clinician to a possible history of drug use. An elevation of total protein relative to albumin may indicate the presence of a polyclonal gammopathy associated with drug injection itself (Brown *et al.* 1974), or with HIV infection when present. A positive syphilis serology, or diagnosis of other sexually transmitted diseases, is suggestive of risky sexual behaviour, itself often associated with drug use. Proteinuria and renal insufficiency may reflect heroin nephropathy.

Overlapping symptoms and syndromes

A challenge that often arises in the course of assessing and caring for the drug using patient is differentiation of symptoms and signs related to drug use itself from those of comorbid medical and psychiatric conditions. Such overlapping presentations are most commonly seen among patients with constitutional or psychiatric symptoms.

Constitutional symptoms are frequently related to drug use and withdrawal, but may also reflect systemic illness. Thus, fever after drug injection may reflect use of an impure drug mixture or the first sign of endocarditis. Myalgias, chills, nausea, vomiting and diarrhea, all hallmarks of withdrawal from narcotics and alcohol, may likewise reflect gastroenteritis or another infectious process. Weight loss is commonly seen in association with heavy cocaine use, yet must also prompt consideration of systemic infection (e.g. tuberculosis), malignancy, or HIV infection. Dyspnea in the crack smoker may be due to chronic pulmonary dysfunction related to drug inhalation (Tashkin *et al.* 1993), or to asthma or to community-acquired or HIV-related pneumonia. Seizures may occur in the context of drug withdrawal (e.g. alcohol or benzodiazepines) or as a result of prior trauma or intercurrent infection.

Psychiatric symptoms among drug users present particular challenges. Clinicians caring for drug users must frequently assess patients for altered mental status and other psychiatric or neuropsychiatric syndromes. It is critical in such cases to investigate the possibility of the acute or chronic effects of substance use, both to avoid misdiagnosis and to identify potentially treatable conditions. As with all such overlapping syndromes, it is important to remember that more than one process may be occurring at once, particularly as psychiatric comorbidity is so prevalent among drug users. Thus, the patient presenting with classic symptoms of depression may have depression, or be suffering from the effects of chronic cocaine use, or both. Agitation may reflect drug withdrawal or anxiety. Cocaine use and mania or bipolar disorder may be indistinguishable in the acute phase. Delerium may result from intoxication or overdose, or from a host of metabolic or toxic encephalopathies (e.g. hypoxia, hypoglycemia, meningitis, etc.). HIV-related central nervous system disorders must always be considered in such differential diagnoses among drug using patients.

A common and challenging clinical scenario is when a user of cocaine or alcohol presents with symptoms of depression. Should one wait until the patient has been abstinent for a period of days or weeks to assess whether the symptoms were related to drug use or to 'primary' depression? How long a period of abstinence is adequate to be sure that persistent withdrawal symptoms (Martin and Jasinski 1969) will not 'cloud' the diagnosis? What if the patient continues to use the drug, as is commonly the case? The best solution in such a case may be to treat for depression despite ongoing drug use, and to observe closely for evidence of a response. The availability of relatively safe and effective antidepressants has simplified the adoption of such a strategy. Waiting until the patient has been abstinent for a extended period before offering treatment for a possible comorbid psychiatric condition may greatly delay or prevent the patient from obtaining needed treatment.

Faced with the challenge of attributing a set of symptoms and signs to drug use or to a comorbid medical or psychiatric disorder, the physician must carefully consider the full clinical presentation. At times, identifying a single process responsible for the patient's condition will not be possible. The severity of the presentation will dictate whether to embark on presumptive treatment for a potentially dangerous medical condition or to opt for a more conservative approach or close observation and follow-up, giving symptoms related to drug use time to subside.

Risk assessment

A critical portion of the assessment of the drug using patient is a determination of the immediate and longer term drug use-related risks he or she may face. HIV infection is particularly important in this regard. It is important to note that for many drug using patients, sexual acquisition of HIV infection is every bit as much of a threat as needle-borne acquisition (Edlin *et al*. 1994, Avins *et al*. 1994). Because of the disinhibiting effects of many drugs, the stimulant effects of others, and the relationship of drug procurement to risky sexual behaviour, drug use is linked to acquisition of HIV infection in many ways other than needle use. For patients known to have been HIV seronegative in the past, or for those unaware of their infection status, drug use and sexual practices must be explored. Are needles being shared? Is sex being exchanged for drugs or for money? What is the extent of the patient's sexual risk for acquiring HIV infection and other sexually transmitted diseases, and how is that risk related to the patient's drug use? The answers to these questions may help determine which interventions are needed most acutely.

Motivational issues

Once data are assembled from the history, physical and laboratory examinations outlined above, the clinician will have substantial information at hand to use in deciding how best to address a patient's substance use. Yet perhaps the most critical piece of information in making such assessments is the extent of the patient's own motivation to address this issue. In the absence of such motivation, any plan developed by the clinician, even with the stated agreement of the patient, is likely to be of little use.

A conceptual model that addresses this issue with particular strength is the 'Stages of Change' paradigm described by Prochaska and Di Clemente (Prochaska and Di Clemente 1992). In this model, five stages are identified that describe a continuum from not dealing with drug use at all to being actively engaged in preventing relapse. The stages are the following: (1) pre-contemplation (no desire to change drug using behaviours is present, and the risks and consequences of such behaviour are denied by the user); (2) contemplation (person is aware that his/her drug use is a problem and is seriously considering addressing it, but has made no internal commitment to do so); (3) determination (intent is present to take action to address drug use); (4) action (modification of behaviour or environment with the goal of reducing or eliminating drug using behaviour or its related harm); and (5) maintenance (active engagement in preventing relapse and maintaining behaviour change over time). While each stage in this model is continuous with the stage before and after it, the model is not unidirectional: over time, patients may move in either direction.

The power of this conceptualization lies in its clinical utility. Presenting a fully-developed treatment plan to a drug user who barely recognizes his behaviour as problematic will prove fruitless. Similarly, treating an addict who has been abstinent for 5 years as if he has little regard for his health will quickly alienate the patient from care. Other examples of stage specific interventions are outlined in Table 8.1. Ultimately, the role of the clinician may be seen as assisting the patient in moving from one stage of the continuum along to the next. For a drug user not yet considering his use to be problematic, the most appropriate intervention might be to help the patient understand the link between his use and recent disappointments or medical ills. For someone considering drug treatment, the most

Table 8.1 Stages of readiness to change addictive behaviours and stage-specific approaches

Stage	Patient features	Possible approaches
Precontemplation	Unaware of substance problems	Express concern about health problems, link to substance use
Contemplation	Recognizes problems	Reinforce links between substance use and problems, promote behavioural change
Determination	Decision made to change	Support decision, provide advice about short and long term actions to change behaviours
Action	Change in behaviours	Monitor compliance with advice and outcomes
Maintenance	Continuing new behaviours	Continued follow-up of substance use problems, support behaviour change/treatment efforts, monitor for relapse
Relapse	Recurrence of substance use	Support return to behaviour change problems and/or re-entry into or continuation of treatment, monitor for recurrence of substance use problems

appropriate intervention might be to arrange for the patient to meet with drug users already engaged in treatment, thus reducing a barrier the patient might have to taking this next step. The essence of such work consists of assessing 'where the patient is at' and, while 'meeting' the patient where he may be, at the same time assisting him to move in a healthier direction. Such 'motivational' techniques can be highly effective, and have been described in detail elsewhere (Miller and Rollnick 1991).

Formulating a plan

Once the patient assessment has been completed and data obtained regarding the extent and severity of drug use, the risk of imminent danger relating to drug use, and the user's motivation to address his or her use, the next step is to help the patient formulate a plan for addressing this issue. The primary goal in this process should be to reduce harm to the patient to the greatest extent possible over time. While total and sustained abstinence from all drug use may be the ideal objective in this regard, it cannot always, or even often, be achieved in the short-term with the majority of patients. Thus, the provider should consider a range of strategies, tailored to fit the needs and motivations of the patient as well as the resources available.

A multidisciplinary approach is usually needed to address the wide range of problems the patient may be experiencing. The primary care clinician may provide the majority of care, including screening, brief substance abuse-related interventions, and management of substance use-related medical problems. More severely involved patients such as those meeting criteria for substance dependence or those with significant psychiatric comorbidity may require specialized care from substance abuse or behavioural health specialists. Primary care providers need to be comfortable with, and knowledgeable of, their own capabilities and limitations in managing these patients. Effective referrals depend upon a familiarity with the resources, strengths and limitations of local programmes.

When behaviour change around substance abuse is agreed upon, the overall goals of treatment should be considered and specified. While abstinence is the preferred goal, especially for those who are substance dependent, harm reduction goals that fall short of total abstinence should be pursued as well. These goals might include activities decreasing substance use to safer levels and avoiding high-risk behaviours such as substance use in high-risk situations (e.g. driving), injection drug use and needle sharing.

Matching the patient with the intervention or treatment

A full discussion of the scope of interventions and treatments available to address active drug use is beyond the scope of this review chapter and many are described in more detail in Chapter 9, prescribing for drug users, Chapter 11 which concerns non-medical therapies and Chapter 14 which is about care in the community. Several points, however, deserve emphasis. Giving primary consideration to the patient's immediate needs increases the chances of success. Considerable attention has been given in recent years to tailoring the selection of interventions and treatments to the individual needs of patients. Successful employment of such strategies substantially increases patient engagement in treatment and thus maximizes its impact. The full spectrum of available interventions must always be considered. Thus, while referral to a syringe exchange programme may be the most effective intervention for an active injector just beginning to recognize the dangers of his behaviour, a brief counselling intervention may be better suited to another individual (see below), and referral to methadone maintenance or residential treatment best reserved for others still. Among the factors deserving of strong consideration in developing a plan with a patient are the urgency and acuity of the problem (from patient and provider perspectives), the nature and extent of risks posed by the individual's drug use, the chronicity of the patient's use, the individual's treatment history, the patient's 'location' on the stages of change continuum and his or her motivation to change, and any comorbid medical and psychiatric conditions that may be present.

It is worth noting that the 'science' of 'patient-treatment matching' has progressed substantially over the past 20 years. The standard regimen of in-patient 'detoxification' followed by after-care, common in the 1970s and 1980s, has been replaced by attempts to tailor treatment to patients' individual needs and base treatment on scientific evidence of efficacy. Epidemiological studies have identified a series of treatment matching variables which may be predictive of outcome for some patients in some treatments and may be useful in selecting specific treatments. These 'matching variables' include demographic features (age, gender, ethnicity), addiction features (topology and severity of substance abuse), intrapersonal characteristics (comorbid psychopathology, cognitive function, treatment seeking behaviour, stage of change problems), and interpersonal function (social severity, homelessness) (American Psychiatric Association 1995). There is evidence that each of these variables plays an important role in treatment outcome for different types of substance abuse in defined categories of patients.

Evidence from studies concerning 'patient-treatment matching' has been translated into clinical guidelines or algorithms by at least two major organizations in the United States (American Psychiatric Association 1995, American Society of Addiction Medicine 1997). For example, the American Society of Addiction Medicine (ASAM) Patient Placement Criteria 2 provides separate guidelines for both adults and adolescents. These guidelines describe five levels of service: early interventions, out-patient services, intensive out-patient/ partial hospitalization services, residential/in-patient services, and medically managed intensive in-patient services. While these and similar criteria are based on a combination of scientific evidence and expert opinion, there are few prospective data to verify their appropriateness. Despite this, they represent the 'state-of-the-art' of clinical patient treatment matching and provide useful guidelines to physicians and their patients.

Harm minimization

Considerable attention has been devoted in recent years to the concept of harm reduction or minimization among drug users. In this way of thinking, not unlike the outlook adopted by many physicians in treating the diabetic patient, the goal is to minimize to the extent possible any adverse consequences associated with the condition in question. Despite the fact that a 'cure' (i.e. sustained abstinence) may not be a realistic near-term goal for many drug users, much can nevertheless be done to minimize the impact of drug use on patients' health. Harm reduction is an approach to treatment that aims to reduce the harm associated with drug use through the use of immediate and practical strategies acceptable to the user. Such an approach may be simultaneously more effective and engaging for patient and provider alike.

The concept of harm reduction or risk reduction for drug injectors with or at risk for HIV infection was articulated primarily in Europe in the mid-1980s. In certain cities (e.g. Amsterdam), this approach was introduced even prior to the AIDS epidemic to prevent hepatitis B transmission. The basis for such a strategy has always been an attempt to minimize drug use-related harm to drug users and their contacts, without waiting to find out whether illicit drug use could be eliminated altogether. In the context of the AIDS epidemic, the major harm reduction interventions have included education and outreach (including condom distribution and sexual risk reduction education), needle disinfection and hygiene, needle and syringe exchange, and increased availability of treatment for drug use. Strategies to reduce drug use-related harm span a continuum from safer needle use to total abstinence from drug use.

Numerous studies from around the world have demonstrated drug users' awareness of their risk for HIV infection and AIDS, and that some behaviour modification has resulted from this knowledge (Becker and Joseph 1988, Brettle and Leen 1991, Des Jarlais *et al.* 1994). The most commonly reported changes in behaviours include disinfection of injection equipment, reductions in needle sharing, reduction in the number of needle-sharing partners, and cessation of high-risk activities such as 'shooting gallery' use. The practice of needle disinfection has most commonly involved the use of household bleach with needles that are being reused. Although this practice is appealing in its simplicity, and has been proposed in areas where increased access to sterile injection equipment is impractical, several studies suggest that bleach use practices may not be consistent or rigorous enough to protect against HIV transmission (even though undiluted bleach inactivates HIV in the laboratory setting) (Gleghorn *et al.* 1994, McCoy *et al.* 1994, Titus *et al.* 1994). Another simple intervention, skin cleaning with alcohol swabs before injection, may result in decreased incidence of skin infections and possibly of endocarditis.

Needle and syringe exchange has been widely promoted as a harm reduction strategy for drug injectors, and exchange programmes now exist in many locations in North America, Europe and Australia. In addition to exchanging needles and providing condoms and related education, these programmes often serve as an important link between active drug injectors and medical and social services. Studies have consistently shown that needle exchange, in addition to improving access to and engagement with needed services, is associated with decreased needle sharing and related high-risk behaviour (Stimson 1989, Stryker and Smith 1993, Watters *et al.* 1994, Schoenbaum *et al.* 1996). For example, data from a needle exchange and research programme in New Haven, Connecticut, suggest that the prevalence of HIV infection in used syringes in that city declined steadily since the programme was introduced. The likelihood of HIV transmission via contaminated needles may have been reduced by as much as one-third in this environment as a result of the increased availability of sterile needles though the needle exchange programme.

Stabilization of HIV infection rates has been observed in recent years in some drug using populations, although it is not known definitively whether this reflects adoption of safer drug-using practices (Gleghorn *et al.* 1994). In New York City, for example, after a rapid rise in HIV seroprevalence during the late 1970s and early 1980s, seroprevalence levels among drug injectors have since remained close to 50%. This plateau has coincided with the increased use of syringe exchange programmes and, among some users, a switch to non-injected forms of heroin use (e.g. intranasal use). It must be noted that stabilization in HIV seroprevalence does not imply the absence of new infections, since high rates of loss from the drug using population of HIV infected persons (e.g. through illness, disability, or death) suggest that transmission must still be occurring if infection levels remained stable. The observation that HIV infection may be acquired relatively early in drug injection careers (Vlahov *et al.* 1990), and that drug treatment programmes generally serve older and more experienced injectors (McCusker *et al.* 1994), emphasizes the importance of continued HIV prevention, especially in high-risk younger populations of drug users. Finally, while risky drug using behaviours may have decreased, there has been little change in the sexual risk behaviour of drug injectors, which has critical implications for heterosexual transmission of HIV (Brettle and Leen 1991, Watkins *et al.* 1994).

Harm minimization strategies encompass the full range of treatment interventions. Compelling evidence of this is provided by studies of the effects of drug treatment on HIV-related risk behaviours and HIV infection incidence. It has been clearly demonstrated that methadone treatment results in decreased heroin injection, overall improvement in health status and social functioning, and reduced risk of HIV infection among opioid addicts (Ball and Ross 1991, Hartel *et al.* 1995, Novick *et al.* 1990, Office of Technology Assessment 1990, Schoenbaum *et al.* 1989). Several studies have suggested that drug injectors in long-term methadone maintenance treatment are less likely to have or acquire HIV infection than those out of treatment. Thus, one recent study from Philadelphia documented an HIV seroconversion rate of only 3% among drug injectors in treatment, as opposed to a rate of 22% in an out-of-treatment comparison group (Metzger *et al.* 1993).

Brief interventions

As primary care providers increasingly attempt to address substance use issues in their practices, attention has focused on a range of brief interventions that may be deployed in the office setting. Brief interventions typically consist of short, focused interactions with patients designed to help modify specific behaviours. Components of brief interventions include education, feedback and advice concerning substance use behaviours, and may require 5 minutes or less to administer. Some brief interventions have been demonstrated to be effective tools (especially for tobacco and alcohol users) in primary

Table 8.2 FRAMES Counseling strategy for brief interventions

Feedback:	Review the problems experienced by the patient because of alcohol use
Responsibility:	Emphasize that changing alcohol use is the patient's choice and responsibility
Advice:	Advise the patient to cut down or abstain from alcohol
Menu:	Provide menu of options and strategies for changing
Empathy:	behaviour
	Use a warm, empathic and understanding approach with the
Self-efficacy:	patient
	Encourage optimism about likelihood and benefits of changing behaviour

care settings (Barnes and Samet 1997, Bien *et al.* 1993, Wilk *et al.* 1997).

The basic counselling strategy of brief interventions is outlined by the FRAMES acronym (Table 8.2). In this approach, the patient is given reflective feedback concerning his or her substance use, including the degree to which it deviated from the norm and the specific medical, psychological and social effects it is having on them. When advice is given, it is specific. Similarly, the menu of options presented to the patient must be specific and appropriate to the patient's level of motivation and stage of readiness to change. A supportive approach from the physician that is characterized by empathy and promotion of the patient's self-efficacy is critical to the success of such an approach.

A recent randomized trial of a brief intervention illustrates the specific components and efficacy this approach may have. Fleming and colleagues enrolled 723 'problem drinkers' identified in 17 community-based primary care practices in Wisconsin, USA. Subjects were randomized to an intervention or control group. The intervention group received structured advice and counselling about their drinking in two brief (15 minute) physician visits. This advice and counselling included: workbook with feedback on health behaviours, review of the prevalence of problem drinking and adverse effects of alcohol, work sheet on drinking cues, a drinking agreement and 'prescription' and a drinking diary. In addition, patients received a phone call from a nurse 2 weeks after the physician visit. After one year of follow-up, the intervention group had significant improvements in drinking behaviours, including number of drinks per week and episodes of binge drinking. In addition, male patients who received the intervention experienced decreased hospitalization for medical problems. Thus, a relatively simple intervention administered within the physician's office can have a significant impact on drinking behaviours and other health outcomes.

Health promotion

In addition to minimizing the harm related to drug use, clinicians must make every effort directly to promote the health of their drug using patients. Comprehensive primary care must include vaccinations, screening for infectious diseases (including tuberculosis, STDs, viral hepatitis and HIV), annual health maintenance examinations, and care of comorbid medical and psychiatric conditions (O'Connor *et al.* 1994). A variety of models exist for delivering such care (Samet *et al.* 1995). Most important is that treatment be delivered in a comprehensive and coordinated fashion, with tight integration between care for the drug use and general medical components of the services the patient receives.

References

American Psychiatric Association 1995: Practice guideline for the treatment of patients with substance use disorders: alcohol, cocaine, opioids. *American Journal of Psychiatry* **152** (11s): 1–80.

American Society of Addiction Medicine. 1997: *Patient placement criteria for the treatment of substance-related disorders,* 2nd edn. American Society of Addiction Medicine.

Avins, A.L., Woods, W.J., Lindan, C.P., Hudes, E.S., Clark, W., Hulley, S.B. 1994: HIV infection and risk behaviors among heterosexuals in alcohol treatment programs. *Journal of the American Medical Association* **271**, 515–18.

Ball, J.C., Ross, A. 1991: *The effectiveness of methadone maintenance treatment.* Springer-Verlag, New York.

Barnes, H.N., Samet, J.H. 1997: Brief interventions with substance-abusing patients. *Medical Clinical Journal of North America* **81**, 867–79.

Becker, M.H., Joseph, J.G. 1988: AIDS and behavioral change to reduce risk: a review. *American Journal of Public Health* **78**, 394–410.

Bien, T.H., Miller, W.R., Tonigan, J.S. 1993: Brief interventions for alcohol problems: a review. *Addiction* **88**, 315–35.

Brettle, R.P., Leen, C.L.S. 1991: The natural history of HIV and AIDS in women. *AIDS* **5**, 1283–92.

Brown, S.M., Stimmel, B., Taub, R.N., Kochwa, S., Rosenfield, R.E. 1974: Immunologic dysfunction in heroin addicts. *Archives of Internal Medicine* **134**, 1001–1006.

Caiaffa, W.T., Vlahov, D., Graham, N.M., Astemborski, J., Solomon, L., Nelson, K.E., Munoz, A. 1994: Drug smoking, *Pneumocystis carinii* pneumonia, and immunosuppression increase risk of bacterial pneumonia in human immunodeficiency virus-seropositive injection drug users. *American Journal of Respiratory Care Medicine* **150**, 1493–8.

Cherubin, C.E., Sapira, J.D. 1993: The medical complications of drug addiction and the medical assessment of the intravenous drug user: 25 years later. *Annals of Internal Medicine* **119**, 1017–28.

Coulehan, J.L., Zettler-Segal, M., Block M., McClelland, M., Schulberg, H.C. 1987: Recognition of alcoholism and substance abuse in primary care patients. *Archives of Internal Medicine* **147**, 349–52.

Daley, D.C., Marlatt, G.A. 1992: Relapse prevention: cognitive and behavioral interventions. In: Lowinson, J.H., Ruiz, P., Millman, R.B., Langrod, J.G. (eds). *Substance abuse: a comprehensive textbook*, 2nd edn. Williams & Wilkins, Baltimore, pp. 533–42.

Des Jarlais, D.C., Friedman, S.R., Sotheran, J.L., Wenston, J., Marmor, M., Yancovitz, S.R., Frank, B., Beatrice, S., Mildvan, D. 1994: Continuity and change within an HIV epidemic. Injecting drug users in New York City, 1984 through 1992. *Journal of the American Medical Association* **271**, 121–7.

Edlin, B.R., Irwin, K.L., Faruque, S., McCoy, C.B., Word, C., Serrano, Y., Inciardi, J.A., Bowser, B.P., Schilling, R.E., Holmberg, S.D. 1994: Intersecting epidemics – crack cocaine use and HIV infection among inner-city young adults. *New England Journal of Medicine* **331**, 1422–7.

Gleghorn A.A., Doherty, M.C., Vlahov, D.D., Celentano, D.D., Jones, T.S. 1994: Inadequate bleach contact times during syringe cleaning among injection drug users. *Journal of Acquired Immune Deficiency Syndrome* **7**, 767–72.

Hartel, D.M., Schoenbaum, E.E., Selwyn, P.A., Kline, J., Davenny, K., Klein, R.S., Friedland, G.H. 1995: Heroin use during methadone maintenance treatment: the importance of methadone dose and cocaine use. *American Journal of Public Health* **85**, 83–8.

Kamerow, D.B., Pincus, H.A., MacDonald, K.I. 1986: Alcohol abuse, other drug abuse, and mental disorders in medical practice. *Journal of the American Medical Association* **255**, 2054–7.

Lieber, C.S. 1995: Medical disorders of alcoholism. *New England Journal of Medicine* **333**, 1058–65.

Martin W.R., Jasinski, D.R. 1969: Physiological parameters of morphine dependence in man – tolerance, early abstinence, protracted abstinence. *Journal of Psychiatric Research* **7**: 9–17.

Mayfield, D., McLeod G., Hall, P. 1974: The CAGE questionnaire: Validation of a new alcoholism instrument. *American Journal of Psychiatry* **131**, 1121–3.

McCoy, C.B., Rivers, J.E., McCoy, H.V., Shapshak, P., Weatherby, N.L., Chitwood, D.D., Page, J.B., Inciardi, A., McBride, D.C. 1994: Compliance with bleach disinfection protocols among injecting drug users in Miami. *Journal of Acquired Immune Deficiency Syndrome* **7**, 773–6.

McCusker, J., Willis, G., McDonald, M., Lewis, B.F., Sereti, S.M., Feldman, Z.T. 1994: Admissions of injection drug users to drug abuse treatment following HIV counseling and testing. *Public Health Report* **109**, 212–18.

McLellan, A.T., Alterman, A.I., Cacciola, J., Metzger D., O'Brien, C.P. 1992: A new measure of substance abuse treatment: initial studies of the Treatment Services Review. *Journal of Nervous Mental Disorders* **180**, 101–10.

Metzger, D.S., Woody, G.E., McLellan, A.T., O'Brien, C.P., Druley, P., Navaline, H., De Philippis, D., Stolley, P., Abrutyn, E. 1993: Human immunodeficiency virus seroconversion among intravenous drug users in- and out-of-treatment: an 18-month prospective follow-up. *Journal of Acquired Immune Deficiency Syndrome* **6**, 1049–56.

Miller, W.R., Rollnick, S. 1991: *Motivational interviewing: preparing people to change addictive behavior.* Guilford Press, New York.

Novick, D.M., Joseph, H., Croxson, T.S., Salsitz, E.A., Wang, G., Richman, B.L., Poretsky, L., Keefe, J.B., Whimbey, E. 1990: Absence of antibody to human immunodeficiency virus in long-term socially rehabilitated methadone maintenance patients. *Archives of Internal Medicine* **150**, 97–9.

O'Connor, P.G., Selwyn, P.A., Schottenfeld, R.S. 1994: Medical care for injection drug users with human immunodeficiency virus infection. *New England Journal of Medicine* **331**, 450–59.

Office of Technology Assessment. 1990: *The effectiveness of drug abuse treatment: implications for controlling AIDS/HIV infection.* US Government Printing Office, Washington, DC.

Prochaska, J.O., Di Clemente, C.C. 1992: Stages of change in the modification of problem behaviors. *Programs of Behavior Modification* **28**, 183–218.

Samet, J.H., Stein, M.D., O'Connor, P.G. 1995: Models of medical care for HIV-infected drug users. *Substance Abuse* **16**, 131–9.

Schoenbaum, E.E., Hartel, D., Selwyn, P.A., Klein, R.S., Davenney, K., Rogers, M., Feiner, C., Friedland, G. 1989: Risk factors for human immunodeficiency virus infection in intravenous drug users. *New England Journal of Medicine* **321**, 874–9.

Schoenbaum, E.E., Hartel, D.M., Gourevitch, M.N. 1996: Needle exchange use among a cohort of drug users. *AIDS* **10**, 1729–34.

Schorling J.B., Buchsbaum, D.G. 1997: Screening for alcohol and drug abuse. *Medical Clinical Journal of North America* **81**, 845–65.

Stimmel, B., Vernace, S., Schaffner, F. 1975: Hepatitis B surface antigen and antibody: a prospective study in asymptomatic drug abusers. *Journal of the American Medical Association* **234**, 1135–8.

Stimson, G.V. 1989: Syringe-exchange programmes for injecting drug users. *AIDS* **3**, 253–60.

Stryker, J., Smith, M.D. 1993: *Dimensions of HIV prevention: needle exchange.* Henry J. Kaiser Family Foundation, Menlo Park, CA.

Tashkin, D.P. 1990: Pulmonary complications of smoked substance abuse. *Western Journal of Medicine* **152**, 525–30.

Tashkin, D.P., Simmons, M.S., Chang, P., Liu, H., Coulson, A.H. 1993: Effects of smoked substance abuse on nonspecific airway hyperresponsiveness. *American Review of Respiratory Disorders* **147**, 97–103.

Titus, S., Marmor, M., Des Jarlais, D., Kim, M., Wolfe, H., Beatrice, S. 1994: Bleach use and HIV seroconversion among New York City injection drug users. *Journal of Acquired Immune Deficiency Syndrome* **7**, 700–704.

Vlahov, D., Munoz, A., Anthony, J.C., Cohn, S., Celentano, D.D., Nelson, K.E. 1990: Association of drug infection patterns with antibody to human immunodeficiency virus type I among drug users in Baltimore, Maryland. *American Journal of Epidemiology* **132**, 847–56.

Warner, E.A. 1993: Cocaine abuse. *Annals of Internal Medicine* **119**, 226–35.

Watkins, K.E., Metzger, D., Woody, G., McLellan, A.T. 1994: High-risk sexual behaviors of intravenous drug users in- and out-of-treatment: implications for the spread of HIV infection. *American Journal of Drug and Alcohol Abuse* **18**, 389–99.

Watters, J.K., Estilo, M.J., Clark G.L., Lorvick, J. 1994: Syringe and needle exchange as HIV/AIDS prevention for injection drug users. *Journal of the American Medical Association* **271**, 115–20.

Wilk, A.I., Jensen, N.M., Havighurst, T.C. 1997: Meta-analysis of randomized control trials addressing brief interventions in heavy alcohol drinkers. *Journal of General Internal Medicine* **12**, 274–83.

9 Prescribing for drug users

Judith Bury and Carl Bickler

Introduction

People who misuse drugs usually have a range of needs and this may include the prescription of drugs at certain times in their drug using career. A number of health and social care professionals are often involved with the drug user and prescribing may be part of an integrated strategy for their management.

Prescribing for drug users has a controversial history. There are many issues that have been the subject of debate, including the role of prescribing in the management of drug users, which drugs should be prescribed and who should prescribe them. Although the controversy continues, there is now a large body of evidence and a great deal of experience to support substitute prescribing in the management of opiate misuse (Sorenson 1996, Farrell *et al.* 1994, Ward *et al.* 1992).

As heroin use and particularly heroin injecting has been the major public health anxiety in the drugs field during the last three decades in the USA, Europe and Australasia, most information and research comes from this field. In addition, the specific substitute drug methadone has been developed as the mainstay of opiate treatment policy, particularly in the USA and Australia.

This chapter will deal primarily with opiate prescribing, but reference will also be made to other drugs. In addition, other issues such as prescribing for withdrawal symptoms and prescribing analgesia for opiate users will also be addressed.

The other major drug causing concern has been cocaine for which, despite attempts to find a suitable substitute, there is still no specific pharmacological alternative (Fulco *et al.* 1995). Thus drug prescribing is not an appropriate intervention in the management of cocaine users and will therefore not be dealt with in this chapter but the general comments on support and counselling refer to all dependency problems including cocaine. Many of those dependent on cocaine are often also dependent on other drugs including opiates. It is important in the management of all drug users, including those who use cocaine, to pay attention to the range of problems presented.

There are a number of approaches to the treatment of drug dependency, including detoxification, rehabilitation, relapse prevention and long-term substitute prescribing. All of them share the broad aims of a reduction in illicit drug use and the progression from a more to a less chaotic state. One reason for a shift in attitudes to substitute prescribing has been an increasing emphasis on the concept of harm minimization, stimulated particularly by the recognition of HIV among drug users in the mid 1980s.

During the 1960s and 1970s there had been a rapid increase in the numbers of drug injectors in the USA with a resulting huge investment in methadone treatment in many centres. In the UK and Europe the increase in the numbers of drug injectors during the 1960s and 1970s threatened to overwhelm existing specialist services and there was a move towards community-led services (ACMD, 1982). The arrival of HIV concentrated responses on the risks of rapid spread in injecting drug users and their sexual partners. There was now an imperative to reduce drug injecting or at the very least to reduce needle and syringe sharing. For example, the UK Advisory Council on the Misuse of Drugs, in their first report on AIDS and Drug Misuse in 1988, concluded that:

'HIV is a greater threat to public and individual health than drug misuse. The first goal of work with drug misusers must therefore be to prevent them from acquiring or transmitting the virus. In some cases this will be achieved through abstinence. In others, abstinence will not be achievable for the time being and efforts will have to focus on risk-reduction.' (ACMD, 1988)

Prior to this, many health workers worked exclusively in an abstinence model – they would support drug users to come off drugs, but would not consider substitute prescribing. Harm minimization on the other hand acknowledges that many drug users are not ready to come off drugs, but can be supported to reduce the harm that the drugs may cause them while they are still using them. In the case of injecting drug users, the provision of an oral substitute has the obvious benefit of reducing the risks associated with injecting. This concept has also been extended to prescribing substitute drugs for oral drug users where the benefits may be more difficult to demonstrate.

Working with drug users raises difficult issues. Some health workers believe that using drugs is always wrong and that helping to reduce the risks associated with drug use condones drug using behaviour. Others take the view that the problems associated with drug use are self-inflicted and should therefore not consume time and other costly resources, while others view drug misuse as a social problem that should not involve medical resources. Some physicians refuse to prescribe for drug users because they find their behaviour difficult or because they feel sceptical about the possibility of change.

It is acknowledged that working with drug users is time consuming and can be difficult. In this chapter the view is taken however that the health risks of drug use make it a valid area of concern for doctors and that most drug users have the potential for change. Experience shows that if drug users are managed in a firm but considerate manner, the work can be satisfying and rewarding, with minimal disruption to the working environment and with both physical and emotional benefits for the drug user.

It is important for healthcare workers to be realistic when working with drug users and to understand that drug use is a chronic relapsing condition which may continue for many years and is sometimes lifelong. To avoid disillusionment it is important that healthcare workers do not expect their intervention, whether prescribing or any other intervention, to result in dramatic improvement or to produce quick results.

Prescribing substitute drugs for drug users can be associated with a number of pitfalls for healthcare workers, for drug users, for their families and for the community as a whole. Working with drug users is time consuming and can be stressful. Drug users can cause disruption and may display threatening and aggressive behaviour. This can have an effect on the healthcare worker, colleagues, the working environment and other patients. By prescribing drugs of addiction, doctors may be seen to be condoning drug use. If drug users can obtain prescriptions for the drugs they want, they may have less incentive to give up their drug use than if they have to cope with the problems of obtaining drugs illegally. There is also considerable concern about the fate of the drugs prescribed. There is no doubt that some drug users take some of their prescribed medication and sell the remainder while a few request drugs not for their own use but so that they can sell them for profit. It has been argued that making oral drugs more available in this way has some benefits as it may reduce the demand for injectables, but it also has considerable disadvantages including the risk that the drugs might be taken by those for whom they might be dangerous, even lethal, including opiate naive adults and children (Farrell *et al.* 1994).

Most of these pitfalls can be reduced if substitute drugs are prescribed in a controlled and responsible way, but some concerns undoubtedly remain. It is therefore essential that those involved in this field continue to weigh up the benefits and pitfalls of any action that they take.

Dole and Nyswander (1965) were the first to provide evidence of the benefits of methadone as a substitute drug for injecting opiate users and since then other research has confirmed their findings (e.g. Gunne and Gronbladh 1981, Ball and Ross 1991). It has been estimated that about a quarter of a million drug users worldwide are now receiving methadone treatment (Farrell *et al.* 1994). Prescribing methadone to opiate injectors reduces the risk of opiate injecting and of needle sharing and reduces the need for criminal activity to buy street drugs (Dole and Nyswander 1976). By providing a regular supply of medication and reducing withdrawal symptoms, it offers opiate users an opportunity to stabilize their drug intake and their lifestyle. Prescribing also helps to keep drug users in contact with health services with the potential for offering physical health care and counselling (Ball and Ross 1991, Farrell *et al.* 1994).

Opiate misuse has been prevalent in many parts of the world for a long time but in recent years misuse of other drugs, either alone or in combination with opiates, has been increasing. Substitute prescribing for other drugs of misuse has been less well researched but there is some support for the use of substitute benzodiazepines for those dependent on these drugs even if they are not injecting (Seivewright *et al.* 1993, Robertson and Treasure 1996). On theoretical grounds

there might also be a case for prescribing amphetamines to amphetamine users but there is as yet little evidence of its benefits (Mattick
and Darke 1995).

It is important not to see prescribing in isolation. Much of the
research on the effects of methadone prescribing emphasize that,
while prescribing itself brings some benefits, the drug user may also
benefit from other help such as counselling (Ball and Ross 1981, Ward
et al. 1992, McLellan *et al.* 1993). In some methadone clinics, the
emphasis is on providing methadone for as many drug users as
possible and this is achieved with minimal human interaction. It
would seem to make sense that the user benefits from the regular
human contact involved in being seen on a regular basis and that this
may be enhanced by enquiries and concern about health issues and
by some attempt at goal setting and regular reviews of progress. Such
a relationship can be developed in a drug service or in a primary care
setting and it achieves more than the simple provision of methadone.
Many drug users will also have practical problems with which they
may need help or advice such as problems with accommodation,
employment, finance or the legal system. Once drug users begin to
stabilize their lives on a substitute prescription, they may be in a
position to address some of the emotional issues that led them to use
drugs and the prescriber might wish to offer them counselling or to
refer them for counselling elsewhere to address these issues. However, such counselling should not be a condition of treatment, as this
can be time consuming, costly and ultimately pointless as drug users
are unlikely to benefit from counselling unless they have identified
the need to work on a problem themselves (Ward 1992).

A further issue of debate is whether substitute prescribing is better
managed by a specialist service or whether it can be managed
successfully in primary care. There is good evidence that, with
appropriate training and support, primary care physicians can do this
work and that it does not always have to be carried out by specialist
workers (Wilson *et al.* 1995, Gruer *et al.* 1997). In fact, primary care
physicians bring to this work the advantages of being more familiar
with the environment in which the drug user is living, often knowing
the family of the drug user and being able to offer care of their drug
use in the context of their general health care. In addition, some
research among drug users suggests that drug users themselves
prefer to be seen in primary care rather than by a specialist service
(Bennett and Wright 1986).

In some areas it has been possible to develop a shared care
approach with primary care physicians receiving the support of a
specialist service (Greenwood 1990, Gruer *et al.* 1997). At first, as with
any specialist area, primary care physicians may need a great deal of
advice and support about each individual patient. Over time, as they

gain more experience and confidence, they may be able to deal with more straightforward cases without the help of a specialist service and may choose to refer only those patients who present more complicated problems or who do not respond to simple interventions.

In general, healthcare workers caring for drug users in the community will find this work easier and will feel less isolated in their work if they familiarize themselves with and make use of the range of other services that might be available to support them in their care of drug users. These may be local or it may be necessary to look further afield. Such services may include:

- urine toxicology – essential for assessment and for reviewing progress
- specialist drug service – for assessment of drug users and advice about management or for general advice and support if not local
- counselling services – this may be a drug counselling service or a general counselling service (see above)
- detoxification unit – these are usually residential
- rehabilitation unit – these are usually residential
- voluntary drug agencies – offer support about practical issues, including counselling, information and advice for drug users and their families or carers.

In general, it is likely that the care of most drug users will, at times, involve more than one healthcare provider and it is important that providers cooperate to ensure that the drug user receives an optimal level of care. This cooperation must involve some degree of networking so that those offering care can ensure that they share knowledge and a common vision about their objectives. It may involve a more formal shared care structure which requires agreement on management guidelines or protocols. Above all, effective communication between providers is essential. This is discussed in more detail in Chapters 13 and 14.

General issues of substitute prescribing

The main functions of a substitute prescription of oral drugs are:

- to reduce the risk of injecting and needle sharing
- to help maintain contact with the drug user
- to reduce or prevent withdrawal symptoms
- to reduce the need for the drug user to engage in criminal activity to buy street drugs
- to offer the drug user an opportunity to stabilize their drug intake and lifestyle.

...iption for substitute drugs should be considered only if ...er is dependent on the drug he or she is taking. Thus there ...some evidence that the drugs are being taken daily and ...n they are not taken daily, the drug user experiences with... val symptoms.

Goal setting

Substitute drugs should only be prescribed if the drug user is motivated to change the way that they use drugs. Otherwise there is a danger that they will use the prescription to supplement their street supply, with the possibility of escalating use and its associated dangers, including the risk of overdose. It is therefore important to discuss with the drug user what changes he wishes to make to the way he uses drugs and/or to other aspects of his life and in what way a substitute prescription might help him to achieve these changes.

Many drug users will start by saying they want to stop using drugs, often because they believe that this is the only way they are likely to receive help. In practice, drug users who have been using drugs for some time may be quite unable to imagine how they could manage without drugs and might feel anxious at the prospect. It is therefore important to support the drug user to distinguish between long-term goals, which might include coming off drugs, and short-term goals which may include necessary steps on the way to abstinence. In the light of short-term changes that the drug user would like to make, it is then possible to set some mutually agreed and realistic goals to be achieved within a few months of starting the substitute prescription. For example, the drug user may wish to reduce and stop his drug injecting or to reduce and stop using drugs bought from the street. He may agree that he wishes to be intoxicated less often or that he wishes to improve relationships with his partner or family.

It is important to support the drug user to set short-term goals that are realistic and achievable. For example, it is unrealistic to expect someone who has been using drugs for a long time to come off drugs quickly and stay off, or who has been unemployed for a long time to find employment within a few months. If the goals are unrealistic and the drug user fails to achieve them, both drug user and healthcare worker will feel the drug user has failed and both will become disillusioned. On the other hand, if appropriate short-term goals are achieved, the confidence and self-esteem of the drug user may be boosted and both drug user and healthcare worker feel that progress is being made. It is important to remember that drug use is a chronic relapsing condition and there may be times when little progress can be made and the focus must be on trying to minimize the harm of the current behaviour, whereas there are other times when more progress can be made. Sometimes the drug user may reject the help that is on offer and stop attending and the healthcare worker may be able to do no more than remain available for a time when the drug user is ready to accept help again. In general, it is important for healthcare workers to set realistic goals for themselves and accept that they cannot help a drug user unless they are wanting to change.

Choice of preparation, dose and dispensing arrangements

It is best to choose an oral preparation that cannot easily be injected, that has little street value and that is longer acting rather than shorter acting. Shorter acting drugs are associated with more frequent withdrawals and with a tendency to increasing tolerance. Drug users are far more likely to comply and to achieve stability on a drug that has to be taken no more than twice a day than one that has to be taken every few hours.

The prescriber is aiming to find the level of drug that prevents withdrawal symptoms and reduces the need for the drug user to take additional street drugs. It is often difficult to assess the correct dose from the beginning and it is usually better and safer to start by prescribing a low dose, accepting that the drug user will continue to use street drugs for a while, and gradually increase the dose until a sufficient level is reached. Drug users are often unable to distinguish between the withdrawal symptoms that they experience when using shorter acting drugs and symptoms of anxiety and insomnia which may coexist. A drug diary, by recording the pattern of drug use during the day, may help to clarify this.

Drug users almost always have problems with controlling their intake of drugs. It is therefore unrealistic to give them more than one day's supply of drugs at a time and expect them to divide it up and take the right amount of drug each day. Once they are more stable they might manage to do this, but at first it is more supportive to arrange for the user to receive only one day's drug at a time, except perhaps at weekends. Ideally, the consumption of this drug should be supervised, but this is only realistic in the case of drugs such as methadone that can be taken once a day and where there are supervision programmes available (Gruer *et al*. 1997).

Information and agreements

It is important to give information to the drug user about the drug that is being prescribed and its dangers and also about other supports and services that are available. Such information can be prepared

---

Model Agreement

Name: .... Date: ....

Doctors, Staff and many Patients have been upset by the behaviour of some Surgery attenders. Many of these people are attending for prescriptions of addictive drugs. You are now receiving a regular prescription for addictive medication and we require you to accept these rules.

Behaviour
1. I agree to attend appointments promptly and quietly.
2. I agree not to upset the Receptionists or other patients in the Waiting Room.
3. Due to restriction of space in the Waiting Room, I agree to attend my appointments unaccompanied whenever possible.

Behaviour outside these limits may result in the Receptionists or Doctors asking you to leave the Surgery premises. If necessary, the Police will be called and you may be removed from the Practice List and no longer be seen at this Surgery.

Prescription, Medication and Appointment
1. I agree to be responsible for making my appointments and checking that my appointment is correct in our appointment book.
2. I accept responsibility for turning up for my appointment on time.
3. I agree to attend only the Doctors mentioned below, on tihs form, and to discuss my prescription only with them.
4. I agree not to use emergency appointments or housecalls to discuss my prescription.
5. I agree to be responsible for my prescription and medication and recgonize that these cannot be replaced.
6. I agree that no alteration will be made to my prescription without my own Doctor's permission.

My Doctor is Dr: .... His/her half day is: ....

In his/her absence I will consult Dr: ....

I have read the above rules, I understand what they mean, I agree to abide by them and realise that if I do not, my prescription may be stopped and that I may be removed from the Doctor's medical list.

Signature: .... (Patient) Date: ....

Signature: .... (Doctor) Date: ....

Figure 9.1 Model Agreement

with the help of a local drug agency. It is also important to address issues raised by partners and other family members.

The behaviour of drug users is often a cause of concern. It may be helpful to link the issuing of a substitute prescription to an agreement that sets out a code of behaviour expected from the drug user and with a clear indication of the sanctions that will apply if the drug user behaves in an unacceptable way. The agreement can also include a clause that encourages the user to accept responsibility for the fact that they are to receive addictive medication. An example of an agreement is shown in Fig. 9.1. Applying an agreement in a firm but considerate manner may be beneficial not only for the running of the practice but also for the maturational process of the drug user.

Review

Drug users on a substitute prescription should be reviewed at regular intervals in order to:

- assess their general progress
- find out if they are using drugs over and above their prescription and if so, why
- assess whether their dose of substitute drugs needs adjusting
- assess what has been achieved since the last review, review any goals that were set and set new goals if appropriate
- find out if there are other problems that need to be addressed.

At each review the doctor can encourage progress and provide or repeat information about safer drug use and about other help available.

The frequency of the review will depend on the stage of the drug problem. When first established on a substitute prescription, drug users may need to be seen at least once a week but, if stable on a maintenance dose, although they will need to be seen every month or two to issue a new prescription, they may not need to be reviewed in a more formal way more than two or three times a year. Such regular reviews remain essential even for those who have been on a maintenance prescription for some time.

If the healthcare worker has access to toxicological testing of urine, it is useful to check a urine sample at random at review visits to verify that the drug user is taking the drug prescribed and to find out whether any other drugs are being taken. It is important to use urine testing as a way to encourage the drug user to talk openly about problems that he is having rather than using it as a check which leads to punishment if the drug user has been found to have lied.

In setting goals and assessing progress, it is important to remember that the principle of harm minimization is to minimize harm at

Table 9.1 Steps of harm minimization

- Reduce dangers of sharing injecting equipment
- Reduce and stop sharing
- Reduce and stop injecting
- Stabilize oral drug use
- Reduce oral drug use
- Abstinence

whatever stage the drug user has reached. Many people working with drug users become disillusioned if they feel that progress is not being made and this is particularly likely to happen if they see abstinence as the only worthwhile goal but if a drug user is still injecting, he or she can be helped to inject more safely, if still using drugs chaotically, she can be helped stabilize her drug use and then gradually to reduce. The steps of harm minimization are described in Table 9.1 and can be summarized as 'safer, more stable, less drugs, abstinence and continued abstinence'.

Prescribing for withdrawal symptoms

In view of the need to assess each drug user before starting a prescription for substitute drugs, it is rarely appropriate to initiate a substitute prescription when the drug user is first seen. Many prescribers adopt as a rule that they will not initiate a substitute prescription without a full assessment. Some doctors may find this difficult, particularly if the drug user is clearly suffering from withdrawal symptoms, but it may be more appropriate to prescribe in order to ameliorate the withdrawal symptoms, rather than start a substitute prescription. Similarly, if a drug user has lost their prescription or run out of their substitute medication before a new prescription is due, it may be better to prescribe for the withdrawal symptoms rather than replace the substitute medication. Another occasion when it may be helpful to prescribe for withdrawal symptoms is when a drug user is experiencing withdrawal symptoms during a reduction regime.

Table 9.2 Indications for prescribing for withdrawal symptoms

- During assessment
- If prescription has been lost
- If drug user has run out of medication early
- During a drug reduction

Opiate withdrawal

Symptoms of opiate withdrawal can include abdominal cramps, muscle aches, rhinorrhoea, lacrimation, diarrhoea, restlessness, insomnia, profuse sweating, vomiting, and pilo-erection. The only objective sign of opiate withdrawal is dilated pupils. However, even this is not entirely reliable as some opiate users do not have dilated pupils even when they are very withdrawn.

There are a number of drugs which can ameliorate symptoms of opiate withdrawal and they can be prescribed singly or in combination.

- Lofexidine is an alpha-2 adrenergic agonist which is related to clonidine, but is more effective at reducing the adrenaline/ noradrenaline related symptoms of opiate withdrawal such as sweats and abdominal cramps and has less hypotensive action. It is only available in some countries and is rather expensive. Although marketed mainly to aid in-patient detoxification from opiates, it can be used in small doses on an out-patient basis. One or two lofexidine 0.2 mg tablets taken every 4 to 6 hours up to a maximum of six daily usually ameliorates most of the symptoms of opiate withdrawal. Lofexidine can be prescribed for 4 days; it should be dispensed daily and the patient advised not to take more than two tablets at a time. It does not affect some opiate withdrawal symptoms such as muscle aches and insomnia.
- Lomotil (diphenoxylate hydrochloride with atropine sulphate) may be more effective than lofexidine at controlling the diarrhoea associated with opiate withdrawal. Diphenoxylate is a mild opioid but it has low addictive potential. Use two tablets four times a day.
- Mebeverine 135 mg tablets can be used to reduce abdominal pain, cramps and diarrhoea. Use one tablet three times a day.
- Thioridazine 25 mg tds or 50–100 mg nocte may reduce the agitation or insomnia associated with opiate withdrawal.

Benzodiazepine withdrawal

The symptoms of benzodiazepine withdrawal are sometimes difficult to distinguish from those of opiate withdrawal as both can involve anxiety or agitation, insomnia, sweating and even crampy abdominal pain but these are usually less severe and yet may be more prolonged after stopping bezodiazepines than after stopping opiates. If benzodiazepines are stopped abruptly there is a danger of withdrawal fits.

Other symptoms of benzodiazepine withdrawal include dizziness, confusion, blurred vision, increased sensitivity to light and sound, paraesthesia, hyperactivity, feelings of depersonalization.

If the doctor decides to prescribe a benzodiazepine for a few days to prevent withdrawal fits, it is important to remember that 30 mg diazepam is sufficient to prevent withdrawal fits in the vast majority of cases, even if the dose of benzodiazepines being taken was much higher than this. Alternatively the doctor can prescribe carbamazepine 100 mg b.d. for a week to prevent withdrawal fits (M. Bruce, personal communication). If something is required for insomnia or daytime agitation, a non-benzodiazepine hypnotic or anxiolytic should be considered.

Substitute prescribing for opiate users

The opiate that is most commonly misused is heroin, usually by injection, but there is a wide range of other opiates that may be misused including morphine, codeine, dipipanone, dextromoramide, buprenorphine and dihydrocodeine. Substitute opiate medication can be offered to those misusing any of these drugs.

Many drugs have been used as substitute medication for opiate users e.g. methadone, dihydrocodeine, buprenorphine. The main advantages of methadone mixture are that it is less likely to be injected (as it is unpleasant and difficult to inject) and that it is longer acting than other opiates. If given in the right dose it can prevent withdrawal symptoms for 24 hours and usually without giving any stimulant effect or 'buzz' after it is taken. This can support drug users to achieve some stability in their life which then allows other problems to be tackled. Its long duration of action means that it is easy to titrate to get the dose correct and it is practical to supervise its consumption. The other advantages of methadone are that it is less likely to be sold than shorter acting tablets which are more easily transportable and which give more 'buzz', that if given in adequate doses it blocks the euphoriant effects of heroin, and that its use has been well researched (Farrell *et al.* 1994, Ward *et al.* 1992) The main disadvantage of methadone is that its long duration of action makes it more dangerous in overdose. A longer acting form of methadone (LAAM) which can be taken every 2–3 days is under investigation (Prendergast *et al.* 1995) but is not yet available for general use.

Advocates of shorter acting drugs would argue that they are less dangerous in overdose and that those misusing dihydrocodeine and buprenorphine are sometimes unwilling to change on to methadone. Thus a willingness to prescribe these shorter acting drugs may make substitute medication with its associated benefits available to those who might otherwise be excluded. Although there is need for more research in this area, experience suggests that widening the range of substitute drugs that are made available may increase the number of opiate users attracted into treatment programmes. However, less experienced workers are well advised to stick to the better researched option of oral methadone until they have gained more experience in this area and refer those who are unsuitable for this treatment to a specialist centre.

It has been argued that a willingness to prescribe injectables (injectable methadone or heroin) will also bring into treatment those who might otherwise be excluded (Farrell *et al.* 1994, Martin 1997). There is little doubt that some injecting drug users are sufficiently attracted to injecting that they are unwilling to stop this and therefore reject substitute medication with oral drugs. Making injectables available will therefore extend the proportion of drug users that can be offered substitutes. One experienced worker has argued that it is not justifiable to prescribe something that drug users do not want (which might anyway be sold in order to buy the injectable that they do want) or to persuade someone to stop injecting until they choose to do so (Martin 1997). The counter argument is that the majority of injecting drug users are willing to change to an oral substitute if one is made available and that condoning injecting dilutes the harm reduction message. There is also the risk that prescribing injectables may increase the frequency of injecting (Farrell *et al.* 1994). There is currently little evidence that those prescribed injectables eventually move onto oral substitutes (Farrell *et al.* 1994).

The prescribing of injectables should be reserved for exceptional cases where oral substitutes have been tried and failed and this prescribing should be undertaken by specialists. Primary care physicians should avoid prescribing injectables unless they have had considerable experience in working with drug users and in prescribing oral substitutes.

Substitute prescribing of methadone

A prescription for methadone as a substitute opiate should only be considered if, after full assessment:

- opiates are present in the urine
- opiates are being taken daily
- there is convincing evidence of dependence including objective signs of withdrawal (e.g. dilated pupils)
- the drug user seems motivated to stabilize their drug use

- the prescriber and the drug user are clear that a substitute prescription could help to achieve certain goals.

In prescribing methadone as a substitute opiate, the prescriber should be aiming to:

- find the level of methadone that prevents opiate withdrawal symptoms and reduces the need for the drug user to take additional illicit opiates
- support the drug user to achieve a level of stability where other issues can be tackled by the drug user, alone or with the support of the prescriber or other agencies
- keep the drug user in contact with the health care physician so that their health can be monitored.

In the light of the changes that the drug user would like to make to the way he uses drugs and/or to other aspects of his life, it is important to set some mutually agreed and realistic goals to be achieved within a few months of starting the substitute prescription.

The aim is to prescribe the lowest dose of methadone that will prevent withdrawal symptoms, prevent injecting and reduce the need for additional street drugs. There is evidence that higher doses of methadone (60 mg and above) are more effective than lower doses in reducing the risk of continued use of illicit opiates (Ball and Ross 1981, Caplehorn et al. 1994). As long as the prescriber can be confident that the user is not oversedated and is not selling the medication, then there is no advantage in keeping the dose at a level that leaves the drug user feeling uncomfortable. It is important to remember that many opiate users experience psychological withdrawal symptoms before they experience physical withdrawal symptoms.

Calculating the starting dose

During assessment, the drug user should be asked to complete a drug diary, recording the amount of drugs and the time of day they are taken every day for at least a week. From this the average daily intake of opiates can be assessed. In discussion with the user, it is usually possible to establish the level of opiates that will prevent withdrawals. Using a conversion table (Table 9.3), the equivalent methadone dose can then be calculated. It is advisable to start a little lower than this as it is often possible to achieve stability on a lower dose of methadone and, if not, it is easy to increase the dose. In addition, there is always the risk that the drug user has been exaggerating their intake of drugs.

EXAMPLE

Drug user claims to be taking 25–30 tablets of 30 mg dihydrocodeine per day. He acknowledges that 20 tablets per day would probably be sufficient to prevent withdrawals. The equivalent dose of methadone is 60 mg. Start on 40 mg and increase as necessary.

Table 9.3   Conversion table: opiate/opioid equivalents

Drug	Dose	Equivelant methadone dose
Street heroin	Cannot be estimated accurately due to variations in purity of street drugs. Start at 40 mg and increase as required	
Pharmaceutical heroin	10 mg ampoule or tablet	20 mg
Pethidine	50 mg tablet or ampoule	5 mg
Morphine	10 mg ampoule or tablet	10 mg
Dipipanone (Diconal)	10 mg tablet	4 mg
Dextramoramide (Palfium)	5 mg tablet	5–10 mg
Buprenorphine (Temgesic)	200 microgram orally / 200 microgram injected	2.5 mg / 5–10 mg
Dihydrocodeine	30 mg	3 mg
Codeine phosphate	15 mg tablet	1 mg
Codeine linctus	5 ml	1 mg

The process of calculating the starting dose is easier if the opiate user has been taking pharmaceutical drugs such as buprenorphine, dihydrocodeine, dipipanone or dextramoramide than if the user has been injecting or snorting street heroin. In the latter case the user may be started on a prescription for 40 mg methadone a day which can subsequently be increased according to the response.

Although the assessment process should eliminate those who are not already dependent on and tolerant to opiates, this will not always be the case. To avoid the danger of overdose in an individual who is not already opiate tolerant, the starting dose of methadone should not be above 40 mg, regardless of the amount the user claims to have been using. The dose can subsequently be increased until an adequate dose is reached.

Preparations of methadone available vary from one country to another. One of the most convenient preparations is methadone mixture 1 mg per ml. This is a green liquid containing methadone hydrochloride, colouring (tartrazine and Green S), glucose syrup and chloroform water. A sugar-free preparation of methadone is available in some countries and a longer acting form of methadone (LAAM) is under investigation. Methadone (e.g. Physeptone) tablets should be avoided as they are more likely to be injected (Preston 1996).

In many countries methadone is a controlled drug which has implications for how a methadone prescription must be written. For example, in the UK, prescriptions for methadone must be written in the doctor's own handwriting and amounts must be written in words as well as figures. In the USA, prescriptions for methadone must be written in triplicate and in the USA, Australia and New Zealand, doctors must be licensed to prescribe methadone.

The primary care physician will usually have an arrangement for the dispensing of drugs prescribed and this is often done by a local dispensing pharmacist. The pharmacist can be contacted to confirm that he is willing to dispense methadone for this patient and to confirm the dispensing arrangements.

Supervised consumption

It is advisable to arrange for methadone consumption to be supervised for the first few days to ensure that the full dose is taken by the patient and is not diverted and to ensure that the dose is neither too high nor too low. Consumption can be supervised by a drug agency, in the doctor's premises or on pharmacy premises.

- If a *local drug agency* is able to offer this service, primary care physicians can refer patients to the agency to start them on methadone until they feel they have acquired the experience and confidence to do this themselves.
- If consumption is to be supervised *in the doctor's premises*, give a prescription for one day's methadone to the patient and ask him to collect this from the pharmacy and return. The patient should be observed taking the medication, kept under observation for approximately half an hour to check he does not vomit and then reviewed after 4 to 6 hours when maximum blood levels will have been reached, to check that he is not intoxicated or drowsy. This check is only required after the first dose or if the dose has been increased by more than 10 mg per day.
- If the primary care physician wishes consumption of the methadone to be supervised *on pharmacy premises*, the pharmacist should be approached to ask if he is willing to do this. It should be

specified on the prescription that supervision is requested ('*Please supervise consumption*') and the patient should be told that the daily dose is to be consumed in the pharmacy. The patient should be asked to return to the surgery 4 to 6 hours after the first dose of methadone to check that he is not intoxicated or drowsy. The pharmacist may be willing to supervise the consumption of methadone for a few days or for longer (Gruer *et al.* 1997) in which case he may develop a set of rules to be explained to the patient at the outset, e.g. time of day to attend, behaviour to be expected in the pharmacy. The pharmacist can be asked to withhold the daily dose and contact the prescribing doctor if the patient is intoxicated or his behaviour is unacceptable.

The primary care physician and the pharmacist can work effectively as a team by collaborating and communicating effectively and by being aware of each other's roles and guidelines. It may also be helpful for them to clarify their separate responsibilities and discuss any difficulties that might arise.

Titrating the dose and dispensing arrangements

Methadone should usually be taken in the morning in a once daily dose. The patient should be seen after 2 days of methadone before the third morning dose to see if he is withdrawn. If there is evidence of withdrawals, the methadone dose should be increased by 5–10 mg. This process can be repeated until a level of methadone is reached which holds the patient for 24 hours without significant withdrawals but does not make him drowsy.

Even if the methadone dose is insufficient, the opiate user may feel well for some hours after taking the morning dose but will begin to feel withdrawn (sweaty, agitated) later in the day or during the night, thus affecting his sleep. The earlier he experiences these symptoms, the more the dose needs to be increased. This can be done in steps and the dose should not be increased by more than 10 mg per day in one step without close supervision.

Many opiate users progress better, and in particular are less likely to inject or to use additional street drugs, if they are on more than the minimum amount needed to prevent physical withdrawals (Farrell *et al.* 1994, Ward *et al.* 1992). If the user continues to feel uncomfortable on the prescribed dose or continues to use additional street opiates, the dose of methadone should be increased. This can be done safely as long as he is seen not to be drowsy 4 to 6 hours after the daily dose has been consumed under supervision.

Methadone should be dispensed daily to begin with until the drug user is settled on a satisfactory dose level. If consumption is to be supervised, then obviously it must continue to be dispensed daily. Otherwise the dispensing arrangements will depend on the stability of the drug user. At first they will usually be tempted to take more than their daily dose each day and daily dispensing will prevent them running out of medication before their next prescription is due. As they become more stable, the dispensing intervals can be increased to alternate days and then to twice weekly. Once very stable, they might manage one week's supply at a time, but few can manage more than this. If their drug use becomes chaotic again – often demonstrated by returning early for a prescription, reporting loss or theft, or last minute holiday arrangements – it is usually supportive to return to daily dispensing, although this change will often be resisted.

Once stable on methadone, it is important to review the drug user from time to time, e.g. two or three times a year to assess progress and review goals (see above). It is particularly important to review the dose of methadone. If he is buying extra drugs this may be because the prescribed dose is too low.

Patient information

When giving a prescription for methadone, the doctor should warn the drug user that, although the methadone is safe for them, it could be dangerous for anyone who is not opiate tolerant, so the user has a responsibility to keep his medication in a safe place.

The user should also be warned that, as a CNS depressant, methadone will have an additive effect with other drugs causing CNS depression including alcohol, benzodiazepines and tricyclic anti-depressants.

In addition the drug user should be warned that, if they are on medication that makes them drowsy, they should not drive. They should also be advised to notify the authorities, if appropriate (*see* Legal issues, page 243).

It is also helpful to give the user written information about methadone. 'The Methadone Handbook' is a useful publication obtainable from ISDD, Waterbridge House, 32–36, Loman Street, London SE1 0EE.

Substitute prescribing for benzodiazepine users

There is much less evidence for the benefits of substitute prescribing for benzodiazepine users than for opiate users. There are a number of differences between benzodiazepines and opiates that have implications for substitute prescribing:

- benzodiazepines can usually be obtained legally whereas heroin cannot
- benzodiazepines are not usually injected
- there are few objective signs of benzodiazepine dependence and withdrawals, making assessment more difficult
- benzodiazepines may be more difficult to come off than opiates
- there is no evidence for the safety of long-term benzodiazepines.

Some drug workers hold the view that it isn't appropriate to prescribe benzodiazepines to drug users, mainly because it is felt that drug users can withdraw from these drugs themselves and because it is difficult to control the abuse of prescriptions. However, if one considers the main functions of substitute prescribing (see page 219 above), prescribing substitute benzodiazepines has the potential to achieve all these functions apart from reducing the risk of injecting and needle sharing (Sievewright *et al.* 1993). In addition, substitute prescribing of benzodiazepines has the advantage of preventing the convulsions which may be associated with benzodiazepine withdrawals (Robertson and Treasure 1996), although such withdrawals can also be prevented by the use of carbamezepine (see page 226).

If a substitute prescription for benzodiazepines is considered, it is important to remember that it may be more difficult to come off long-term benzodiazepines than opiates, and that long-term use may cause problems. Doctors should therefore be wary of initiating a prescription for a benzodiazepine until other approaches have been tried and should aim to prescribe for a short time only. It is often found that if a drug user is using opiates and benzodiazepines, the benzodiazepine may be being used to cope with the withdrawals from the opiate and that, if enough methadone is prescribed, then the drug user may not need benzodiazepines at all or may be able to reduce and come off them quite quickly.

If a drug user is taking large amounts of benzodiazepines, e.g. more than 60 mg diazepam or its equivalent, then it is worthwhile encouraging the user to reduce the amount that they are taking themselves. A drug diary can be helpful in assessing the pattern of drug use. If the user is taking all their daily dose in one go in the morning, sometimes for its stimulant effect, then it is worthwhile encouraging the user to divide the daily dose leaving some to be taken at night. If they continue to be 'stoned' or drowsy on their benzodiazepines, then they should not receive a prescription as they are clearly not motivated to stabilize their drug use and there is a danger that they might continue to buy and take drugs from the street in addition to their prescribed benzodiazepines.

If the decision is taken to prescribe benzodiazepines, then the same principles should apply as when prescribing opiates; that is, a prescription should be considered only if:

- benzodiazepines are present in the urine
- benzodiazepines are being taken daily
- there is convincing evidence of dependence, e.g. from the drug diary or from a description of withdrawal symptoms when the supply of benzodiazepines is unavailable
- the drug user is motivated to stabilize their drug use (see above)
- the doctor and the drug user are clear that prescribing a substitute benzodiazepine could help to achieve certain goals.

Which drug and how much?

Only one benzodiazepine should be prescribed even when the user has been taking more than one. Although different benzodiazepines have different qualities (in particular, some are more effective as tranquillizers and some as hypnotics), in practice there is not sufficient difference between their action in use to justify the use of more than one substitute benzodiazepine. In addition, it is difficult to achieve stability on shorter acting drugs such as temazepam. Therefore a longer acting benzodiazepine such as diazepam is the drug of choice (see Table 9.4).

There is still a lack of certainty about how much to prescribe. Aim for the lowest dose that will prevent withdrawal symptoms. This is usually considerably less than the amount the user claims to be taking.

It is rarely appropriate to start above 40 mg diazepam, regardless of the amount that the drug user claims to be taking and a lower starting dose may be sufficient.

The daily dose should be divided, leaving some to be taken at night. If after 2 weeks the patient is not coping and is experiencing withdrawals or is continuing to take extra drugs, it may be necessary

Table 9.4 Benzodiazepine equivalents

Drug	Dose
Diazepam	10 mg
Temazepam	20 mg
Nitrazepam	10 mg
Chlordiazepoxide	20–30 mg
Loprazolam	1 mg
Lorazepam	1 mg
Oxazepam	30 mg

to increase the dose in 5 to 10 mg steps to a maximum of 60 mg diazepam. The user should be encouraged gradually to reduce their use of additional benzodiazepines obtained elsewhere.

If the drug user continues to use extra benzodiazepines while on a prescription for 60 mg diazepam, it is best to seek a specialist opinion as to whether a larger dose is required to achieve stability or whether the drug user perhaps lacks motivation to stabilize and come off the benzodiazepines. It is also important to help the drug user to distinguish between withdrawal symptoms and coexistent symptoms of anxiety or insomnia.

Dispensing should, if possible, be daily for at least the first few weeks. Once the user is stable, the dispensing arrangements can be changed to three times weekly and then twice weekly or weekly if appropriate.

If insomnia remains a problem, a non-benzodiazepine hypnotic such as chloral hydrate mixture or thioridazine can be given for 2 to 3 weeks. Similarly, thioridazine can be prescribed short term for daytime anxiety.

Substitute prescribing for amphetamine users

There is little research evidence on the merits or otherwise of prescribing amphetamines as a substitute for those users whose problems centre round its use (Mattick and Darke 1995).

Prescribing substitute opiates has been seen as useful in attracting opiate users into therapeutic environments. It is well recognized that amphetamine users are unlikely to venture into drug units, clinics or even drop in centres, therefore limiting their opportunities for receiving a harm reduction message (Klee 1992). Concern is further heightened with the findings that injecting amphetamine users have high rates of needle sharing and high numbers of sexual partners (Darke et al. 1995). The conclusion is that the harm reduction message may be even more important for this group.

If these issues are to be addressed by using a prescribing model it is important to examine the issues that substitute prescribing tries to address. Most of this chapter has been concerned with opiate substitute prescribing. Opiate use is addictive and substitute prescribing of opiates has well-documented success in reducing harm. Discussions on benzodiazipine substitution can be seen to follow a similar pattern. Oral substitute benzodiazepines are prescribed to reduce the harm associated with more risky street use, although the lack of evidence for the effectiveness of prescribing benzodiazipines discussed earlier raises some doubts as to the merits of this approach.

Amphetamine use tends to follow a different pattern in that its use is usually recreational and non-addictive. Whether a prescribing model is appropriate for amphetamine users is therefore in great doubt. However some heavy amphetamine users, especially those who inject, may experience tolerance, craving and withdrawal symptoms. Some clinicians have suggested that substitute prescribing may have a role in caring for such heavy users (Fleming and Roberts 1994) but there is currently insufficient evidence to support this (Mattick and Darke 1995). Such prescribing is best undertaken by those with experience in the field.

If the case for substitute prescribing for amphetamines is yet to be proved, other appropriate interventions for these users must be considered. Harm reduction advice, information and the offer of support remain important. Many drug users experience psychological problems and insomnia, anxiety and depression may all be associated with misuse of any type of drug. However, psychological illness seems to be more prevalent in amphetamine users. The use of non-addictive psychotropics may be appropriate to manage depression, insomnia or anxiety and the use of beta-blockers can be successful in the treatment of the physical manifestations of anxiety.

Antidepressants such as desipramine or fluoxetine may also have a role in reducing symptoms of withdrawal and craving in amphetamine users (Sievewright and McMahon 1996).

Drug reductions

Reduction of dosage with a view to eventual abstinence is usually seen as the goal of drug treatment programmes, but it may take months or even years for a drug user to reach the stage where a reduction in his or her prescribed drugs can be considered and some may never be able to achieve total abstinence. In the case of benzodiazepines, there may be good reasons to attempt a drug reduction as the effects of long term use are uncertain, but maintaining a drug user on methadone long term may do more good and may cause less harm than reducing the dose of methadone before the drug user is ready. If a reduction regime is imposed on the drug user, it can lead to a return to street drugs and unsafe injecting (Ward et al. 1992).

Starting a reduction often causes anxiety for the drug user who will need encouragement and support. It is often best to negotiate each separate step in the reduction. If the drug user starts with a small reduction, further reductions can then follow when he feels confident and stable on the new dose. If he doesn't cope with the reduction, a return to the previous level may be necessary and the reduction can be tried again at a later date, perhaps in smaller steps.

The advantage of this approach rather than using a fixed reduction regime is that reductions can be planned to take account of other circumstances in the drug user's life and he will be able to focus on each small reduction rather than feeling anxious about eventually having to cope without drugs, with the result that he is more likely to succeed in eventually getting off drugs and staying off.

- If the user is being prescribed two drugs, it is best to reduce one at a time and if on a benzodiazepine and an opiate, it is usually best to reduce the benzodiazepine first.
- If a user has been on drugs for more than a year, it is rarely appropriate to attempt to make reductions in the dosage more frequently than fortnightly. If a more rapid reduction is required this is usually best achieved in a detoxification unit (see above).
- The size of each reduction will depend on the drug and the dose that is being taken and what the drug user thinks they can cope with.

Methadone maintenance or reduction

The term 'methadone maintenance' is used differently in different countries. For example, in Australia, the term is used to mean a methadone prescribing regime, regardless of the dosage, whereas in the UK the term is used to refer to a programme where no attempt is made to reduce the dose of methadone.

It is important to keep in mind the goals of methadone prescribing (*see* goals, p. 220 above). The evidence suggests that these goals are more likely to be achieved with higher rather than lower doses of methadone and by 'having a treatment goal of successful ongoing maintenance rather than abstinence' (Farrell *et al.* 1994). Doctors often feel they are failing in some way if the drug user has not reduced their methadone dose, but the important question is whether or not the user has achieved any change since going on methadone and whether a reduction is likely to achieve more harm than good. In other words, the focus should be on reducing harm rather than on aiming for abstinence.

It is important to remember that, although most opiate users eventually come off drugs, a substantial minority do not. One study suggests that those who continue opiate use into their late 30s may continue to use long term (Hser *et al.* 1993). The reduction of harm continues to be an important goal as long as drug use continues.

If the drug user wishes to reduce their methadone, this can be done in the community. It is best to reduce by small amounts at a time (usually no more than 10% of the current dose) and by separately negotiated steps (see above), at intervals of no less than fortnightly and often much longer, depending on the circumstances of the user.

Withdrawal symptoms are sometimes a problem 2 to 3 days after each reduction and they can often be treated symptomatically, e.g. simple non-opiate analgesia for muscle cramps, anti-diarrhoeal preparations and anxiolytics, but these should be used with caution and only for a few days after each reduction to reduce the danger of the user transferring their dependence onto the new drug. If withdrawal symptoms continue to be a problem, smaller reductions might be preferred or an alpha-2 adrenergic agonist such as lofexidine can be prescribed in low dose for a few days (see page 225 above).

Benzodiazepine reductions

Always convert to diazepam and stabilize on this first.

- If stable on 60–100 mg diazepam, reduce by 5–10 mg at a time
- If stable on 40–60 mg diazepam, reduce by 5 mg at a time
- If stable on 20–40 mg diazepam, reduce by 2–5 mg at a time
- If stable on less than 20 mg diazepam, reduce by 2 mg at a time.

It is rarely necessary to give any other medication for withdrawal symptoms, although a short course of chloral hydrate mixture up to 20 ml nocte or thioridazine 25–50 mg nocte may help with insomnia. Thioridazine 10–25 mg tds may help with day-time anxiety. It is important to check for associated depression and consider appropriate treatment which may include antidepressants (see Chapter 5).

The use of naltrexone

Naltrexone is a potent competitive opiate antagonist that works by blocking opiate receptors. It is highly effective against high doses of opiates and therefore effectively prevents re-addiction to opiates if taken regularly. As with disulfiram in relation to alcohol, it works most effectively if its administration is supervised and this usually involves a member of the family (Brewer 1996). Naltrexone comes in tablet form and has few side effects (Brewer 1996). It is useful for those who have come off opiates completely and need support to prevent them returning to opiate use. It is not used widely in Britain but would seem to have an important role in supporting opiate users to remain abstinent.

Naltrexone can also be used for rapid detoxification from opiates, usually in association with clonidine (Gerra et al. 1995). This is usually done as an in-patient in a specialist centre.

Management of overdose

Physicians are sometimes called to drug users who are thought to have taken an overdose. If the drug user is unconscious, he or she should be placed in the recovery position, the airway should be checked and cleared and then pulse, respiration and pupils checked. It is then essential to obtain as much information as possible from others, from bottles or other evidence lying around and by examining the patient, about:

- what drug or drugs have been taken?
- how taken (oral or injected)?
- how much?
- how long ago?
- could anything else be contributing to the physical state, e.g. alcohol, head injury?

If there is the slightest suspicion of opiate ingestion, e.g. small pupils, give naloxone hydrochloride (Narcan).

Use of naloxone

Given intravenously, naloxone acts within 2 minutes of injection. It should be given intravenously (rapid onset of action) and intramuscularly immediately afterwards (less rapid onset of action but lasts longer). The initial dose should be 400 micrograms by intravenous injection and 400 micrograms intramuscularly. If there is no improvement or only slight improvement after a few minutes, the dose should be doubled and repeated, both intravenously and intramuscularly. If there is still no response, the diagnosis of opiate overdose should be questioned.

The duration of action of methadone may exceed that of naloxone, even if given intramuscularly, and repeat injections may be necessary. If is therefore worthwhile trying to insert a 'butterfly' needle so that further injections can be given more easily.

Doctors caring for drug users should consider having naloxone, an airway and butterfly needles available for use in such emergencies.

Prescribing analgesia for opiate users

Some opiate users have become addicted to opiates that were originally prescribed for analgesia. As they develop tolerance to the opiate, they also develop tolerance to the analgesic effects. If they try to reduce the opiates, they may find it difficult to distinguish between a recurrence of the original pain and pain due to withdrawals, especially if the original pain was in the legs or abdomen.

When managing an opiate addict who continues to experience pain, it is important to separate out the need for analgesia from the addiction and to deal with each separately. The opiate user should be encouraged to acknowledge that they now have a problem with opiates in addition to their pain and they should be offered a different analgesic, preferably a non-opiate, for their pain rather than increasing the dose of their opiate medication. Sometimes a non-steroidal anti-inflammatory drug such as ibuprofen might be useful. Small doses of tricyclic antidepressants and certain anti-epileptics are sometimes used for their analgesic properties in chronic pain. Further investigation or advice about pain management may be worthwhile.

If opiate users experience acute pain such as toothache, it is important to advise them that additional opiates will usually be relatively ineffective in relieving the pain, so that there is little point in increasing the dose of methadone or taking other opiates such as dihydrocodeine or codeine. Using simple analgesia such as paracetamol or aspirin may be more effective and aspirin or another non-steroidal is advisable if there is an inflammatory element.

Prescribing for drug users with HIV/AIDS

In some areas such as Edinburgh, some parts of Italy and Spain, New York, parts of Asia and the Far East (Des Jarlais *et al.* 1992) a significant proportion of drug users are infected with HIV. The coexistence of HIV infection with drug misuse will, in many instances, have no effect on the management of the patient, but there are a number of issues to consider.

A drug user who is diagnosed HIV positive may or may not be motivated to reduce or come off drugs. It is important for the healthcare worker not to make assumptions but to assess each person individually. There is nothing to be gained medically by forcing any patient to come off drugs if they are not wanting to and this applies particularly to those who are infected with HIV or hepatitis C. There is a risk that they might respond by returning to using street drugs which may worsen their medical condition. There is also the risk that they may return to injecting with associated risks for them and the risk that they might share their injecting equipment and transmit the infection to others.

Nevertheless, if an infected drug user chooses to reduce or come off drugs, they should be supported in doing so.

There is some evidence that methadone may have an impact on the metabolism of zidovudine (AZT) so that lower doses of zidovudine can be used (Burger *et al.* 1994). Many of the newer antiviral drugs have significant interactions with a number of other drugs including drugs of addiction. This underlines the need for good communication between health professionals involved in the care of drug users with HIV/AIDS.

The focus of drug users may change as they become ill, away from drugs and towards their illness, with the result that problems about their drugs and prescriptions may lessen. Those on a substitute prescription may have difficulty in collecting their prescription from the pharmacist as they become ill, and special arrangements may need to be made. It is also important to remember to cancel their prescription if they are admitted to hospital. More chaotic users may continue or return to injecting as they become ill and it may be wise to leave a sharps box in the house for the safe disposal of injecting equipment.

When someone is close to death, it is common practice to increase their opiate medication for symptom control. This can be a problem with end-stage HIV disease as it is more than usually difficult to predict when the end-stage has been reached. Difficulties may arise where medication has been increased and then the patient has recovered and their increased medication has been a problem. Although this situation cannot always be avoided, it is important to be aware of this pitfall when deciding to increase medication.

Many people dying from HIV disease have distressing symptoms which are sometimes ignored in the search for a cause or cure. Many of these symptoms can be helped with appropriate treatment. It is important to keep the management of the drug problem separate as far as possible from the need for symptom control, especially in relation to analgesia and sedation.

There is a common misunderstanding, especially among hospital workers, that drug users on opiates do not need analgesia. In fact, opiate users are usually tolerant of the analgesic effects of opiates and may need more opiates than other people to control their pain.

It is often better to give different medication for pain control rather than increase the dose of substitute opiate medication. For example, if a drug user is on methadone, give a different opiate for analgesia such as morphine, rather than increasing the dose of methadone. It may be better to offer sedation with drugs such as thioridazine rather than by increasing the dose of opiates.

Prescribing on release from custody

Many drug users, especially younger drug users, are at particular risk of increased and chaotic drug use and of accidental overdose in the first few weeks after release from custody. This is particularly dangerous in relation to opiates because of reduced tolerance. Many drug users continue to use drugs in gaol, but the supply is usually irregular and the doses are likely to be less than prior to custody.

If consulted by a drug user on release from custody, it is important to warn the drug user of the dangers of overdose due to reduced tolerance. If the drug user is requesting a prescription and it seems likely that they will continue to abuse drugs, it may be appropriate to prescribe substitute drugs but this should be in a lower dose than prior to custody – the dose can subsequently be increased if necessary. If prescribing methadone, do not start above 40 mg daily; arrange for the drugs to be dispensed daily at least for the first few weeks and consider supervision of consumption (*see* page 227 above) for the first few days.

Prescribing and young people

There is evidence of widespread drug use among young people in many parts of the world. For example, a recent survey in England found that 55% of 16–19 year olds had 'ever used' drugs (McNeill and Raw 1997). Most young people do not progress from recreational use of cannabis, ecstasy or amphetamines to more addictive drugs such as benzodiazepines or opiates, although there is some evidence of young people using benzodiazepines or opiates to 'come down' from the stimulant effects of ecstasy or amphetamines and then becoming addicted to these. A minority of young people progress on to using more addictive drugs such as benzodiazepines and opiates on a regular basis and some may become involved in injecting.

It is not appropriate to prescribe substitute medication unless a drug user is dependent on the drug they are taking, is experiencing withdrawals when they are not taking the drug and, most importantly, is motivated to change the way they use drugs. It is unwise to prescribe for a drug user who is wanting drugs to be 'stoned'. It is usually more effective in these circumstances to offer support and advice, but to refuse to prescribe until they are motivated to stabilize their drug use. Thus, they should be supported to stabilize and begin to reduce their intake of drugs themselves before a prescription is considered.

If it is decided to start the young drug user on a prescription, it is important to have clear goals in mind which are agreed with the user and are recorded. As with more mature users, it is best to start on a low dose and encourage them to reduce their intake of additional drugs down to this level. Unlike with more mature users, it is often helpful to have a fixed reduction programme.

Although there is no absolute lower age limit for considering a substitute prescription, in general, the younger and less mature the drug user, the more reluctant the health professional should be to start them on a prescription and the more rapidly the reduction should occur.

Women

Most drug services in the UK, Australia and the US report that about a third of those who seek help are women, although there is some reason to believe that women are under-represented among those who seek help and that the true proportion of women drug users in the community may be greater. Women may be less likely to seek help than men as they may fear greater censure and may fear that their children will be removed from their care. There is some evidence that making drug services more accessible and sympathetic to women (e.g. by employing more women workers, by having women only sessions and by providing crêche facilities) leads to an increase in the likelihood that women will seek help (Henderson 1990).

Women who use drugs are more likely than men to have associated emotional difficulties or personality disorders. Evidence is also emerging that a significant proportion of women who use drugs have been sexually or physically abused in the past (Porter 1994). This has implications for prescribing substitute drugs because once stabilized on substitute medication, the woman may experience a return of the feelings associated with the past abuse and may return to using street drugs in addition to the prescribed medication in order to blot out these feelings and memories.

There is no evidence that women use significantly different drugs from men, nor that they require different substitute medication, either of type or of dose. They are however more likely to require and benefit from counselling in addition to their prescription, for reasons stated. The many issues associated with pregnancy in drug users are discussed in Chapter 12.

Legal issues

The legal issues involved in prescribing substitute drugs will vary from one country to another but there are a number of issues to consider.

In some countries, health professionals are required by law to notify drug users to the authorities. This was the case in the UK until

May 1997 when the Home Office Drug Addicts Register was withdrawn. Notification to local drug misuse databases is still advised but is not a statutory requirement.

In some countries there are restrictions on which drugs can be prescribed and whether or not a licence is required. For example, in the UK a doctor requires a license to prescribe heroin (diamorphine), cocaine or Diconal to a drug user, but any doctor can prescribe methadone. In some countries, e.g. USA, Australia and New Zealand, doctors require a licence to prescribe methadone. In most countries, there are special requirements for writing prescriptions for controlled drugs and methadone is usually included in this requirement. It is important for prescribing doctors to familiarize themselves with the local legislation.

Different countries have different laws governing which drugs and what doses can be exported from and imported into the country. If a patient on a substitute prescription wishes to travel abroad it is important to check on and comply with these restrictions and provide the patient with a letter 'to whom it may concern', outlining which drugs they are carrying and why, to assist them at customs.

The prescribing doctor has a responsibility to warn drug users of the dangers of driving if they are drowsy from the effects of their substitute medication. In the UK it is up to the driver to declare 'any disability likely to affect safe driving' which would include the use of benzodiazepines or opiates. Doctors do not have a responsibility to notify but should inform the drug user of the legal position. This position differs in some countries and once again it is important for prescribing doctors to familiarize themselves with the local situation.

In some instances, people prescribed addictive drugs have subsequently blamed health professionals for their addiction. It is wise to obtain evidence of addiction such as urine toxicology before starting someone on a prescription and to record fully details of the assessment.

Confidentiality

Modern medical practice usually involves teams of both clinical and non clinical workers, many of whom may become involved in the care of drug users. To optimize the quality of this care it is often essential to pass on confidential information between members of the team. Patients have a right to expect information that doctors hold about them to be treated confidentially, and they must give informed consent to allow such information to be released to others. Professionals involved with the care of drug users should encourage drug users to be truthful and open, encouraging patients to allow the sharing of information between those offering care and support. It is advisable therefore for prescribers to tell drug users that, although issues of confidentiality will be respected, it may be in their interest for certain issues to be discussed with other members of the larger team, e.g. for further practical support such as counselling. It is also worth reminding drug users that other doctors in the practice, receptionists and some other clinical workers may have access to information through clinical records, correspondence etc.

The issue of confidentiality is often highlighted in smaller communities where there may be little choice of dispensing pharmacist and the patient may well know, or even be related to, pharmacy staff. The patient may have similar relationships with a member of the healthcare team. Such circumstances need to be handled delicately and supportively to allow the patient to take the opportunities of all treatment options available, for example by helping the patient to see that the advantages of a substitute prescription may outweigh the embarrassment or difficulties of using a pharmacist in which a friend or relative is working.

As previously stated, the management of drug users and the issues of substitute prescribing cannot be considered in isolation. The misuse of drugs affects not only drug users themselves but also their family, friends and usually the wider community. Prescribing policies will therefore impact on this wider community often encompassing police, legal and penal systems, social/welfare and statutory and non-statutory agencies and others. Requests for the disclosure of information of a confidential nature should, however, always be treated with suspicion, and great care taken. Police and legal officers, for example, are often interested in information on drug users. The patient's permission, or the permission of someone properly authorized to act on their behalf, must always be obtained. It is always worth checking on the authenticity of such a request, and confirming that the patient has given such permission. Exceptions to this rule are when disclosure is in the patient's medical interest and in certain judicial or other statutory proceedings. The General Medical Council (1995) provides excellent information regarding the issue of confidentiality.

References

Advisory Council on the Misuse of Drugs 1982: *Treatment and rehabilitation*. HMSO, London.

Advisory Council on the Misuse of Drugs 1988: *AIDS and drug misuse*. HMSO, London.

Ball, J.C., Ross, A. 1991: *The effectiveness of methadone maintenance treatment: patients, programs, services and outcome.* Springer-Verlag, New York.

Bennett, T., Wright, R. 1986: Opiate users' attitudes towards and use of NHS clinics, general practitioners and private doctors. *British Journal of Addiction* **81**, 757–63.

Brewer, C. 1996: On the specific effectiveness, and under-valuing, of pharmacological treatments for addiction: a comparison of methadone, naltrexone and disulfiram with psychosocial interventions. *Addiction Research* **3** (4), 297–313.

Burger, D.M., Meenhorst, P.L, ten Napel, C.H.H., Mulder, J.W., Neef, C., Koks, C.H.W., Bult, A., Beijnen, J.H. 1994: Pharmacokinetic variability of zidovudine in HIV-infected individuals: subgroup analysis and drug interactions. *AIDS* **8**, 1683–9.

Caplehorn, J., Dalton, S., Cluff, M., Petrenas, A.-M. 1994: Retention in methadone maintenance and heroin addicts' risk of death. *Addiction,* **89**, 203–7.

Darke, S., Ross, J., Cohen, J., Hando, J., Hall, W. 1995: Injecting and sexual risk-taking behaviour among regular amphetamine users. *AIDS Care* **7**, 19–26.

Des Jarlais, D.C., Friedman, S.R., Choopanya, K., Vanichseni, S., Ward, T.P. 1992: International epidemiology of HIV and AIDS among injecting drug users. *AIDS* **6**, 1053–68.

Dole, V.P., Nyswander, M. 1965: A medical treatment for diacetylmorphine (heroin) addiction. *Journal of the American Medical Association,* **193**, 80–84.

Dole, V.P., Nyswander, M. 1976: Methadone maintenance treatment: a ten-year perspective. *Journal of the American Medical Association,* **235**, 2117–19.

Farrell, M., Ward, J., Mattick, R., Hall, W., Stimson, G.V., Des Jarlais, D., Gossop, M., Strang, J. 1994: Methadone maintenance treatment in opiate dependence: a review. *British Medical Journal* **309**, 997–1001.

Fleming, P.M., Roberts, D. 1994: Is the prescription of amphetamine justified as a harm reduction measure? *Journal of the Royal Society of Health* 127–31.

Fulco, C.E., Liverman, C.T., Earley, L.E. (eds). 1995: *Developments of medications for the treatment of opiate and cocaine addictions: issues for the government and private sector.* National Academy Press, Institute of Medicine, Washington, DC.

General Medical Council 1995: *Duties of a doctor.* General Medical Council, London.

Gerra, G., Marcato, A., Caccavari, R., Fontanesi, B., Delsignore, R., Fertonani, G., Avanzini, P., Rustichelli, P., Passeri, M. 1995: Clonidine and opiate receptor antagonists in the treatment of heroin addiction. *Journal of Substance Abuse Treatment* **12**, 35–41.

Greenwood, J. 1990: Creating a new drug service in Edinburgh. *British Medical Journal* **300**, 587–9.

Gruer, L., Wilson, P., Scott, R., Elliott, L., Macleod, J., Harden, K., Forrester, E., Hinshelwood, S., McNulty, H., Silk, P. 1997: General practitioner centred scheme for treatment of opiate dependent drug injectors in Glasgow. *British Medical Journal* **314**, 1730–35.

Gunne, L.-M., Gronbladh, L. 1981: The Swedish methadone maintenance program: a controlled study. *Drug and Alcohol Dependence* **7**, 249–56.

Henderson, S. (ed.) 1990: *Women, HIV, drugs: practical issues.* Institute for the Study of Drug Dependence, London.

Hser Y, Anglin D, Powers K. 1993: A 24-year follow-up of California narcotics addicts. *Archives of General Psychiatry* **50**, 577–84.

Klee, H. 1992: A new target for behavioural research – amphetamine misuse. *British Journal of Addiction* **87**, 439–46.

Martin, E. 1997: Prescribing injectable opiates. *Substance Misuse Management in General Practice* Newsletter issue no. 4.

Mattick, R.P., Darke, S. 1995: Drug replacement treatments: is amphetamine substitution a horse of a different colour? *Drug and Alcohol Review* **14**, 389–94.

McLellan, A.T., Arndt, I.O., Metzger, D.S., Woody, G.E., O'Brien, C.P. 1993: The effects of psychosocial services in substance abuse treatment. *Journal of the American Medical Association* **269**, 1953–9.

McNeill, A., Raw, M. 1997: *Drug use in England: results of the 1995 National Drugs Campaign Survey.* Health Education Authority, London.

Porter, S. 1994: Assault experience among drug users. *Substance Misuse Bulletin* **8**, 1–2.

Prendergast M.L., Grella, C., Perry S.M., Anglin, M.D. 1995: Levo-alpha-acetylmethadol (LAAM): clinical, research and policy issues of a new pharmacotherapy for opioid addiction. *Journal of Psychoactive Drugs* **27** (3), 239–47.

Preston A. 1996 *The methadone briefing.* Martindale Pharmaceuticals, London. Distributed by ISDD, Waterbridge House, 32–36, Loman Street, London SE1 0EE.

Robertson, J.R., Treasure, W. 1996: Benzodiazepine abuse – the nature and extent of the problem. *CNS Drugs* **5** (2), 137–46.

Sievewright, N., Donmall, M., Daly, C. 1993: Benzodiazepines in the illicit drugs scene: the UK picture and some treatment dilemmas. *International Journal of Drug Policy* **4** (1), 42–8.

Seivewright, N., McMahon, C. 1996: Misuse of amphetamines and related drugs. *Advances in Psychiatric Treatment* **2**, 211–18.

Sorensen, J.L. 1996: Methadone treatment for opiate addicts. *British Medical Journal* **313**, 245–6.

Ward, J., Mattick, R., Hall, W. 1992: *Key issues in methadone maintenance treatment.* New South Wales University Press, Kensington, New South Wales.

Wilson, P., Watson, R., Ralston, G.E. 1995: Supporting problem drug users: improving methadone maintenance in general practice. *British Journal of General Practice* **45**, 454–5.

10 Detoxification and achieving abstinence

Roy Robertson and Brian Wells

Introduction

While complete abstinence from the drug of use is seen as the ideal goal of most drug treatment services which offer detoxification, the reality is often different. Most patients who have used drugs for any length of time have had periods of abstinence due to serious attempts to help themselves or lack of availability of the drug. Successful detoxification is often followed by relapse. This is such a common outcome that most drug therapists expect it to happen. The resulting approach of most agencies is to select patients carefully, support and counsel them before entry into treatment and expect stabilization and reduction in drug intake rather than abstinence. As relapse is common it is not considered to be a sign of treatment failure. Other common measures of effectiveness are therefore required and include improved employment status, reduced criminal activity and a wide variety of psychosocial indicators. Improved perinatal outcome or parenting abilities are similarly regarded as successes of such therapeutic input (McCaffrey 1996).

Detoxification programmes may be residential, in-patient or most commonly out-patient facilities. Over many years the effectiveness of various types of programmes have been debated, but long-term studies have been few and the enormous diversity of approaches makes it difficult to determine the successful ingredients.

At least one authoritative report has concluded that detoxification is not a viable method of treatment so much as an important gateway into treatment (Gerstein and Lerwin 1990) and that it may usually be undertaken on a residential, partial day care, or ambulatory basis. We now know that addictions are highly treatable conditions and that many powerful treatments exist. Detoxification is a precursor to treatment, the beginning of treatments that are aimed towards abstinence. Detoxification is what people do when they want to become drug-free, whether or not they have medical or other support and is essentially the easy part of the process of achieving the longer term objective of lasting abstinence. This chapter examines the distinction between detoxification and abstinence and the process of passing from one to the other rather than merely achieving a usually short-term, period of the drug-free state. An understanding of the nature of the dependency syndrome and its natural history is essential and this is discussed in Chapter 1. Through other chapters the remitting and relapsing nature of drug dependency is discussed in different contexts and the paradigm shift in recent years from cure to damage limitation or harm minimization brought about by the apparent failure of the traditional abstinence orientation treatment model. The need for detoxification, however, has never gone away and in any mature drug treatment culture is an essential requirement which is often underfunded and sometimes undervalued. The reasons for this and the way treatment services have evolved are the subject of this chapter.

Principles of detoxification

Current medical and social rehabilitation practice demands a high level of concern for adequate support in any detoxification programme. The following list of requirements and insights indicate the large range of considerations which must be given to embarking on such a treatment.

- detoxification alone is rarely adequate treatment for alcohol and drug dependencies
- when using medication regimens or other detoxification procedures, clinicians should use only protocols of established safety and efficacy

- providers must advise patients when procedures are used that have not been established as safe and effective
- during detoxification, providers should control patient's access to medication to the greatest extent possible
- initiation of withdrawal should be individualized
- whenever possible, clinicians should substitute a long-acting medication for short-acting drugs of addiction
- the intensity of withdrawal cannot always be predicted accurately
- every means possible should be used to ameliorate the patient's signs and symptoms of alcohol and drug withdrawal
- patients should begin participating as soon as possible in follow-up support therapy such as peer group therapy, family therapy, individual counselling or therapy, 12-step recovery meetings, and alcohol and drug recovery educational programmes.

Assessment

The importance of a detailed and professional assessment cannot be overstated. Without knowledge of the medical history of the patient proper facilities cannot be selected or safety guaranteed. Knowledge of the individual's domestic situation and previous experiences, and response to, treatments are crucial to predicting the benefit or hazards of any treatment modality, but perhaps most of all the use of detoxification facilities. In many centres, the inadequacy or absence of detailed selection processes may account for the high failure rates. Proper assessment is therefore essential and should include the following factors:

- is in-patient or out-patient treatment required?
- which drug(s) are being used and what level of dependence is present?
- is medical supervision required? (depends on a number of factors but principally upon the drug type and social conditions)
- what are the follow-up arrangements or situations?
- what are the other factors present? (such as psychiatric comorbidity and presence of HIV or chronic symptomatic liver disease).

Assessment includes matching detoxification facility for drug type. For example, medical supervision may be required for alcohol or sedative/hypnotic withdrawal. The effect of withdrawal from alcohol and short to intermediate acting hypnotics must be considered in the patient assessment as the risk of seizure and delirium begins at 24 hours after the last dose and peaks within the next 48 hours. Other practical issues can be critically important in the outcome of any attempted detoxification programme. These can include such easily ignored issues as, care of children, preparation of relatives, agreement at outset of expectations and levels of supervision and monitoring. The suitability of the programme and the timetable and the action to be taken in the event of relapse are all issues which should be discussed before starting.

Barriers to success/short-term relapse

Careful attention to the preparations outlined above are essential to the success and failure of any treatment programme and experience shows this to be especially true of detoxification attempts. Embarking on a formal detoxification schedule is likely to be a major event for any drug-dependent patient and he or she often arrives at this juncture in a state of some emotion. This may be after resolving to make a serious lifestyle change and may follow a period of marital or relationship trauma, court appearances or other life events of a confrontational nature. The individual may well need careful preparation and require considerable support. Lack of preparation frequently leads to failure and the majority or relapses occur because of unrealistic expectations, lack of preparations in personal practicalities and inadequate support when things get tough or go in an unpredicted direction. Many studies have identified coping strategies in patients undergoing detoxification and often conclude that prior therapy to train them in the use of such strategies is likely to improve the rate of success (Madden *et al.* 1995).

Recurrent attempts/long-term relapse

As the failure rate is high on the first detoxification attempt many projects expect that failure and representation at a later date is almost the normal course of events. Depending upon the type of intervention planned, a failed attempt is to be seen as part of a learning process in the life of a dependent patient. This can easily be built upon at future attempts and lessons learned from previous failures. Many projects will have a protocol for dealing with relapse and make efforts to reassure the client that this is not a major problem or indeed unexpected. This will encourage further attempts and possibly better preparation in the future as discussed the relapse is to be seen as part of the essential learning process towards longer lasting abstinence and recovery.

Long-term relapse is the return to damaging drug use after a period of months or even years of absolute or comparative abstinence. This might be the resumption of drug taking after a period of abstinence from all drugs, the relapse into more damaging use such as injecting after a spell on oral drugs only or resumption of serious drug use in response to an adverse life event. All these events are unpredictable, but the better the education process and support after the detoxification programme the more likely that this will be prevented. Evidence shows that the likelihood of relapse decreases as the length of the abstinent period increases, although relapse into drug use can of course occur at any time for a variety of reasons (Daley and Marlatt 1997).

Self-detoxification

Most drug-dependent patients are experienced in withdrawal symptoms although not always with the full range and severity of consequences of withdrawing from longer acting opiates or sedatives and hypnotics. Younger, more recently dependent individuals may be less experienced and therefore less realistic about the potential for achieving the drug-free state easily. By the time most drug using patients come into any contact with treatment services they are likely to have had, sometimes sustained, periods of abstinence. These abstinent episodes may be short or long and may have been initiated by several factors such as lack of available drugs, family problems, positive developments in their personal life or a determined effort to effect a self-cure. Perhaps obviously there must be a large group of ex-drug dependents who have achieved and continued the abstinent state with little or no obvious help or support (Waldorf 1983).

Rapid detoxification

Various techniques have been used to induce rapid detoxification. Clonidine and lofexidine are drugs used in medical detoxification programmes and both act on the central nervous system to alleviate symptoms of withdrawal. The opiate antagonist naltrexone blocks the actions, including the euphoria, of opioids and is given to former addicts as an aid to relapse prevention. Induction of rapid withdrawals has also been achieved in an attempt to detoxify using naloxone, a rapid acting opioid antagonist.

A treatment known as rapid anaesthetic–antagonist detoxification was originally used by Loimer and others in Vienna and has been used in the USA and other European centres since then. The technique involves quick detoxification of a patient by administration of opiate antagonist drugs such as Naltrexone whilst under general anaesthetic. A variety of techniques are described ranging from intramuscular and oral sedation to intravenous sedation, paralysis and intubation (Bartter and Gooberman 1996). The process claims to accelerate the withdrawal process and complete the process within 24 hours.

Several authors have suggested that the technique is unnecessarily dangerous and has no significant advantages over slower withdrawal techniques that would make it useful or indeed justifiable in a population already at high risk of anaesthetic complications (Mattick and Hall 1996). Perhaps most important is the risk that the apparent simplicity of this technique may lead drug users, their families and carers to fail to appreciate the longer term nature of their problem (Strang *et al.* 1997)

Models of treatment and types of facility

Treatment facilities for detoxification come in a variety of forms and have evolved in various directions over the last few years and decades. Although there are considerable overlaps and variations in agencies and countries, or even within the same country, there are some types of services which emerge wherever there is a substantial drug problem.

- In-patient medical detoxification (short stay)
- Out-patient medically supervised detoxification
- Short stay residential detoxification facility
- Rehabilitation facility, longer stay of therapeutic community approach
- Concept or religious based house.

The more traditional detoxification or rehabilitation facilities are often based on the Alcoholics Anonymous model and exist largely in the non-statutory sector of healthcare provision. From this base the establishment of the therapeutic community and more recently residential 'concept' houses and religious houses have emerged. This evolution over the last 30 years has left a variety of establishments providing a range of approaches from the non-residential Narcotics Anonymous with a philosophy adapted from Alcoholics Anonymous and the 12-step model (Minnesota model – Table 10.1) (Wells 1994) to the residential abstinence based therapeutic communities and the less rigid and more flexible concept houses. The last two involve considerable periods of residential rehabilitation in a closely structured environment (Toon and Lynch 1994).

For present requirements, this chapter will concentrate less on historical models which have, since the awareness of the risks of transmission of blood-borne viruses, changed many of their more inflexible regimens to shorter more issue-centred practices. In many European and North American centres of drug use, the essential requirement is the adequate provision of economical therapeutic approaches which take into account polydrug use, HIV and hepatitis, prevention, patients from marginalized groups, women and children

Table 10.1 The 12 steps of Narcotics Anonymous

1. We admitted that we were powerless over our addiction, that our lives had become unmanageable.
2. We came to believe that a power greater than ourselves could restore us to sanity.
3. We made a decision to turn our will and our lives over to the care of God as we understand him.
4. We made a searching and fearless moral inventory of ourselves.
5. We admitted to God, ourselves and to other human beings the exact nature of our wrongs.
6. We were entirely ready to have God remove all these defects of character.
7. We humbly asked Him to remove our shortcomings.
8. We made a list of all persons we had harmed, and became willing to make amends to all of them.
9. We made direct amends to all such people wherever possible, except where to do so would injure them or others.
10. We continued to take personal inventory, and when we were wrong promptly admitted it.
11. We sought through prayer and meditation to improve our conscious contact with God, as we understood Him, praying only for knowledge of His will for us, and the power to carry it out.
12. Having had a spiritual awakening as a result of these steps, we tried to carry this message to addicts and to practice these principles in all our affairs.

of drug users and contemporary attitudes to continued drug use. This last requirement has brought about considerable change in the approach to treatment. Only a few years ago the provision of any facilities was controversial, whereas the modern recognition of the greater risk done to society of not treating drug dependency has allowed rapid development in this sector.

Recent changes in the field of alcohol detoxification practice have begun to have the effect of changing attitudes towards the provision of services for those wishing to detoxify from other drugs. These changes come from a recognition that most alcohol-dependent patients can withdraw in safety with little or no formal medical supervision. This has led to a dramatic change in the need for in patient beds and staff which has been replaced by home detoxification supervision (Mattick and Hall 1996).

Medical model programmes

There is considerable variation in provision of medical supervision and provision of medical support between different detoxification and residential facilities (Wesson 1995). In-patient programmes in hospitals have usually a large medical support and capability. Medical model programmes are those that have been devised by a physician or another medical doctor such as a psychiatrist and are carried out in an in-patient or a closely supervised out-patient arrangement by healthcare personnel. Some residential treatment programmes are loosely affiliated with a medical centre and some out-patient programmes are located within or closely linked with a hospital or medical centre. In recent years funding issues have distracted attention, and financial support, from hospital to the community resulting in a decrease in-patient facilities and an increase in out-patient care. The huge increase in methadone maintenance in Europe has given rise to a reduction in demand for the traditional type of detoxification programme.

Social model programmes

Social model treatment programmes concentrate on providing psychological services. A variety of workers from social work or healthcare training backgrounds provide services in a range of environments. Such support therapies include individual and family counselling, coordination of care and a large variety of diversion activities. Patients who need medical care are referred to a nearby medical resource and some programmes have a visiting physician who can provide detoxification medications. Social model programmes concentrate on non-pharmacological management of withdrawal and usually counsellors do not have prescribing capabilities. Programmes vary enormously, but increasingly have the ability to manage medications in order to stabilize intake to that agreed upon and to pursue a negotiated series of reductions in medications. The patient's medications must be observed and supervised and more or less strict controls are imposed in order to prevent additional self medication occurring from other sources.

Social model programmes require that patients are properly assessed before entry and that they are not heavily dependent on alcohol or hypnotic drugs as withdrawal from these can precipitate a medical crisis.

Multimodal programmes

Multimodality programmes offer a variety of services (Jaffe 1973, Kleber 1989). These include in-patient treatment, medical care, out-patient brief treatment, vocational training, education for adolescents, family therapy, therapeutic community approaches, methadone treatment, group psychotherapy, individual psychotherapy, drug education and stress coping techniques. The ability to select and match patients to the most appropriate treatment modality is dependent on the availability of multiple resources and requires skilled assessment and knowledge of the patient. The pursuit of abstinence or rapid drug-free state is more than often appropriate and the chance of success may be enhanced with a progressive approach through other treatment options.

In-patient or out-patient programmes

Detoxification may occur in an in-patient or an out-patient setting. Both types or settings initiate recovery programmes that may include referrals for problems such as medical, legal, psychiatric and family issues. There are various advantages and disadvantages to both types of setting (Alling 1992).

In-patient treatment

- The patient is in a protected setting where access to substances of abuse is restricted.
- The withdrawal process may be safer, especially if the patient is dependent upon high levels of sedative or hypnotic drugs since the clinician can observe him or her closely for serious withdrawal symptoms and medications can be adjusted.
- Detoxification can be accomplished more rapidly than it can be in an out-patient setting.

Out-patient treatment

- It is much less expensive than in-patient treatment.
- the patient's life is not as disrupted as it is during in-patient treatment.
- the patient does not undergo the abrupt transition from a protected in-patient setting to the everyday home and work setting.

Detoxification may be achieved in a variety of programme types. These include residual and non-residual and social or those with a medical support.

Outpatient detoxification treatment may be divided into several types:

- Intensive out-patient programmes
- Non-intensive out-patient programmes
- Methadone maintenance programmes.

Intensive out-patient programmes offer professionally directed evaluation and assessment in a structured environment. Examples include day or evening programmes in which patients attend a full spectrum of programming. Some provide medical detoxification and some have established links through which they may refer patients to behavioural and psychosocial treatment. One strength of such pro-grammes is the daily contact between patient and staff.

In non-intensive out-patient programmes, patients attend sched-uled sessions which are professionally directed and supervised. Some offer only assessment, in others counselling may last for a year or longer. The majority provide one or two sessions a week, and may deliver psychiatric or psychological counselling and other services such as referral or management. Many combine counselling with 12-step recovery (Table 10.1).

Maintenance pharmacotherapy or methadone maintenance clinics may provide supervised withdrawal for patients who do not want to enter maintenance treatment, but who want to use methadone reduc-tion in order to detoxify from illicit opiate use. In Europe the distinction between those on a maintenance programme is less important than in the USA where licensing from the Food and Drug Administration and State regulatory agencies are more restrictive. Many opiate dependent patients use methadone reduction in a pro-tracted process of detoxification over many months. This may even-tually lead to a drug-free state or progress to a state of confidence which allows a short more intensive course of detoxification as an in-patient.

Entry into treatment

Accident and emergency departments of acute treatment hospitals are often the gateway through which drug dependent patient in a state of serious withdrawal enter treatment. This contact may be brief and only attempt to deal with the acute consequences of the medical nature before discharge or may form a link with a structured de-toxification facility. Patients presenting in this way are often poorly prepared for serious attempts at becoming drug-free, and require further preparation and support before entering such a facility. For the patient who has overdosed or has a medical complication of drug misuse, the emergency department is often the point of contact with the health services system. It serves as a source of identification and referral to alcohol and drug detoxification programmes. The accident and emergency department staff of any hospital should be familiar with and have clinical expertise in dealing with patients with a variety of drug-related medical emergencies. The patient should, after stabilization and assessment, be referred to a more suitable depart-ment for detoxification if this is seen as appropriate. More often the referral to a support worker who is able to make a further assessment is the course of action agreed by the doctor and patient. Frequently the opportunity is not taken up by the patient and repeated presenta-tion to the emergency services occurs.

Another major entry into treatment is through community care. This may be through primary medical care services or the criminal justice system or some social programme to which the client presents. All these agencies are aware of the wide variety of circumstances surrounding presenting patients, some of a compulsory nature. The importance of these agencies having a system for dealing with new presentations as well as repeated presentations of known individuals cannot be over-emphasized.

Therapy used in programmes

Therapy in this sense is a blanket term which can cover a huge variety of interventions. Drug abuse treatment can take place in hospitals, long-term residential treatment programmes, walk-in clinics and counselling centres, psychotherapists' offices and church basements. The choice and setting and types of treatment selected by or mandated for the individual depends on such factors as the drugs of addiction, the history of drug use and the previous drug treatment, social needs criminal record, economic status and personality characteristics. In both the drug treatment and the treatment research communities there is a broad consensus that drug abuse treatment works. However, identifying the most effective type of treatment and for whom it is most effective continues to be a difficult task. In this climate of managed care it is more important than ever to determine which treatment will work best for which patient. The surest way to make this effective is through rigorous evaluation of treatment modalities, treatment programmes and patient outcomes. In this complicated world of treatment options the variety is enormous and poorer programmes exist as well as effective ones. Patients may select well the service which they need, or use a variety at any one time or may expect a physician or representative to select therapies for them. This is an important part of the treatment procedure. Many agencies concentrate on special areas of treatment or offer a specialized therapy. Drug-free treatments clearly differ from those with the prescribing capability and concept houses based on religious doctrine differ from secular organizations. Residential and non-residential are other clear divisions. Within these broad categories treatments may be specific or general or targeted at particular gender issues, ethnic minorities or age groups. Recent offenders may find some agencies more appropriate than others and new or recently starting drug users may find group work with long-standing patients traumatic and threatening. Selection of treatment and understanding of the variety of treatment modalities is critical to the success of the outcome.

Selection of treatment programme

It has been frequently observed that detoxification is best seen not as a treatment in itself, but as a gateway into ongoing treatment or recovery processes. The repeated nature of detoxification for many, if not most drug dependants, is not necessarily repeated failure but a learning process during which valuable personal insights occur and from which progress can be developed even if return to drug use occurs. The programme selected depends, critically, therefore on past successes or failures, expectations of the patient and carers and the facilities available. Unfortunately the latter consideration is all too often the directing force and the choice may be limited to a small number of options some or all of which may be totally unsuitable. Purchasers' interests in economic factors are unfortunately having a major impact on these decisions particularly on the length of stay in residential facilities and the speed with which entry into this type of treatment may be available. Repeated entry may be prevented because of a lack of understanding of the relapsing nature of the problem and the belief that repeated requirement for detoxification represents failure by patient or programme.

For some patients a period of hospital admission may be recommended if other approaches have failed. Traditionally 3 to 4 weeks were considered normal, but in recent years and with the advent of managed care, in-patient stay may be as little as 3 days. Criteria for hospitalization are as follows:

- users whose drug compulsions are uncontrollable, especially heavy cocaine and intravenous drug users
- users with physical dependence on a number of drugs
- users with severe medical or psychiatric complications
- users with severe psychosocial impairment
- users who have failed in out-patient treatment.

Re-establishment in the community and aftercare

Increasing numbers of programmes offer aftercare facilities. These may be in the form of a key worker who carries out a number of follow-up counselling sessions, or a period of further in-patient stay to reinforce the gains achieved and the resolutions made during the main treatment package. This recognizes the difficulties inherent in returning to the normal environment of living after treatment ceases. This is likely to include return to the temptations and support systems previously maintaining the individual in drug taking. Support care in the community involves carers and relatives as their needs may be considerable, as well as their importance in preventing relapse of the drug user. Periodic individual or group counselling, 12-step meetings, self-help and relapse prevention strategies can be used for months or years after a period of abstinence-orientated treatment.

Special populations

Not surprisingly there are individuals or groups of individuals who require special consideration. This may be because they have additional, complicated or unique problems or situations. Attention to individual requirements can be part of the assessment process described above or inherent in the situation presented. The following list includes several areas of difficulty in which normal detoxification procedures may be compromised or require additional expertise:

* those in custody
* polydrug users
* women
* pregnant women
* adolescents
* elderly persons
* patients who are HIV antibody positive
* patients with other medical conditions
* patients with known or suspected psychiatric comorbidity.

Detoxification in prison

Treatment of those in custody is notoriously problematic and has challenged many national authorities. The attraction of the detoxification approach has been severely limited by lack of successful outcome and the tendency to harm reduction and in some cases methadone maintenance (Mahon 1997) indicates the lack of success of the coercive approach. However, controlled prospective studies in a few well-established therapeutic communities in prisons with strong links to therapeutic community treatment programmes indicate that therapeutic communities in prisons can reduce rates of re-arrest (but not necessarily other measures of recidivism) by 10 to 20% (Gerstein and Lewin 1990).

Detoxification in prison is not well-described and very few examples are available of serious attempts to address the treatment of long-term drug users entering custody. This is despite the possibility of providing organized medical supervision for people with a disordered life. The high turnaround of prisoners, the overcrowded facilities, the illicit drug use and the non-consensual sexual activity and the reduction of resources to the minimum all make the prison environment unbelievably hostile (Levy 1997). Such an experience is unlikely to be constructive and the attempts to liaise with community agencies on discharge are notoriously lacking. Prison statistics exclude health data and performance indicators are limited to suicide rates (Biles and Mc Donald 1992). Experiments with harm minimization are limited and controversial (Jutta and Stover 1996). Detoxification is often claimed to be provided in systematic format, but its content has been criticized (ACMD 1996) and its success unevaluated.

Alcohol and polydrug dependence

Since most persons who have a substance abuse disorder are addicted to a combination of alcohol and or other drugs (polydrug abuse), detoxification often involves withdrawal from more than one drug. Although alcohol dependency represents one of the problem areas for those providing detoxification, attitudes are changing as to the best type of treatment. It was, until recently, accepted practice that alcohol withdrawal needed in patient medical supervision because of the risk of convulsions and possible asphyxiation.

It was estimated in 1990 that 100 000 admissions occurred in the USA for the purpose of detoxification of alcohol (Gerstein and Harwood 1990). Since that time a huge change has taken place towards the provision of out-patient detoxification supervision. It is now often seen as unnecessary to hospitalize patients unless there is severe coexisting sedative or hypnotic dependence or concurrent medical or severe psychiatric problems. Detoxification from alcohol and other drugs can therefore usually take place in a non-hospital residential, partial day care or ambulatory basis (Stockwell et al. 1986). Instruments for assessing the severity of alcohol dependence are available and the Clinical Institute Withdrawal Assessment instrument measures the severity of alcohol withdrawal by rating ten signs and symptoms. These are: nausea; tremor; autonomic hyperactivity; anxiety; agitation; tactile, visual and auditory disturbances; headache and disorientation (Sullivan et al. 1989). The maximum score is 67 and those with a score of 20 or over may require admission for observation (Saitz et al. 1994). This score can be used repeatedly and treatment adjusted accordingly. The regimen most commonly used is benzodiazepine prescription when withdrawal is taking place, but when bezodiazepine use is also a problem this is not suitable. Treatment regimens for those with multiple dependencies often involves a staged process to reduce those substances causing most damage first, followed by a gradual reduction of other substances. Several admissions or prolonged out-patient sessions may be required, in some cases extending to many months or years. Signs and symptoms of the acute phase of alcohol withdrawal may include the following:

• Restlessness, irritability, anxiety, agitation
• Anorexia, nausea, vomiting
• Tremor, elevated heart rate, increased blood pressure
• Insomnia, intense dreaming, nightmares
• Impaired concentration, memory and judgment
• Increased sensitivity to sounds, alteration to tactile sensations
• Delirium (disorientation to time, place and situation)
• Hallucinations (auditory, visual or tactile)
• Delusions (usually paranoid)
• Grand mal seizures
• Elevated temperature

The coexistent use of a variety of other drugs and substances may modify all these symptoms or mimic many of them, and the distinction between the effects of chronic use of cocaine and amphetamines and withdrawal from alcohol and other sedative type drugs is often not easy to make. Indeed, as is discussed in detail in Chapter 5, serious psychiatric syndromes are included in the differential diagnosis in severe manifestations of many of these states. Additional use of cannabis, nicotine, hallucinogens and solvents can add to the difficulties in defining a cause for individual or combined symptoms or signs (West and Gossop 1994).

Opiate withdrawal

For many years the opiate withdrawal syndrome has been recognized to be unpleasant but not life-threatening. It is characterized by various signs and symptoms including eye-watering, running nose, sweating excessive sweating, which occur 8–12 hours after the last dose of opiate. This is followed by increasing restlessness, dilated pupils, tremor, piloerection, irritability, anorexia, muscle and joint pains and colicky abdominal cramps. Symptoms peak at 48–72 hours with intensification of all symptoms and subside thereafter largely disappearing after 7–10 days. There seems to be a longer protracted syndrome characterized by malaise, fatigue, decreased well-being, poor tolerance of stress, and a craving for opiates which seems to last for some months during which time there is a high rate of relapse into opiate use. The requirement for any medical facilities or other supervision is therefore based on the need to encourage the individual in the continuation of an unpleasant process and to use the opportunity to provide sympathetic counselling and supportive care with a view to continuation of abstinence.

Options for medical withdrawal therapy for opiate dependants

A Opiate substitution and detoxification using methadone, codeine, buprenorphine or other opiate of patient's choice.

B Clonidine alone, with an opiate antagonist, following methadone, via a patch or as an adjunct.

C Detoxification using other medications such as neuroleptics, diphenoxylate, beta-adrenoreceptor blocking drugs, sedative hypnotics.

D Auricular acupuncture.

(Chang and Kosten 1997)

Cocaine/amphetamine withdrawal

Central nervous stimulants such as cocaine and amphetamine rarely require in-patient hospitalization or supervision.Withrawal from this group of drugs is characterized by the opposite effects of there stimulant activity and individuals experience hypersomnia, depression, fatigue and apathy. Reports of life-threatening depression and the requirement for brief hospitalization and antidepressant medications are in a minority. Improvements in symptomatology have been reported with the use of acupuncture (Lipton *et al.* 1994). Both cocaine and amphetamines are used most commonly in intermittent and binge patterns. Following a 2 to 3 day binge, stimulant users are dysphoric, exhausted and somnolent for 24–48 hours. Because other drugs such as heroin, cannabis and alcohol are used to reduce irritability, multiple dependency may be present.

The rapid rise and apparent rapid decrease in dependent cocaine use in the USA during the late 1980s and mid 1990s indicates the possibility of effective self-withdrawal and abstinence. In the absence of widespread facilities for treatment for this form of addiction the possibility of spontaneous abstinence, at least among a sector of the population, is high. Information from the Drug Use Forecasting programme (National Institute of Justice 1991) indicates a declining trend in cocaine use among younger cohorts in Manhatten, although not in Miami, in the late 1980s and early 1990s. Although there is no specific therapy for stimulant use, the ingestion of massive amounts may require heavy sedation and treatment of chronic dependency may require mild sedation with phenobarbital, chloral or benzo-diazepines. Treatment of less heavy use includes reassurance that unpleasant symptoms will pass; patients should be advised after stopping drug use to drink lots of fluids (excluding alcohol), to exercise, and to eat three meals a day.

Behavioural research has concentrated on a variety of packages for treating cocaine dependent patients for withdrawal symptoms. In the absence of significant success in finding a suitable pharmacological agent to treat withdrawal symptoms, behavioural therapy has included intensive programmes using incentives and reward systems in order to prolong periods of abstinence. The importance of treating associated drug problems such as alcohol abuse at the same time as developing coping features for abstinence from cocaine has been shown to improve outcome. High doses of cocaine and/or prolonged use can trigger paranoia. Smoking crack cocaine can produce a particularly aggressive paranoia behaviour in users, and when addicted individuals stop using cocaine they often become depressed. This may also lead to further cocaine use to alleviate depression and treatment in the withdrawal state is frequently associated with the need for specific pharmaco therapy for the depressive episodes. Several samples of drug dependent individuals entering treatment have shown a high proportion with cocaine as a primary drug of abuse. Other studies indicate that over a third had used cocaine or crack cocaine within 30 days prior to admission for treatment, although this drug was not indicated as the primary drug of abuse (Higgins *et al.* 1994).

In the California Drug and Alcohol Treatment Assessment Study (CALDATA 1992) treatment for problems with crack cocaine and powdered cocaine was found to be just as effective as treatment for alcohol problems and more effective than treatment for heroin problems. Short-term and long-term medications have been studied for their potential to reduce symptoms of cocaine withdrawal and longer term craving for the drug. None of these agents has been accepted for widespread use, but fluphenthixol, which is an antidepressant with antipsychotic properties, has been shown to help withdrawals and improve retention in treatment.

Hypnotic/sedative withdrawal

In contrast to opiate and stimulant withdrawal, detoxification from sedatives including alcohol require careful medical consideration. Potential medical complications which may constitute an emergency are fits and delirium which can give rise to sudden death if untreated in some situations. Onset of withdrawal depends on the type of drug and its length of action. Short-acting barbiturates and benzodiazepines may result in withdrawals 12–16 hours after last ingestion whereas longer acting drugs such as diazepam may not result in withdrawal symptoms until 7–10 days after cessation. Symptoms include:

- *Anxiety symptoms*: anxiety, sweating, insomnia, headache, shaking, nausea, feelings of panic
- *Disordered perception*: feelings of unreality, abnormal body sensations, abnormal sensations of movement, hypersensitivity to stimuli, fear
- *Major incidents*: psychosis and epileptiform seizures.

Depending upon the length of time dependent, the type of drug used, and the tolerance of the patient, gradual reduction of the dose can allow successful detoxification without the use of any other pharmacotherapy.

High/low dose withdrawal

When the patient has been dependent on a high dose of the drug for a prolonged period, then reduction should be gradual. This is considered to be the case if the dose of diazepam, or equivalent, has been 40 mg or more for more than 8 months. Such patients should be tolerance tested as described in Chapter 9 and reduced by 10% per day under supervision. If serious withdrawal symptoms occur on dose reduction then this dose should be maintained until the symptoms improve.

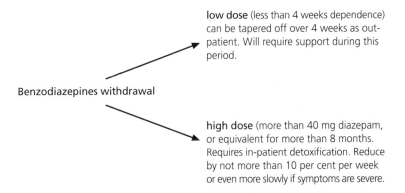

low dose (less than 4 weeks dependence) can be tapered off over 4 weeks as outpatient. Will require support during this period.

Benzodiazepines withdrawal

high dose (more than 40 mg diazepam, or equivalent for more than 8 months. Requires in-patient detoxification. Reduce by not more than 10 per cent per week or even more slowly if symptoms are severe.

Figure 10.1 High/low dose benzodiazepines withdrawal

Table 10.2 Approximate equivalent doses of diazepam 5 mg

Drug	Dose
Chlordiazepoxide	15 mg
Lorazepam	500 mcg
Oxazepam	15 mg
Temazepam	10 mg
Nitrazepam	5 mg
Flunitrazepam	2 mg

In benzodiazepine withdrawal treatment, antidepressants and antipsychotics should be avoided and reduction in the speed of withdrawal considered instead.

Conclusions

Detoxification is an easily conceived concept, but a complicated process. It can be carried out successfully with no medical or other support in the same way as alcohol detoxification is known to many who misuse this drug. Most individuals who have a drug dependency problem have experienced withdrawal symptoms and have detoxified themselves many times. These episodes may be when drugs were not available or when social and domestic pressures encouraged abstinence. The problem for most drug dependent patients is not achieving abstinence, but maintaining it (Newman 1987, 1983). Early on in any drug using career this is unclear to patients and relatives as it is to inexperienced clinicians and carers. The result is repeated disappointment and a consequent deterioration in domestic and professional relationships.

Detoxification can at times be associated with medical complications and social problems and is frequently a recurring event in the life of a drug user. Facilities for assisting detoxification are various, often reflecting the variety if individuals who come forward for treatment. These types of programmes are often suitable for individuals lacking in support from family or relatives and with less than adequate social circumstances. The high failure rate and return to drug taking is associated with these lack of resources, but is also inherent in the nature of the addiction process. Detoxification should not therefore be seen as a single treatment episode, but part of a bigger picture of treatment. This longer term process involves repeated detoxification episodes and coordination with preparatory work in selecting and patient/treatment matching and the vital process of follow-up care and reassessment. The need for accurate diagnosis of associated problems, both social and medical, can prevent failure, maximize success and minimize cost.

References

ACMD. 1996: *Drug users and the criminal justice system. Part 3: Drug misusers and the prison system – an integrated approach.* HMSO, London.

Alling, F.A. 1992: Detoxification and treatment of acute sequelae. In: Lowinson, J.H., Ruiz P., Millman, R.B. (eds)., *Substance abuse: a comprehensive textbook.* Williams & Wilkins, Baltimore, MD, pp. 402–15.

Bartter, T., Gooberman, L.L. 1996: Rapid opiate detoxification. *American Journal of Drug and Alcohol Abuse* **22** (4), 489–95.

Biles, D., McDonald, D. (eds). (1992): Deaths in custody in Australia, 1980–1989. Australian Institute of Criminology, Canberra.

CALDATA 1 1994: *California drug and treatment assessment.* US Department of Health Services.

Chang, G., Kosten., T. 1997: Detoxification. In: Lowinson, J.H., Ruiz, P., Millman, R.B., Langrod, J.G. (eds). *Substance abuse: a comprehensive textbook,* 3rd edn. Williams & Wilkins, Baltimore, MD, pp. 377–82.

Daley, D.C., Marlatt, G.A. 1997: Relapse prevention. In: Lowinson, J.H., Ruiz, P., Millman, R.B., Langrod, J.G. (eds). *Substance abuse: A comprehensive textbook,* 3rd edn. Williams & Wilkins, Baltimore, MD, 458–68.

Gerstein, D.R., Harwood, H.J. 1990: The effectiveness of treatment. In: *Institute of Medicine, treating drug problems.* National Academy Press, Washington DC, **1**, 32–199.

Gerstein, D.R., Lewin, L.S. 1990: Treating drug problems – a special report. *New England Journal of Medicine,* **323**, 844–8.

Gossop, M., Battersby, M., Strang, J. 1991: Self-detoxification by opiate addicts: a preliminary investigation. *British Journal of Psychiatry* **159**, 208–12.

Gossop, M. 1988: Clonidine and the treatment of the opiate withdrawal syndrome. *Drug and Alcohol Dependence,* **21**, 253–9.

Higgins, S.T., Budney, A.J., Bickel, W.K. 1994: Applying behavioural concepts and principles to the treatment of cocaine dependence. *Drug and Alcohol Dependence,* **34** (2) 87–97.

Jaffe, J.H. 1973: Multimodality approaches to the treatment and prevention of opiate addiction. In: Fisher, S., Freedmen, A.M. (eds). *Opiate addiction: origins and treatments.* Winston and Sons, Washington DC.

Jutta, J., Stover, H. 1997: Shoot out in Germany: Prisons take charge. *Druglink* **12**, 4–9.

Kleber, H.D. 1989: Treatment of drug dependence: what works? *International Review of Psychiatry* **1**, 81–100.

Levy, M., 1997: Prison health services. Should be as good as those for the general community. *British Medical Journal* **315**, 1394–5.

Lipton, D.S., Brewington, V., Smith, M. 1994: Acupuncture for crack cocaine detoxification: experimental evaluation of efficacy. *Journal of Substance Abuse Treatment,* **7**, 205–15.

McCaffrey, B.L. 1996: Treatment protocol effectiveness study. Office of the National Drug Control Policy, Executive Office of the President.

Madden, C., Hinton, E., Holman, C.P., Mountjouris, S., King, N. 1995: Factors associated with coping in persons undergoing alcohol and drug detoxification. *Drug and Alcohol Dependence* **38** (3), 229–35.

Mattick, R.P., Hall, W. 1996: Are detoxification programmes effective? *Lancet* **347**, 97–101.

National Institute of Justice 1991: *Drug use forecasting: drugs and crime.* 1990 Annual report. US Department of Justice, Washington, DC.

Newman, R.G. 1983: The need to redefine 'addiction'. *New England Journal of Medicine* **308** (18), 1096–8.

Newman, R.G. 1987: Methadone treatment: defining and evaluating success. *New England Journal of Medicine* **317**, 447–50.

Saitz, R., Mayo-Smith, M.F., Roberts, M.S., Redmond, H.A., Bernard, D.R., Calkins, D.R. 1994: Individualized treatment for alcohol withdrawal: a randomized double blind controlled trial. *Journal of the American Medical Association* **272**, 519–23.

Stockwell, T., Bolt, E., Hopper, J. 1986: Detoxification from alcohol at home managed by general practitioners. *British Medical Journal* **292**, 733–5.

Strang, J., Bearn, J., Gossop, M. 1997: Opiate detoxification under general anaesthesia. *British Medical Journal* **315**, 1249–50.

Sullivan, J.T., Sykora, K., Schneiderman, J., Naranjo, C., Sellers, E. 1989: Assessment of alcohol withdrawal: the revised Clinical Institute Withdrawal Assessment for Alcohol Scale (CIWA-Ar). *British Journal of Addiction* **84**, 1353–7.

Toon, P., Lynch, R. 1994: Changes in therapeutic communities in the UK. In: Strang, J., Gossop, M. (eds). *Heroin addiction and drug policy: The British System.* Oxford Medical Publications **17**: 231–9.

Waldorf, D. 1983: Natural recovery from opiate addiction: some social-psychological processes of untreated recovery. *Journal of Drug Issues* **13**, 237–80.

Wells, B. 1994: Narcotics Anonymous in Britain. In: Strang, J., Gossop, M. (eds). *Heroin addiction and drug policy. The British System.* Oxford University Press, pp. 240–47.

Wesson, D.R. 1995: Consensus panel chair. *Detoxification from alcohol and other drugs.* Treatment improvement protocol (TIP) Series 19. US Department of Health and Human Services. Centre for Substance Abuse Treatment, Rockville, MD.

West, R., Gossop, M. 1994: Overview: a comparison of withdrawal symptoms from different classes of drugs. *Addiction* **89**, 1483–9.

Psychosocial and support treatments

Annette Dale-Perera and Fiona Hackland

Introduction

Drug misusers are not a heterogeneous group. Drug misuse can affect a wide variety of people from a range of cultural and ethnic backgrounds. Though some kinds of drug misuse are more prevalent in areas of social deprivation, namely, heroin use (Ramsay and Percy 1996), psycho-social drug treatment options need to be able to reflect this range in order to meet the needs of such diverse groups. The report of the recent review of treatment in England (Department of Health 1996) is based upon a systematic review of national and international research, and the National Treatment Outcome Study (NTORS). This study followed the progress of 1100 drug misusers through treatment and found that there were no 'magic bullets' to cure drug problems. Indeed it stated that drug misuse was a 'chronic, relapsing condition', which required treatment packages matched to individual client needs. Further, most clients would require several attempts at drug treatment before any significant reductions in harm were accrued. However, this report, concluded that drug 'treatment which embraces social care and support as well as clinical interventions, can be notably effective in reducing (drug-related) harm'. Similar conclusions have been reached in the USA and are reflected in influential documents (Gerstein and Lewin 1990).

Different kinds of drug treatment, particularly psychosocial treatment options, have a range or hierarchy of goals. The NTORS study identified six goals which service providers commonly cited:

- reduction in psychological, social or other problems directly related to drug use
- reduction of the psychological, social or other problems not directly due to drug use
- reduction of harmful or risky behaviour associated with the use of drugs (e.g. sharing injecting equipment)
- attainment of controlled, non-dependent or non-problematic drug use
- abstinence from main problem drug(s)
- abstinence from all drugs.

The Effectiveness Review, as the Department of Health report is known, reported that these goals may be interrelated and depend on the motivation and circumstances of each individual. The report recognizes that abstinence is not always achievable or realistic for some drug misusers and that harm minimization, or the pursuit of intermediate treatment goals to reduce harm to the individual, is 'the best option'. Models of this pragmatic approach are pursued in various countries and the Dutch system is described in detail in Chapter 3.

Psychosocial treatment options have themselves been developed by a range of professional disciplines, self-help groups of ex-drug users, religious and church groups, and committed individuals. They have developed in the UK in response to trends in drug use, new funding initiatives, guidance such as that by the Advisory Council on the Misuse of Drugs and developments in generic health and social care.

Addressing a serious drug problem, may entail a total lifestyle change for an individual. It may be necessary to change friends or sever relationships, to change one's environment (home, leisure haunts), to find employment or change employment, to change the way one has related to friends and family, and to deal with underlying emotional problems which may have been masked by drug use for many years. The breadth of support a person may require may range from psychological help for underlying personal difficulties to employment training, from housing support to long-term relapse prevention.

This chapter models the main types of initiatives currently practised under the remit of drug treatment drawing mainly on contemporary UK experience. In reality, a clinician may utilize several of the options described below in one treatment package, or an individual may receive a variety of interventions sequentially, over the course of their drug using career. Much of the information presented is gathered by SCODA (The Standing Conference on Drug Abuse).

The Standing Conference on Drug Abuse (SCODA) seeks to reduce the harmful effects of drug use through informed debate and through the promotion of best practice and effective comprehensive services. It is an independent membership organization, providing a voice for drug services and others concerned about the effect of drug use on individuals or communities.

Advice and information initiatives

Telephone helplines

In the UK there are a number of local and national telephone helplines for drug users which are accessible 24 hours a day, 7 days a week. These include the national Drugs Helpline and local agency or areas-based lines. Most community-based services will provide advice and support by telephone during office hours.

Information leaflets

Drug services also produce a range of written materials aimed at drug users from different backgrounds. Many information packs are produced in a variety of languages utilizing images from different cultures. Information is targeted at different groups of drug users such as the safer dancing campaigns aimed at drug users on the rave music scene. An example of this is the harm-minimization material produced by the Lifeline organization in Manchester which is aimed at young drug users. They have been developed using research with this group to assess which images and methods would be most accessible to this group. Cartoon images, local slang and images reflecting local youth cultures, together with strong harm minimization messages were used.

Needle exchange schemes

Needle exchange and harm reduction services are key elements of many non-residential services. Needle exchange and other harm reduction services aim to reduce the transmission of HIV, hepatitis and other infectious diseases and also help to maximize service user health. They are low threshold and accessible and provide the service user with the opportunity to engage with other services such as counselling or legal advice (Stimson *et al.* 1988).

There are needle exchange schemes in most localities in the UK, as there are in many European centres. They fall into four basic models:

- stand alone services
- those run from community-based drug services, either in-house or outreach services
- pharmacy-based schemes
- General Practitioner-based services.

All offer a supply of new injecting equipment including a range of syringes, disposal containers and condoms, together with advice on safer drug use and safer sex. Most community-based services offer needle exchange as part of core work and many offer needle exchange within the contexts of outreach into other generic services (peripatetic needle exchange). Some pharmacy and detached schemes use ready made packs distributed during detached or street outreach work, for example with homeless drug users. Pharmacy based needle exchange schemes have grown rapidly over the past 5 years with most areas having a network of retail pharmacists distributing packs of injecting paraphernalia – sometimes with support from a co-ordinator.

Counselling

Many services described here report that counselling is an approach they use extensively in their work with service users. The recent Compass Report (1996) reported that 94% of community drug agencies surveyed listed counselling as a key treatment. The Effectiveness Review (1996) reported that 'drug misusers present with a wide range of problems associated with their pattern of drug misuse . . . counselling is a technique flexible enough to offer some response to this wide variety of problems. However, this very flexibility means it can be difficult to clarify the purpose of counselling and to evaluate it objectively'.

The Effectiveness Review found two approaches to counselling commonly employed by drug services, counselling itself, and the provision of advice and support. The two were often not distinguished by agencies.

The process of defining and differentiating between these approaches has recently been undertaken by the Advice, Guidance, Counselling and Psychotherapy Lead Body (1992) which is charged with devising occupational standards for this area of work. Standards and qualifications already exist for advice and guidance, with standards for counselling in development. The work of the Lead Body offers clear definitions which differentiate between advice-giving and counselling, as well as providing vocationally-based qualification routes for workers in drug services. Advice is defined as 'a brief consultation to provide someone with appropriate and accurate information', and give 'suggestions about how to act upon that information'. Counselling as being 'the principled use of relationship to provide someone with the opportunity to work towards living in a more satisfying and resourceful way'. The relationship takes place within agreed boundaries. . . . 'The counsellor's role is to facilitate the client's work in ways which respect the client's values, personal resources and capacity for self-determination'.

Clarity about the structure and method of each approach will assist services to:

- define good practice
- provide information to clients and purchasers which clearly outlines the nature of the service and expected outcomes
- identify current levels of skill and any training or staff development needs.

The Effectiveness Review (1996) concluded that counselling carried out by a trained and supervised counsellor is the key element in successful outcomes, with the degree of structure within which counselling being significant to its success.

Three counselling models

The Effectiveness Review cited three specific approaches to counselling: non-directive counselling; cognitive behavioural approaches;

and 12-step addictive counselling. Non-directive counselling, derived from the work of Carl Rogers, encourages clients to find their own solutions to problems. Cognitive behavioural approaches, developed by clinical psychologists, include motivational interviewing and relapse prevention. These are used to promote abstinence or achieve gradual control of drug misuse. The Effectiveness Review could not describe the extent of relapse prevention groups in England, but did not find them to be widespread. They found that this form of counselling focuses on teaching cognitive and behavioural techniques which enable drug misusers to resist drug use and related behaviours. Specific training in these techniques is essential if they are to be carried out and evaluated effectively.

Finally, 12-step addiction counselling is underpinned by a strong ideological and theological theoretical base. This is derived from a disease model of addiction, in which the consequences and problems of drug use are seen to be only avoidable by life-long total abstinence. Consistent abstinence can be achieved through following the 12-step model advocated by Alcoholics and Narcotics Anonymous. Counselling techniques are used to support the 12-step programme; these are often psychodynamic and provided by addiction counsellors, many of whom are former addicts.

In reality, many methods of counselling are used in drug treatment. Some community-based drug services provide time-limited, focused counselling which may last six sessions, with clear goals set during an initial assessment.

Residential care

For some drug misusers, a period of residential care, away from a familiar environment, may prove the most effective means of tackling a drug problem. The community or home environment may sometimes be difficult places to resist drugs, even for motivated individuals. Continued access to drugs, pressure from local drug dealers, drug using friends and peers, may make abstinence near impossible. Additionally, some drug users will not have stable or supportive living arrangements which enable them to cope with community-based treatment options in the first instance. The NTORS study found residential drug treatment to be more effective than non-residential treatment in achieving lasting abstinence. Indeed NTORS has found that residential rehabilitation of drug users pays for itself several times over in savings to local communities through the reduction of crime alone. There are currently some 100 residential drug services listed for England and Wales (SCODA 1997a). These residential agencies tend to fall into two categories, high support residential rehabilitation units and lower support (semi-supported or move on) units.

Residential rehabilitation units: core components

The 'Effectiveness Review', named three different types of residential rehabilitation units:

* the therapeutic community
* '12-step' or Minnesota Method houses
* general houses, including many with a strong Christian philosophy.

The therapeutic community approach grew from at least two strong traditions, the Maxwell Jones approach which developed in England, as a model of dealing with behavioural or psychiatric problems, and the Synanon or Concept House approach which developed in the USA in the addiction field. Therapeutic communities tend to be drug-free and highly structured with an emphasis on psychotherapeutic group work facilitated by a staff team. In the Maxwell Jones model, a democratic approach tends to be taken with residents having a say or a vote in some of the decision-making of the community. In both approaches, peers are encouraged to support and confront each other in a constructive manner to enable and facilitate behaviour change. Residents are generally required to take part and be responsible for the daily upkeep of the house in a team. Responsibilities include domestic chores (shopping, cooking, cleaning, maintenance of the house, gardening and repairs). Residents gain status throughout their stay in the house. Initially they are generally confined to the house or not allowed out without an escort (to prevent relapse into drug use). Gradually they acquire more responsibilities, privileges and freedom as they prepare for re-entry into the outside world. In the latter stages of a placement they may engage in voluntary work or education. Examples of these therapeutic communities include Phoenix Houses (concept houses) and the Richmond Fellowship Crescent House (democratic approach). Many Concept Houses have modified their approaches over the last 10 years or so, mainly due to the impact of HIV, because of which a less stressful atmosphere was advocated to minimize the risk of the onset of AIDS, and to the increased emphasis on clients' rights and individual care-planning required by Community Care legislation (Wells 1994).

The '12-step' or Minnesota Method originated in the USA and is the largest self-help network for people with drug and alcohol problems. There is a large network of 12-step residential units in England, across Europe and north America. This approach views drug and alcohol misuse as a 'disease affecting mind, body and soul'. Progress through 12 steps aims to improve health and amend attitude and lifestyle with an ultimate goal of abstinence from drugs and alcohol. In a residential unit, residents learn about and sequentially follow the 12 steps. As in other types of residential units there is a strong emphasis on self help group work. Most of the staff in these units tend to be ex-drug and alcohol users who follow the same philosophy and who provide counselling and mentoring to the residents.

Other residential units, such as Christian Houses use group work, counselling and community living as a basis for changing a drug using lifestyle.

In a national survey of residential care (SCODA 1997a) increasing diversity and innovation was found, particularly in relation to target group specific work. Over a hundred rehabilitation units were surveyed with a 65% response rate. These results showed that in addition to traditional therapeutic programmes of group work and counselling, many units had diversified. Diversifications were found in pre-care and induction packages, crisis interventions, prescribing and detoxification packages, education and training, and aftercare.

Crisis interventions

Drug users requesting residential care are often in a state of crisis. They may require or have undergone detoxification and be at risk of relapse.

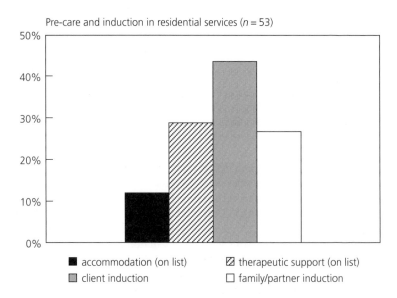

Figure 11.1 Pre-care and induction in residential services

Clients experiencing a medical or drug-related emergency may be treated within the context of a hospital or specialist NHS drug inpatient unit. Some residential rehabilitation units are now offering a similar service, either in a dedicated unit or separate facilities within wider residential services. This sort of service is intended for clients whose drug misuse has critically impaired their health, or has led them into other life-threatening situations such as threat of physical attack. Detoxification models and theory are described in Chapter 10.

Drug users in crisis usually require rapid access and speedy assessment and placement are therefore essential. Services may need to be block-funded to side-step lengthy community care assessment and funding requirements and to allow for fast tracking mechanisms to be developed.

EXAMPLE: Specialist Crisis Unit, City Roads

Located in central London, City Roads offers a 3 or 4 week long programme for clients before referral to other agencies which can offer longer term support. This includes detoxification, primary healthcare, psychiatric assessment, alternative therapies, food and rest, intensive care planning, help to sort out outstanding legal problems, housing and social care problems.

EXAMPLE: within a network of services: Kaleidoscope

This network of services has a one-bedded self-contained unit for crisis intervention. This accommodation provides asylum enabling respite care for the client. The on-site staff team comprises medical staff and social workers, enabling supervised detoxification and offering help in areas such as housing, financial and legal problems. This is a short-term programme of about 3 weeks, after which clients are able to stay at Kaleidoscope to participate in a longer-term residential programme.

Pre-care and induction in residential units

A small number of units make holding accommodation available to drug users waiting to take up a placement. A slightly larger number of units provide therapeutic support for drug users on a waiting list. This can entail telephone support, counselling or weekly group support for local drug users. Good induction can help clients settle in to a unit more quickly and prevent early drop out from residential care. Increasingly, residential services provide induction support packages which comprise individual support, mentoring, beginners'

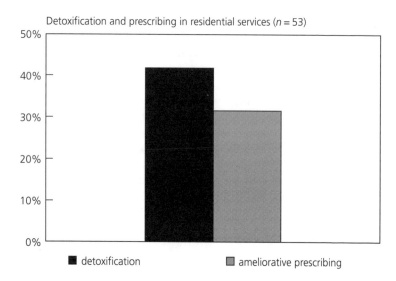

Figure 11.2 Detoxification and prescribing in residential services

groups and clear information packs. Induction for partners or family members is also increasing.

Detoxification and prescribing in residential units

Many residential units no longer require clients to be drug-free on admission. This is a major change from previous practice. Now almost half of those surveyed provide initial detoxification consisting of on-site medical and psychiatric staff providing individually-tailored detoxification regimes or methadone reduction plans. A third of units prescribe medication for the after-effects of withdrawal from stimulant use and some combine this with the use of alternative therapies such as acupuncture.

Ensuring fitness and health

Primary healthcare is essential for drug users because the chaotic life led by some may have disrupted regular health checks. Drug use may also mask lingering or advanced infections and illnesses. Most residential units provide primary healthcare in conjunction with the local General Practice, or as part of an in-house medical facility. Free access to fitness facilities is common with many residential units negotiating minimal rates or free passes to local sports centres. Some even have sports facilities on-site.

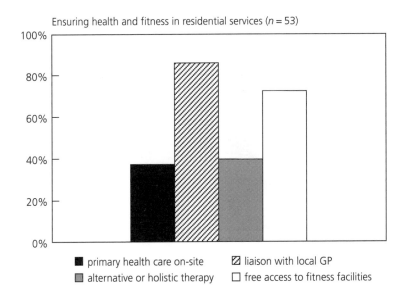

Figure 11.3 Ensuring health and fitness in residential services

Managing stress and anxiety is an important skill for people aiming to live a life without drugs. Alternative therapies are becoming more common as a means of addressing this problem. Residential units usually employ qualified therapists on a sessional basis and acupuncture, shiatsu massage, and visualization are the most commonly offered therapies.

Catering

A healthy diet is essential for drug users who may have become undernourished. It is important to provide for a range of diets. Some units employ cooks who assess residents dietary needs and help guide them in menu planning and cooking. Vegetarian and vegan diets are commonplace. Low-fat and other regimens may be important for clients with liver and kidney problems resulting from drug use or blood-borne diseases such as hepatitis and HIV infection. Many units also take into account religious and cultural preferences such as kosher (Jewish) or halal (Muslim) meat, or the prohibition of pork.

Skills for the wider world

Many drug users benefit from skill development, including numeracy and literacy training. This may be addressed through access to local

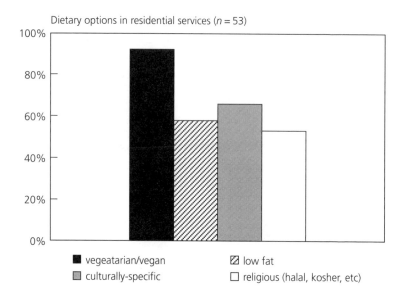

Figure 11.4   Dietary options in residential services

adult education centres or colleges. Most basic education courses in the context of residential units is provided off-site. Residents may be offered help with enrolment, support while attending (including escorts) and encouragement in completing courses.

Increasingly, training for National Vocational Qualifications (NVQs) and other qualifications are becoming available as part of a residential programme. Some residential units are accreditation centres. Popular subjects for training include basic computing, catering, photography, pottery, woodworking. Staff help clients build portfolios so that they can access further education.

Voluntary work placements are well-established in residential rehabilitation units as stepping stones to work or college. Many units have links with local volunteer agencies and employers and encourage clients to undertake some voluntary work during the late stages of their rehabilitation.

Targeting groups with special needs

There are many different types of groups of drug users and, increasingly, residential units are making provision for their special needs. Table 11.1 summarizes the extent of target group specific work reported by residential services in 1996. These are detailed later in this chapter.

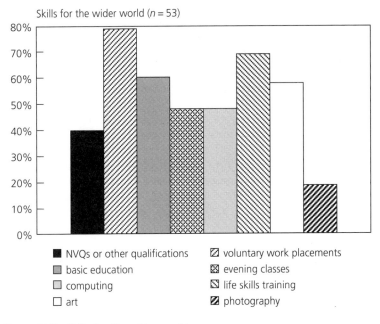

Figure 11.5 Skills for the wider world

Table 11.1 Summary of innovation in target group specific work in residential units

Innovation	%	Number
Drug-using offenders groups	40	21
Black drug user groups	25	13
Young drug users	34	18
Gender groups	42	22
Crack-specific groups	17	9
Narcotics and Alcoholics Anonymous	34	18

Innovation in aftercare support

Just over half of rehabilitation units in the SCODA study had specific responses to the accommodation requirements of those leaving residential care. These comprised drug-free accommodation in the local area, with varying degrees of therapeutic support.

Examples included Crescent House, who own and manage a drug-free six-bedroomed flat with optional day care and Manna Farm who own and manage six three-bedroomed flats. Phoenix House has a supported housing scheme running at two of their sites in London, Waldram Park and Bell Green where residents who have completed residential care programmes have the chance to move towards independent living with full resettlement support. Other units, such as Murray Lodge and Phoenix House (Newcastle) reported having move-on accommodation for ex-residents of their units.

Half of the rehabilitation units in the survey reported having housing nominations to local authorities and local housing associations or trusts. For example, Phoenix House Family Centre in Sheffield has a link with a local housing association called the Thursday Project to find flats and houses for ex-residents of the centre.

Aftercare counselling

Counselling for ex-residents is offered by nearly three-quarters (70%) of residential units. This tends to be time-limited support which is individually-negotiated with each ex-resident and clients are usually required to be drug-free if they attend sessions at the unit itself. At Clouds House, ex-residents can come to individual counselling or to psychotherapy sessions with their families. Just over a third (34%) of units, for example Trevi House in Plymouth, offer domiciliary visits to drug users who have left a residential placement. Generally, this service is provided when a unit is able to obtain funding by an individual contract basis and the frequency of visits is negotiated between the client and a designated outreach worker.

Day care: structured day programmes

Increasingly, residential units report providing day care for clients who have been residents in the unit but who now live locally and still require support. Over a third offer a day programme for drug users. This form of care is usually purchased on a contract basis and varies in intensity according to both individual needs and unit capacity. Some units, like Crescent House in London, link this form of day care with special accommodation in the community such as a drug-free community flat for those who are leaving residential care. Ex-residents are able to negotiate levels of attendance on the day programme, fitting in those structured activities with developing their lives outside of the unit, by means such as educational courses, voluntary or paid work.

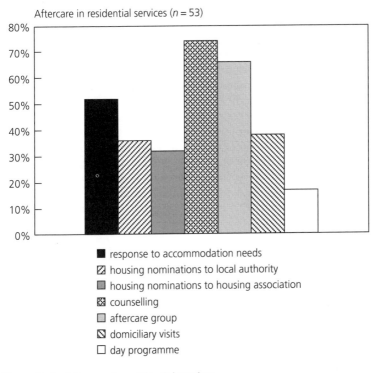

Aftercare in residential services (*n* = 53)

- ■ response to accommodation needs
- ▨ housing nominations to local authority
- ▨ housing nominations to housing association
- ▩ counselling
- ▢ aftercare group
- ◩ domiciliary visits
- ☐ day programme

Figure 11.6 Aftercare in residential services

Nearly a quarter offer other forms of support for drug users leaving residential care. This ranged from *ad hoc* telephone support, to out patient services, formal aftercare services, family therapy, drop-in centres and ex-residents support group.

Example: aftercare business enterprise

At Turning Point unit in Whitley Bay, ex-residents who stay in the local area are able to get involved in the aftercare group cooperative. The group is 16-strong and is self-run, meeting twice a week. The cooperative which they self-manage runs a gardening service and a local market stall at which they sell handmade goods such as candles, silk-screened T-shirts, pottery and woodcrafts.

Conclusions about residential services

SCODA's survey found considerable local innovation and diversity in improving residential care for drug users. Funding changes have resulted in the shortening of treatment programmes since 1993 to 3 to 6 months, sometimes half their original length. As a result residential services in Britain have changed significantly. Increasingly these residential units are forging links with housing, probation and primary healthcare services to make the services they offer more comprehensive and more robust. Evidence from the National Treatment Outcomes Research Study (NTORS) demonstrates the complexity of problems presented by people referred to residential drug treatment services. Further developments are anticipated in services to address that complexity, with more of a partnership approach being adopted between services. Future challenges include addressing more effectively the needs of young drug users, ethnic groups and families, or women with children, with an aim to improving retention rates. Building on achievements in aftercare provision is another key area for development.

Structured Day Programmes

Since 1993, many Structured Day Programmes (SDPs) have emerged, which offer intensive community-based support which mimic a working week or college course. London hosts almost half of these new initiatives (SCODA 1996b). Five models of SDPs are found in London and all have certain characteristics in common: finite length programmes of 3 to 5 days a week; a holistic approach to rehabilitation including life skills and vocational training; a focus on personal independence and responsibility; enabling drug users to maintain family and social support networks; and a very structured approach either through a rolling programme of fixed activities or individually negotiated timetables for each drug user. Some programmes also accommodate both drug-free and active drug users. The five types are:

SDPs for drug using offenders

Specific programmes for drug using offenders are usually funded by probation services and may include probation officers as staff. These programmes tend to have a cognitive approach which targets both drug using and offending behaviour. The Community Drug Project SDP in South London has modified a specific cognitive approach for offenders to address drug use. The Cable Street structured day programme also focuses on drug using offenders, many of who are serving community sentences which stipulate attendance at the programme. This programme also provides vocational training. Government plans for the future include the possibility of sentencing offenders to treatment programmes. This is likely to herald further changes in community facilities.

SDPs for crack cocaine users

London has at the present time two structured day programmes which target crack users. The Blenheim SDP in West London is cognitive in focus and teaches clients relapse prevention techniques. Alternative therapies also provided include auricular acupuncture and 'detox and sleep' homeopathic teas. Vital (part of Newham Drug Project) in East London targets ethnic minority drug users and provides culturally specific group work. It also hosts women and rock sessions targeting female crack users and provides literature for female partners of crack users.

Vocational SDPs

Some SDPs aim to provide drug users and ex-drug users with vocational skills to aid employment and also address drug use. Milton skills centre provides structured day care for both drug-free and non-drug-free clients in separate programmes. Education and training is offered on a range of topics and clients may gain National Vocation Qualifications (NVQs) on a range of subjects. The Base (Cranston Projects) in South London offers a range of activities and skills training together with counselling services within a framework of individual care planning.

12-step SDP

London hosts the only SDP with a 12-step Minnesota method phil-osophy, the Self Help Addiction Recovery Programme (SHARP). Treatment follows the first three steps of Narcotics and Alcoholics Anonymous (NA and AA), and clients are encouraged to use the NA and AA self-help networks of support during and after the pro-gramme.

Aftercare for residential rehabilitation

The final model of SDP is the increasing provision of aftercare by residential units. Ex-residents attend a residential programme on a daycare basis for a limited period of time with the aim of easing transition into independent living. Many of these SDPs are linked with accommodation schemes managed by the rehabilitation unit.

Floating support schemes

Floating support schemes enable drug using clients to live in the community while receiving help from drug specialists. There are two of these schemes.

Specialist drug agencies supporting drug users in public housing

Support, day care and domicilary services for drug users living in the community, have been provided by voluntary sector street agencies and community drug teams for some years. This support has tended to be led by individual needs. Some rehabilitation units are now utilizing public housing to provide accommodation whilst they provide therapeutic support packages for ex-residents. Some community-based services have also been involved in community drug education and involvement schemes such as training for tenants associations and other community groups.

EXAMPLE: The Harbour Project

The Harbour Project provides a specialist non-residential drug service for residents of Plymouth. Part of the project also aims to provide drug education for local people and involve the local community in the care and treatment of those affected by drug misuse.

Case Study: Phoenix Floating Support Scheme

Through its Floating Support scheme, Phoenix House provides broad-based support for tenants who are at risk of losing tenancies because of drug or alcohol misuse problems. This scheme has been set up in partnership with Quadrant housing association and the London housing foundation. The service includes basic advice and debt counselling for clients, with referral to specialists in drug and alcohol misuse and community care assessors, to enable access to appropriate packages of care. Project workers help tenants access other services such as Social Service Departments and educational and health services, and they are able to give advice on issues concerning housing, welfare rights and benefits. Support is given for a time-limited period negotiated between the tenant, the housing association and Phoenix House workers. Usually the three project workers have 14 clients each and report to the scheme manager, who also has a small caseload of clients. The scheme aims to provide fast effective services for tenants helping them to stabilize their tenancies and reducing nuisance for other tenants.

Self-help, peer and family support networks

Narcotics Anonymous

Narcotics Anonymous (NA) is the largest self-help network for ex and current drug users in the UK. NA is one of the 12-step fellowships born out of Alcoholics Anonymous. NA is financially self-supporting, with an estimated London membership of 3000. There are on average 20 meetings held daily in London, 365 days of the year. Members are encouraged to attend support groups daily, or more frequently. Mentoring is also an important tool in enabling newcomers to understand the 12 steps, prevent relapse and provide ongoing support. More details of the 12 steps are included in Chapter 10.

Drug user support groups

Other support groups and services managed by current or ex-drug users include Mainliners. This organization was originally established by users and ex-users affected by HIV, and now provides a network of services including outreach and HIV prevention initiatives, a drop-in service with meals, alternative therapy groups, counselling and group work, training events and a newsletter.

Family

Services for the relatives and carers of drug users tend to be based in the voluntary sector, such as the national self-help network for relatives of drug users, Adfam. Some rehabilitation units provide residential services for drug using couples or parents and their children (for example the Maya Project in South London). Clouds House provides a week long residential programme for non-drug using family members who have been affected by chronic drug use.

Training

The range of service provision described in this chapter necessitates a skilled, competent workforce able to deliver good quality services to all those affected by drug use.

Training requirements vary across the professions. Those working in specialist drug services have distinct training needs from those who occasionally encounter drug users in their work. However, all those who come into contact with those affected by drug use must be able to respond in an effective way.

Training of staff and volunteers underpins the development and delivery of appropriate, good quality services. The training needs of individuals and organizations should be linked to strategic objectives. The planning of training which satisfies these objectives must be linked to overall strategic planning. Training which is established strategically supports service objectives. It helps achieve these more quickly by ensuring that the skills and knowledge required to deliver them are in place (SCODA 1996a).

Training bridges the gap between what a person is required to do and what they are currently able to do. However, training is often viewed as superfluous to the delivery of quality services, not as an investment which will enable such delivery.

The 1990 ACMD review of training states that 'there is a substantial demand for training from those with direct client/patient contact. This is not being adequately met ... in consequence, the quantity and quality of work with problem drug users is undermined and the strategies which have been developed at national, regional and district levels to respond to drug problems cannot be effectively implemented. To ignore this need on grounds of cost will almost certainly prove to be a false economy. Training is a necessity not a luxury. Considerable benefits will accrue from a relatively small investment now. In the longer term it can ensure that better value is obtained from services already provided' (ACMD 1990). Seven years after this statement was first made it continues to be both pertinent and pressing.

Targeting hard to reach groups

Drug using offenders

Drug services are increasingly providing specific treatment and care for offenders in the UK and have in many countries been drawn into contact with the criminal justice system. Community sentencing options with treatment components are used in some SDPs and residential rehabilitation units. Some residential services such as the Langley House Trust provide units specifically for drug using offenders. Other drugs services run specific groups which address drug use and offending behaviour. Most units recognize the importance of diverting motivated drug users from custodial sentences to treatment

settings. Many interview potential clients in prison to develop effective through care. Some services allow courts to bail drug using
offenders to them to carry out extended assessment for rehabilitation
or treatment and local authority funding. Nearly half of residential
units reported running special programmes for drug using offenders
in 1996. Most units for drug using offenders are men-only.

A range of treatment programmes are developing within prisons
including drug-free wings and structured treatment programmes.
Peripatetic outreach is increasing in probation services and bail
hostels.

Structured day programmes for drug using offenders

Specific programmes for drug using offenders are usually funded by
probation services and may include probation officers as staff. These
programmes tend to have a cognitive approach which target both
drug using and offending behaviour. Some have modified a specific
cognitive approach for offenders to also address drug use. These
programmes also tend to provide vocational training, with some
providing vocational programmes for drug users who are unable to
stop using drugs or who are stabilized on methadone.

Criminal justice access schemes

These schemes target drug using offenders and focus on providing
advice and information and, facilitating access to drug treatment and
care. Schemes include arrest referral schemes and bail assessment.
Most rehabilitation units recognize the importance of diverting motivated drug users from custodial sentences to treatment settings.
Many drug rehabilitation units will interview potential clients in
prison if resources allow.

EXAMPLE: Prisoners Resource Service (PRS)

Cranstoun Projects manage a number of residential services across London
as well as the Prisoners' Resource Service (PRS). PRS provides assistance
for both sentenced prisoners and drug users on remand. Prisoners are
offered information, advice and counselling through regular surgeries held
in the prison. The teams liaise with probation officers and solicitors and
negotiate referral to a variety of drugs services (including, but not limited
to, Cranstoun's residential projects). PRS facilitates through care by
securing places for offenders in drug treatment centres as an alternative
to or following custody.

> ### EXAMPLE: Residential bail assessment
>
> The Ley Community in Oxford in conjunction with Probation Services manages a bail assessment scheme. Offenders are bailed by the court to the Ley Community for a 4-week period in which they are assessed for rehabilitation or treatment and for local authority funding. This often facilitates community sentences with conditions to attend a rehabilitation unit or other drug service.

Women

Congruent with the limited empirical research on women, theories of addiction and treatment have also ignored women. The typical alcoholic or drug addict is assumed to be male, and services have been developed to address alcohol and other drug problems so conceptualized (Broom and Stevens, 1991). Services have been created to meet needs as represented in an addiction literature weighted towards the experience of men. These services have then, generally, been presumed appropriate for women. It is assumed that this situation has led to under-utilization of services by women.

Attitudes to women's drug use present another barrier to women's use of services. Broom and Stevens offer the notion of the ' "doubly deviant woman" – someone who has transgressed not only the law or general social convention, but . . . specifically violated the norms of being a "good woman" ' (Broom and Stevens, 1991). Such attitudes not only affect those who may offer services, but also drug using women's expectations of how they will be dealt with by services should they admit their drug use.

Statistics on women's drug use indicate a 3:1 male:female ratio in the UK at the present time (Statistical Bulletin 1997). Babcock explores the notion of convergence, that women are catching up with men's level of drug use as demonstrated in research (Babcock 1996). This is often depicted as an actual increase in women's drug use. However, Babcock argues that research has usually ignored the greater under-reporting of drug/alcohol use in women. . . . and that convergence may be only apparent as this avoidance recedes. Babcock describes a cyclical relationship between indifference to researching women's drug use leading to under-reporting of such use which, in turn, results in indifference to researching women's drug use. A similar cyclical relationship may be described between women's under-use of services, their subsequent absence from addiction research and literature, demonstration of need for women appropriate services, and the design and implementation of such services.

Most research studies which do examine women's access to services and experiences of addiction refer to the scarcity of previous research. Little empirical work has been done which compares women specific with generic treatment and care services. A recent study (Hodgins *et al.* 1997) compares single gender with mixed gender programmes. They conclude that male and female substance abusers report different histories and courses for their disorders and display different needs and characteristics in treatment settings. For women, single-gender groups will lead to greater engagement, retention and self-disclosure than mixed groups.

Pregnant users

A number of models are used when working with drug using pregnant women. Some localities have a liaison nurse specialist who acts as the focal point between drug and alcohol services, antenatal services and health visitors for any drug using pregnant women in the area. The liaison nurse has been responsible for facilitating the local area policy, practice and training of professionals. Other areas have a special clinic service for pregnant women and their partners who express concerns about drug and alcohol use. This model of providing a specialist drugs worker in antenatal services has other examples in other centres. The alternative training of generic antenatal staff to cope with drug users as they present has the attraction of being more flexible and providing a holistic approach to drug use which may be present in many forms in pregnant women.

Innovation in residential care for women

Some units are single sex, women only. Male only rehabilitation units tend to be for drug using offenders or specifically Christian based. Rehabilitation units for women offer a variety of special services such as assertiveness training, understanding and combating eating disorders, problems due to sexual abuse, sexuality, social concerns, physical concerns, child care issues, financial and legal problems. Others target particular groups of women. The Bethany Project in London is a women only residential unit serving the needs of women who are working or have worked in the sex industry. Hope House in London is a women only residential unit for women who have completed the first stages of drug treatment in a Minnesota Method treatment centre. The Pathway project in Bristol offers a post-detoxification, therapeutic environment for women. The Maya Project in Southwark is a women only residential unit which can accommodate and care for the children of clients as well. It gives particular priority to women from black and ethnic minority communities.

Young people

The Health Advisory Service (1996) found a paucity of dedicated drug services for young dependent drug users. Most drug services are still adult orientated and therefore neither suitable nor skilled in working with a younger age group with different (age specific) needs. Services in England for young drug users (18 years and under) are required to operate within the spirit of the Children Act (1989). This necessitates the use of detailed monitoring procedures and the involvement of local area Child Protection Committees and social services child protection teams if a child is deemed at risk of significant harm (Social Services Inspectorate 1997). The Standing Conference on Drug Abuse issue guidelines as 10 key principles (SCODA 1997b) (Appendix 11.1). They will also be issuing in 1998 policy guidelines on working with young drug users. These address some of the many difficulties such as the legal complexities of competency to consent to treatment aid working with young people at risk (SCODA 1998).

Minority ethnic groups

Drug services targeted at different groups of minority ethnic drug using groups are growing. Some drugs agencies actively target black drug users by having ratios of black and minority ethnic staff and positive multicultural images. Others run black drug user groups and provide outreach work into Black and Asian community agencies. One community drug team has a peer education scheme for 40 Bangladeshi youths run by an Asian worker with local connections. Specific drug services are emerging which are solely targeted at specific ethnic and other groups, for example *Asian prescribing services*.

HIV and hepatitis C

Services range from a dedicated respite care unit for those with HIV and AIDS to sessional input by specialists into a residential programme. Over half of residential units reported that they provided health-related services for those who are HIV antibody positive or with an AIDS diagnosis. At some units, for example the Coke Hole Trust, residents who identify themselves as HIV antibody positive are offered specific group work or counselling, often provided in liaison with local specialist organizations and the local medical centre. All rehabilitation units should refer clients for HIV testing and counselling if requested. Many rehabilitation units also reported providing information on HIV, AIDS, and hepatitis, together with special diets, health and safety regimes and the provision of condoms in toilets. Some rehabilitation units refer clients to local medical services for hepatitis B testing and vaccination. Many rehabilitation units also reported holding regular groups on harm minimization. Units had fewer clear policies regarding hepatitis C although this is likely to change rapidly over the next few years.

Some residential units provide emergency leaving packs for those drug users who leave unexpectedly, which contained details of the nearest syringe exchange schemes.

EXAMPLE: Griffin Project

Turning Points Griffin Project in London is a specialist rehabilitation unit dedicated to drug users with HIV and AIDS which offers respite and medical care. An on-site medical team works closely with local prescribing services. The unit is staffed 24 hours a day and has facilities for severely disabled people.

Conclusions

In recent years community development has seen a rapid growth in provision of services for drug users. Those which have been available before the emergence of HIV infection have adapted considerably during the last decade. Internationally similar moves from specialist to generalist services have given rise to expansion in the importance of community care and considerable increase in the range of services required and expected from such organizations. Non-statutory groups are commonly now found to liaise effectively with specialist services and increasingly take responsibility for those discharged from hospital or diverted from an otherwise custodial sentence by the courts. This is an area which will increase as cost savings in the prison and criminal justice system demands community care in the same way as economic considerations have driven the move to community health and social care. The resulting development of more complex agencies requires more expertise in both management and service delivery. Organizations such as SCODA are important in identifying standards and developing models of good care (SCODA 1997c).

Several challenges are evident. The need constantly to adapt to new clinical and organizational demands creates the requirement for flexibility and growth. The emergence of HIV and hepatitis C has required considerable ingenuity and change from drug workers. The increasing use of diversion schemes by the courts is bringing a group of drug dependent clients into contact with community agencies. By definition these clients are present under duress and strategies are required to address their specific difficulties. Modification of pre-existing counselling and support packages to accommodate the requirements of the sentence imposed and the individual client are necessary.

There is inevitably some concern that those sentenced to a period of drug treatment will exclude those on a voluntary waiting list for such therapy.

Finally, the requirement of drug workers and employers of such agencies described in this chapter for training and further education is unending and is expensive.

Appendix 11.1 Policy Guidelines for Working with Young Drug Users – the Standing Conference on Drug Abuse and the Children's Legal Centre

In this Appendix we have distilled what we believe to be the 10 key principles to be applied in working with young drug users. The aim is to bring clarity of focus, and to give some structure to planning and decision making processes – for all those wanting to respond constructively to young people's drug use. We expect that understanding and operating according to these 10 principles will always be the essence of good practice with young people.

1 A child or adolescent is not an adult

Approaches to young people need intrinsically to reflect that there are differences between adults and children, and between children of different ages. In all drug-related interactions and interventions with young people, consideration will need to be given to: differences in legal competence; age appropriateness; parental responsibility; confidentiality; and exposure to, and protection from, risk and harm.

2 The overall welfare of the individual child or young person is of paramount importance

The overarching principle in this document, in accordance with the UN Convention on the Rights of the Child and The Children Act 1989, is that all professionals and agencies that offer a service to young people must have the best interests of the young person as their paramount focus. Each young person is unique and should be worked with on an individual basis. In putting the welfare of the child first, it may be necessary for the interests of workers, parents, services or other adults to come second. Sector loyalties or agency rivalries should not be maintained if the best interests of the young person are best met by joint working.

3 The views of the young person are of central importance, and should always be sought and considered

Practitioners should always explain their roles and boundaries clearly and honestly, and make sure that they are understood by the young person. It must be remembered that the expressed views or opinions of the young person may, in some cases, not be the same as the professional assessment of their best interests.

4 Services need to respect parental responsibility when working with a young person

Providers of services should remember that in the case of virtually every young person there will be an adult with parental responsibility. The involvement and support of parents or carers may be beneficial to successful work with young drug users, and their consent may be required before intervening.

5 Services should recognize and cooperate with the local authority in carrying out its responsibilities towards children and young people

Local authorities have responsibilities to ensure that appropriate services are provided for children in their area who are 'in need', and to investigate and protect children 'at risk of significant harm'. The young person with serious drug misuse problems is quite likely to already fall into one or both of these categories and, therefore, protocols for liaison and joint working will need to be established between the local authority and the young people's substance misuse service, whether it is a statutory or a voluntary sector service.

Where young drug users are not yet known to the local authority as 'in need' or 'at risk', a careful balance must be struck between ensuring that interventions are made appropriately and quickly to protect the present and future safety of the child, and not intervening unnecessarily in the lives of the young person and their family.

6 A multidisciplinary approach is vital at all levels, as young people's problems do not respect our professional boundaries

Multiagency coordination, and integration of policy, need to be achieved at commissioning, planning and contracting levels, linking with Drug Action Teams, Area Child Protection Committees and

Integrated Children's Services Planning structures as key strategic and policy making bodies. Provision of services should also be made through a multidisciplinary approach to meeting the needs of the young person, whether within a team, or as part of a wider team network within the children and family services infrastructure. Professional disciplines that will need to be involved will include child and adolescent mental health, education and youth services, health and social services, and criminal justice agencies.

7 Services must be child-centred

Interactions and interventions must be appropriate to the age, maturity and level of development of the individual child or young person, setting their drug use or misuse within their wider personal, social and cultural context. Services should be attractive to young people, respecting their individual needs, lifestyle, gender, ethnicity, and beliefs. Consideration must be given to how a service accesses young people, in particular: opening times (whether during or after school hours); location (whether separate from adult services and in 'safe' areas); age appropriate publicity and information; and ensuring contact with 'hard to reach' young people.

8 A comprehensive range of services needs to be provided

Service provision in any local area must be able to respond to a range of levels and patterns of drug and alcohol use and misuse by young people, by providing access to a wide range of drug-related interventions, as appropriate to each individual case. These will include: drug education; prevention programmes; advice; counselling; prescription and detoxification; rehabilitation; needle exchange services; as well as information, advice and support for parents. It may also include access to alternative and complementary therapies.

9 Services must be competent to respond to the needs of the young person

The staff team of a young people's substance misuse service will need to incorporate core skills in working with children, adolescents and families, and in working with substance misuse. The competence of the service will also lie in its multidisciplinary approach to meeting complex needs, whether through ensuring a variety of skills within a staff team, or by mobilizing expertise through joint working with other services.

10 Services should aim to operate, in all cases, according to the principles of best practice

This requires that services operate within the current legal framework, particularly in accordance with the underlying philosophy of the Children Act and the UN Convention on the Rights of the Child, and according to accepted, evidence-based effectiveness. Services should take responsibility for ensuring that they are aware of, and practice in accordance with, the latest locally and/or nationally established policy and guidance on working with young drug users.

References

ACMD 1990: *Problem drug use: A review of training*. HMSO, London.

Advice, Guidance, Counselling and Psychotherapy Lead Body 1992: *Report to differentiate between befriending, advice, guidance counselling skills and counselling*. A, G, C & P Lead Body, London.

Babcock, M. 1996: Does feminism drive women to drink? Conflicting themes. *International Journal of Drug Policy* **7** (3), 158–65.

Broom, D., Stevens, A. 1991: Doubly deviant: Women using alcohol and other drugs. *International Journal of Drug Policy* **2** (4), 25–7.

Children Act 1989: HMSO, London.

Compass Report 1996: Compass Partnership, 1995. *Review of community-based drug services*. A report prepared for the Task Force (unpublished).

Department of Health 1996: *The Task Force to review services for drug misusers. Report of an independent review of drug treatment services in England*. Department of Health, London.

Effectiveness Review 1996: *Otherwise known as the Task Force Report to review services for drug misusers. Report of an independent review of drug treatment in England*. Department of Health, London.

Gerstein, D.R., Lewin, L.S. 1990: Treating drug problems. Report from the National Academy of Sciences, Washington. *New England Journal of Medicine* **323**, 844–8.

Health Advisory Service. 1996: Children and young people: substance misuse services: the substance of young need. HMSO, London.

Hodgins, D., El-Guebaly, N., Addington, J. 1997: Treatment of substance abusers: single or mixed gender programs? *Addiction* **92** (7), 805–12.

Ramsey, M., Percy, A. 1996: *Drug misuse declared: results of the 1994 British Crime Survey*. Research and planning unit paper 151. London, Home Office.

SCODA 1996a: *Training for drug action*. SCODA, London.

SCODA 1996b: *Structured day programmes*. SCODA, London.

SCODA 1997a: *New options in residential and social care.* SCODA, London.

SCODA 1997b: *Enhancing drug services: a management handbook for quality and effectiveness.* SCODA, London.

SCODA 1997c: *Involving drug users.* SCODA, London.

SCODA 1998: *National policy guidelines for working with young people.* SCODA and Children's Legal Centre. London (in press).

Social Services Inspectorate 1997: *Young people and substance misuse: the local authority response.* Department of Health, London.

Statistical Bulletin 1997: *Statistics of drug addicts notification to the Home Office, United Kingdom, 1996.* Issue 22/97, Home Office, London.

Stimson, G.V., Alldritt, L., Dolan, K., Donoghoe, M.C., Lart, R. 1988: Injecting equipment exchange schemes: final report. Goldsmith's College, London.

Wells, B. 1994: Narcotics anonymous (NA) in Britain. In: Strang, J., Gossop, M. (eds). *Heroin addiction and drug policy. The British system.* Oxford University Press, Oxford.

Pregnant drug users

Frank D Johnstone

Introduction

Pregnancy provides a very special context in the life history of the drug user. It offers opportunities, as well as risks, and brings into sharp focus all the underlying themes of management. In this chapter a broad view of drug use is taken, to include nicotine and alcohol. This is because the risks of these drugs are particularly well established, and because they are often used in combination with illicit drugs. Although nicotine and alcohol are 'legal', it is important not to confuse legality with safety. Other chapters in this book are all relevant to pregnancy, but this chapter tries to highlight those specific points which are most important. It also concentrates on the particular perspective of community care.

Drug use is important in pregnancy care

First of all, drug use in pregnancy is common (Evans and Gillogley 1991, Buchi 1996). The most important drug at a population level is nicotine, with well-documented adverse effects. One-third of our population smokes during pregnancy. Alcohol is also a commonly used drug (Noble *et al.* 1997), though the serious fetal alcohol syndrome is seen only at very high maternal intakes. Illicit drug use is widespread. Most studies on prevalence come from the United States. The prevalence of use of different illicit drugs is very variable according to time and place. Three population studies suggested that at least 8–14% of women took cannabis, cocaine or opiates during pregnancy (Chasnoff *et al.* 1990, MMWR 1990, Pegues *et al.* 1994). The figures for urban teaching hospitals tended to be much higher (21–32%) (Zuckerman *et al.* 1989, Gillogley *et al.* 1990, Forman *et al.* 1994). In the UK, the only study of anonymous testing in an obstetric population was in inner London, where 8.5% of urines were positive for cannabis and 2% were positive for cocaine or opiates (Farkas *et al.* 1995). Drug use of some sort is now a fundamental part of many women's lifestyle.

Drug use does impact on obstetric and paediatric morbidity and mortality. The effects of specific drugs are highlighted below but there are important associations with congenital abnormality, pre-term delivery, intrauterine growth restriction, neonatal abstinence syndrome and sudden infant death syndrome, as well as the maternal risk. There are worrying and unproven, theoretical risks that prolonged exposure of the developing fetal brain to psychoactive drugs could produce long-term effects on neural organization.

Drug use may also emphasize deficiencies in the organization of care. Although team care is frequently spoken of, there is often poor communication between different components of this care. In addition, drug users may sometimes have disruptive and frightening effects on normal pregnant women and force carers to examine how their system of care is organized.

Drug use is not by itself a very high risk condition compared with many other problems in obstetrics, but because of all the above factors, it is nowadays one of the leading conditions requiring specific guidelines and strategies.

Pregnancy care can be important in the natural history of drug use

Pregnancy may be an important event in the natural history of drug use. Many women, who do not have or acknowledge any problem with their drug pattern may present for the first time within the system of care because of pregnancy. Their requirement is for pregnancy care rather than drug management, but this may present an opportunity for harm minimization or education, or change in their approach towards drug use.

Pregnancy can be a motivator, and a time when patient and carer share the same consistent aim, a healthy, normal baby. Because of this, women may be more cooperative and more open to healthier strategies. This again offers a window of opportunity. It is, of course, not only the woman herself who may be positively affected in terms of the natural drug use history. Her partner and family are integral to any system of care, may themselves be influenced to exert a positive effect on the woman herself, and also to support subsequent childcare and help break the cycle of inter-generational morbidity.

Some effects of drugs on pregnancy

We must all be aware of the generally poor quality of information about drug effects. This is because of a number of recurring confounders, the most important being as follows; bias in selection of women based on dependency clinic attendance, or 'obvious' chaotic drug use so that they are quite unrepresentative of population use; the small numbers studied may be inadequate to study infrequent events, e.g. major congenital anomaly; there may be preferential publication of studies which show harmful effects (Koren *et al.* 1989); there is difficulty in ascertaining and measuring drug use especially where this is illicit; many drug users are polydrug users and this makes it difficult to isolate the effect of one drug; there are major problems in separating the effects of drug use from the other adverse personal, psychological and social circumstances in which drug use is taking place. This may be a particular difficulty in relating specific intrauterine fetal drug exposure to long-term behavioural effects as the child grows up.

The poor quality of data has implications. We should be wary about saying there is no risk because none has been demonstrated and we should be cautious about stating a risk based on small anecdotal clusters. Part of the process of giving accurate information is an indication of reliability and this underlying theme should inform information transfer. But the overall public health message should not be constrained by waiting decades for definitive studies.

Nicotine

The use of nicotine refers to smoking cigarettes. Of the 4000 compounds in tobacco smoke, there is good evidence that nicotine is the key drug of addiction and nicotine, carbon monoxide and cyanide are thought to have the greatest adverse effect on the fetus. Smokers have an increased risk of many pregnancy complications. As always with drugs, the situation is complex because women who smoke in pregnancy have a higher rate than non-smokers of other health risk behaviours, social disadvantage, and emotional disturbance (Stewart and Streiner 1995). Most risk increases are relatively modest (around 1.5–2.5) but this assumes enormous significance in the light of the numbers of pregnancies involved. The excess risks have been well-reviewed (Fredricsson and Gilljam 1992, Bevan and Kenney 1996, Wong and Bauman 1997, Kendrick and Merritt, 1996).

- There are increased risks of spontaneous abortion and ectopic pregnancy (Kline *et al.* 1995)
- Placenta praevia and placental abruption are both more common
- Pre-term premature rupture of the membranes and pre-term delivery are more common
- Birth weight is depressed by about 250 g with an increased risk of significant intrauterine growth restriction. No protective effect can be demonstrated from higher maternal weight, pregnancy weight gain or body mass index (Ellard *et al.* 1996, Zaren *et al.* 1997)
- Intrauterine death in late pregnancy is increased
- About 10% of perinatal mortality is attributable to smoking
- Maternal milk production is reduced by about 30%
- There is a strong relationship with sudden infant death syndrome
- There is a strong effect on respiratory disease and hospital admission in the first year of life, and an effect on respiratory disease in childhood
- There are small effects on physical and mental development of the child, of uncertain clinical significance. This includes poorer reading and language skills (Fried *et al.* 1997, Fried, 1989)
- A relationship between maternal smoking and idiopathic mental retardation has been reported (Drews *et al.* 1996)
- Maternal smoking appears to be a robust independent risk factor for conduct disorder in boys (Wakschlag *et al.* 1997)
- There is no convincing evidence that nicotine causes congenital anomaly, but an association with several specific anomalies, particularly limb reduction defects, has been suggested.
- There is a lower incidence of pre-eclampsia, although the perinatal case fatality rate is higher in those affected.

There are obviously all the risks for the mother herself, with half of all smokers dying because of the habit, one-third of them before the age of 65 (Sell *et al.* 1996).

Alcohol

This drug has the clearest association with teratogenesis. Although the adverse effects have been well documented with high maternal intakes, there may be less complete fetal effects with lesser intakes. Mild or occasional use may be harmless but a safe level of maternal alcohol consumption has not been established.

- Diagnosis of fetal alcohol syndrome (FAS) depends on three specific criteria (growth retardation, CNS involvement and characteristic facial dysmorphology). Whether this is truly specific to alcohol or represents a more general toxic effect is uncertain. It occurs at very high maternal alcohol intakes, and the average in one report was 17 units/day (Oulellette et al. 1977).
- In some western countries, FAS is claimed to be the leading recognized cause of mental retardation (Abel and Sokol 1986).
- A wide range of other alcohol-related birth defects appear to occur with heavy drinking (Pietrantoni and Knuppel 1991).
- There is a high spontaneous abortion rate in alcoholic women and a possible association with lower levels of maternal alcohol assumption (Abel 1996).
- There appear to be adverse effects on birth weight of moderate drinking (around 20 units/week) (Windham et al. 1995, Passaro et al. 1996).
- Alcohol may affect fetal brain development at any gestation. Abnormalities of brain development have been observed at a range of reported intakes and threshold effects on subsequent reading, spelling and arithmetic abilities have been reported at intakes of only 1 unit/day (Goldschmidt et al. 1996, Konovalov et al. 1997).

Problem drinking has longer term risk for mother and child. Alcohol is associated with 80% of suicides, 40% of road traffic accidents, 80% of deaths from fire, 1 in 3 divorces, 1 in 3 cases of child abuse and 20–30% of all hospital admissions (Ashworth and Gerada 1997).

Opioids

Information about opioids is rather limited, particularly on long-term effects on the child. The following observations are available from a growing research literature on the effects of opiates in and after pregnancy.

- There is no convincing evidence that opioids cause fetal abnormality. Because such huge numbers of women have taken these drugs, it seems unlikely that they are major teratogens.
- Opioids probably do have a small effect on inhibiting fetal growth, but this is less than smoking (Johnstone et al. 1996).
- Pre-term labour is more common in women injecting drugs rather than taking them orally. This may be because of an unstable

alternation between intoxication and withdrawal with relatively short-acting injected drugs, rather than a pure drug effect. It is however clinically important.

- Many different pregnancy problems have been described in drug using populations. It is uncertain how much of this is a drug effect rather than due to the effect of other variables and lifestyles. However, modest increases in perinatal mortality, due to prematurity and late pregnancy stillbirth are consistently reported. An increase in meconium staining of the liquor at delivery is also commonly reported, perhaps due to episodes of fetal drug withdrawal (Johnstone 1990, Ellwood and O'Connor 1989).
- There is a high rate of neonatal abstinence syndrome (NAS), ranging from 40–90% in women taking opiates daily. There is a relationship between maternal dose, serum drug levels and severity of NAS but this is not a close one (Doberczak *et al.* 1993, Mack *et al.* 1991, Malpas *et al.* 1995).
- There is good evidence that sudden infant death syndrome is increased. The largest study showed a seven times increased risk with maternal methadone use and a five times increased risk with heroin use. After correction for high risk variables, the relative risks were 3.6 and 2.3 respectively (Kandall *et al.* 1993).
- In contrast, a study based on screening at birth by meconium analysis did not show an excess mortality in babies exposed to drugs prenatally, for the first 2 years of their life (Ostrea *et al.* 1997).
- Information on long-term consequences of *in utero* exposure to opioids is contradictory and inconclusive. Drug effects, and the consequences of an unstable, impoverished environment, are very difficult to disentangle. But this remains an area of concern (Kaltenbach and Finnegan 1984, 1987, 1988).

There are obviously all the risks of non-sterile injecting, overdose, respiratory depression and death for the mother (Tardiff *et al.* 1996, Marzuk *et al.* 1997, Woodburn and Murie 1996, Robertson *et al.* 1994, Morrison, 1995).

Cocaine

There is a huge amount of descriptive evidence that cocaine causes problems for pregnancy. There is also a plausible theoretical mechanism for its action. Its central action is through inhibition of receptors of dopamine in the nucleus accumbens and pre-frontal cortex. But it has important peripheral effects on inhibition of uptake of noradrenalin in pre-synaptic nerve terminals. The resulting high catecholamine levels cause vasoconstriction, tachycardia, hypertension and probably uterine contractility. Most pregnancy complications arise from this peripheral action.

- Studies of cocaine teratogenicity are not conclusive, but the vasoconstrictive properties of cocaine raise the possibility that there might be damage during episodes of fetal ischaemia. The pattern of defects reported, and some animal experiments, are consistent with this. (Non-duodenal intestinal atresia/infarction, limb reduction defects, urinary tract anomalies, and cardiac malformations have been reported.) The overall population risk for users does not seem very high, and this is perhaps because only those with high dosage at key gestations may be vulnerable (Holzman and Paneth 1994, Bingol et al. 1987, Neerhof et al. 1989).
- There is probably a decrease in birth weight based on the consistency of a number of studies in women, and animal studies which show a dose-related decrease in uterine blood flow and decreased fetal size (Holzman and Paneth 1994, Morris et al. 1997).
- Pre-term delivery is more common and, although it is vary difficult to adjust for multiple co-variates, this is probably also a real drug effect.
- Placental abruption, fetal cerebral injury, intrauterine death all seem to be events temporarily related to cocaine use. Population data are not conclusive, and presumably these events are dependent on dose, timing and other co-factors.
- Sudden infant death syndrome appears to be slightly more common but overall there is little evidence of any causal effect.
- Long-term neuro-behavioural follow-up studies have not found any obvious or consistent cognitive impairment or deficit in IQ, but children may be at risk of developing problems of fine motor coordination and attention deficit disorder that could lead to poor school performance (Woods 1996, Nulman et al. 1994, Richardson et al. 1996).

The mother is at risk from rare but dramatic events such as myocardial infarction, cerebro-vascular accident, subarachnoid haemorrhage, hepatic rupture, cardiac arrhythmias, accidental injury and pre-eclamptic like states (Cregler and Mark, 1986, Marzuk et al. 1995, Marzuk et al. 1997).

Cannabis

This very commonly used drug will usually not come to medical attention and, as a result, information on pregnancy is poor. Although commonly used episodically, heavy and frequent use is much less common.

- Most studies have not reported any definite association between prenatal cannabis exposure and morphological abnormalities of the baby.
- Some studies have reported lower birth weight and shorter gestation, but reports are not consistent (Zuckerman *et al.* 1989, Buchi 1996, Linn *et al.* 1983, Fried, 1991).
- Few studies have addressed long-term effects. Negative effects have been reported, including disturbed nocturnal sleep at age 3 years, but data are insufficient to be definitive (Day *et al.* 1994, Richardson *et al.* 1995, Dahl *et al.* 1995).

A summary document from the Australian drugs task force reviewing the literature on the effects of cannabis in pregnancy concluded that, 'the evidence is variable but prudence suggests that until this issue is resolved (the possible risk of birth defects), we should err on the side of caution and recommend that cannabis is not used during pregnancy or when trying to conceive' (Hall *et al.* 1994).

Benzodiazepines

These commonly used drugs have often been studied with low dose use, whereas in some drug users very high doses are involved.

- There have been several reports which have shown the same pattern of abnormalities, particularly cleft lip/palate. However, population data suggest the effects may be quite small, and two studies found no evidence of any increase in abnormalities. At present, it seems possible that there may be an increase in fetal abnormality, but this has not been proved (Pastuszak *et al.* 1996, Altshuler and Szuba 1994, Czeizel 1988, Laegreid *et al.* 1992a, 1992b, Laegreid, 1990).
- There have been concerns about possible dysmorphic change, reduced growth, brain development and long-term outcome, but it is difficult to be categorical about risks at the present time.
- Withdrawal does occur in the neonate, typically with irritability and slowness to feed and respond. There may be poor suck, feeble cry and hypotonia.

Amphetamines

There are reports of reduced birth weight, occipito-frontal circumference and length, and an increased incidence of prematurity. These are plausible effects given that large doses of amphetamines are associated with weight loss in adults. Data currently available do not allow any accurate estimate of risk although at least one study has shown a high perinatal mortality and increased number of malformations (Eriksson *et al.* 1981). Since amphetamines and cocaine have similar central physiological effects, their impact on pregnancies should be similar. Both agents cause vasoconstriction and hypertension, which may result in acute or chronic fetal hypoxia. More information is required and, as with other drugs, advice must be to avoid or at least reduce intake during pregnancy (Finnegan 1979).

Volatile substances

In the UK, it is estimated that 3.5–10% of current adolescents have experimented with solvents, and up to 1% of the secondary school population are currently abusers (Langa, 1993). Between 1981–1990, 605 people aged less than 18 years died of volatile substance abuse (Esmail *et al.* 1993). One hundred and eighty of these deaths were in Scotland. The main mechanism of death is arrhythmia but anoxia, respiratory depression, inhalation of vomit and trauma may contribute. Males are much more at risk than females. The commonest substance is cigarette lighter refills (butane) but there is a wide range of products.

- One study in rats showed that the intermittent acute high concentration of solvent abuse caused a number of differences in the pups, including lower weight gain and developmental delay (Jones *et al.* 1996).
- There is uncertainty about whether there is a discrete fetal solvent syndrome ('toluene embryopathy') (Medrano 1996).
- There is a neonatal abstinence syndrome, the Finnegan score (Table 12.1) is appropriate to assess this, and phenobarbitone appears effective in treatment (Tenenbein *et al.* 1996).

The mother who continues to abuse solvents is at risk of sudden death, or if use is prolonged, of causing permanent damage to the central nervous system, heart, liver, kidneys and lungs. For every ecstasy death, 11 people die of inhaling volatile substances found in domestic consumer products.

'Designer drugs'

A number of analogues of fentanyl, mescaline, amphetamines and phenylcyclidine have been produced. The most widely used drugs at present are amphetamine analogues. 3,4-methylenedioxymethyl amphetamine (MDMA, 'ecstasy') is one derivative related chemically to both amphetamines and hallucinogens. Complications of use are rare, but potentially devastating. There have been fatalities from hyperpyrexia, rhabdomyolysis, disseminated intravascular coagulation (DIC) and hepatotoxicity.

- There is, as yet, no information in the literature about effects in human pregnancy.

Although an attempt has been made to define risks for separate drugs, it is important to remember that many drug users are poly-drug users, intakes depending on availability. There is little enough good information about many drugs and hardly any about particular synergies or potentiations of drug combinations. On general common sense grounds, multiple fluctuating drug use seems likely to be most harmful, but this impression is not evidence based.

Options for drug management

Many women who are not truly dependent on their drug will stop spontaneously as soon as they know they are pregnant. This applies to about 20% of women who smoke, it applies to many women who use ecstasy or cannabis episodically, and it is also true of some controlled users on opiates.

For those women remaining on drugs, there are opportunities for cessation. This is perhaps best demonstrated for nicotine. Nicotine is somewhat different from other drugs in that, although a withdrawal syndrome is recognized, the syndrome is not an important cause of clinical morbidity, and cessation can be encouraged without incurring serious risks for mother or child. Although only about 5% of long-term smokers attempting to become abstinent will remain so at 1 year without help, there is evidence that brief intervention by family doctors is effective in increasing the number of smokers becoming long-term abstainers over the background rate. In pregnancy, advice about smoking cessation has been shown to be effective (Dolan-Mullen et al. 1994, O'Campo et al. 1995). Indeed, this is one of the few interventions in obstetrics proven in randomized controlled trial to be effective. Small but significant gains in birth weight have been reported following such advice. Nevertheless, achieving changes in smoking behaviour in pregnant women is difficult (Kendrick and Merritt, 1996; Walsh et al. 1997; Hartmann et al. 1996). Strongly addicted women may be unable to quit and trying to modify behaviour in late pregnancy, when the baby is found to be growth retarded, may simply increase guilt and anxiety with no benefit. The correct public health approach is to stop young women becoming addicted.

Excessive alcohol intake is such a potential risk for the developing fetal brain that detoxification, under very closely monitored hospital conditions, should be considered and usually advised at any gestation. This needs specialist supervision because of the potential dangers of alcohol withdrawal. It needs attenuation therapy, close fetal monitoring if in later pregnancy, and needs to be slow (Ashworth and Gerada 1997). All women who are drinking heavily should be prescribed multivitamin preparations with particular attention to thiamine. Women should have liver function tests measured, to include prothrombin time. Disulfiram (Antabuse) is contraindicated in pregnancy.

For most other drugs, much of the skill in management lies in planning realistic aims with each individual pregnant woman. Many women say they would like to stop drugs, but in the particular situation at the time in their life, this may not be possible for them. Trying to persuade the woman to stop drugs may simply alienate the patient, lead to return to a more chaotic drug use pattern, and result in non-attendance for antenatal care. Therefore, the different options of detoxification, substitution and maintenance and other aspects of damage limitation need to be considered with full understanding of the woman's aspirations and particular social and psychological circumstances. Drugs may have been taken by the patient for many years and may be an integral part of her lifestyle. She may consequently have no intention of changing or altering and this may be reinforced by friends or relatives who have had babies successfully, even with continued drug use. The woman herself may have had a previous pregnancy while using drugs with no apparent ill effects. Getting the balance of recognizing the inevitability of continued drug use against our professional obligations to advise against any substance abuse in pregnancy is difficult and has to be tailored to the understanding and attitudes of individual patients.

Acute opiate withdrawal is rarely fatal for the mother, and is less serious than withdrawal from alcohol, benzodiazepines or barbiturates, but it is unpleasant. The belief that there is risk for the fetus is based on case reports where violent intrauterine movements immediately preceding fetal death were reported. There were also studies showing high catecholamine levels in amniotic fluid when the mother was withdrawing (Zuspan et al. 1975). Animal research using pregnant ewes shows clear abnormal changes in fetal heart rate, with decreased arterial pH, decreased Po_2 and meconium release, on naloxone precipitated opiate withdrawal. Recurrent naloxone-induced withdrawal is associated in animals with fetal wastage and growth failure (Cohen et al. 1980). Despite all of this, the risks of withdrawal have probably been exaggerated in the past, and can be minimized by appropriate drug therapy to the mother. Detoxification

Table 12.1 Dose equivalent to diazepam 5 mg

Lorazepam	500 μg
Nitrazepam	5 mg
Oxazepam	15 mg
Temazepam	10 mg

can be carried out in the mid trimester quite safely and this has a place in overall management. However, acute detoxification should be avoided in late pregnancy.

Slow reduction may be preferred by many women for opiates, and is necessary for benzodiazepines. The size of each reduction depends on the drug and the dose that is being taken and what the drug user thinks she can cope with. The key issues are that reduction should be *gradual, stepwise* and *tailored* to the woman's response. But withdrawal is only likely to be successful if both doctor and patient are fully committed to a withdrawal plan. A common strategy for reduction is to substitute diazepam for shorter acting agents (Table 12.1), and to reduce by small amounts, not more than 5 mg/week, until withdrawal symptoms emerge, or until the drug is stopped, the process taking at least 3 months (Okacha, 1995). The woman should be warned that sleep may be disturbed for some days until a normal rhythm is re-established. For methadone reduction, one plan is if stable on 40–90 ml methadone, reduce by 5 ml at a time; if stable on 20–40 ml, reduce by 2–5 ml at a time; below 20 ml, reduce by 1–2 ml at a time. It is not usually appropriate to reduce more often than weekly or fortnightly, but with strong motivation and starting early in the second trimester, it may be possible to achieve dosages which are unlikely to cause significant neonatal abstinence syndrome (for example, a dose of less than 20 mg of methadone).

For most women who are dependent and who have a long-standing habit, substitution and maintenance is usually the preferred option for opiates. This has the advantage of allowing a more stable lifestyle, without the need to raise money for street drugs (Farrell *et al*. 1994, Mattick and Hall 1996). It may remove the need for prostitution or criminal behaviour and it reduces injection with all its dangers. It is very important to emphasize that substitution should be prescribed as part of a package including social and psychological support. For pregnancy, the drug of choice is methadone linctus. This cannot be injected and, because it lasts for 24 hours, it offers stability of drug levels. The risk of overdose and potentially death if other drugs are taken, and the likelihood of neonatal abstinence syndrome, must be understood by the woman.

Care with methadone prescriptions is essential during pregnancy and in the postnatal period. Some studies of pregnant women receiving methadone have shown that plasma levels decrease during pregnancy because of an increased fluid space and a large tissue reservoir. There may also be altered metabolism of the drug by the placenta and fetus. These results suggest that the pregnant woman may require an increase in methadone during gestation and that lowering the dose to avoid complications may be inappropriate. Similarly, in the postnatal period, a reversal of these effects may lead to increased plasma levels of methadone with potential toxic effects (Finnegan and Kandall 1997).

Other interventions include prolonged inpatient stay in a drug-free environment. This is effective in the short term and may be extremely important for individuals at critical points. However, it is too expensive to be widely used, and it may also be counterproductive, by simply putting off the evil hour of facing up to problems in the community. A number of drugs may have a place in non-pregnant withdrawal and maintenance of abstinence (Seivewright and Greenwood 1996, Schuckit 1997, Mendelson and Mello 1996) but the unknown effects in pregnancy will limit their use for some time.

Much of the management of drug misuse is damage limitation rather than cure, and in patients who continue to inject, it is essential to ensure that they have access to clean equipment. This is preferably achieved by needle exchange. The least desirable option, or in an emergency, is the use of bleach. Injection equipment can be sterilized by drawing up washing up liquid or household bleach into the needle and syringe, flushing it away (not back into the receptacle) repeating that three times, and then flushing though with cold water three times.

It is very important for each care agency to be able to offer a full range of options for drug management. It is also essential that a full range of help is available for housing, financial and psychological problems. The immediate priorities of attracting into treatment and retaining in treatment mean that help has to be offered, not only with stabilizing drug use but with stabilising lifestyle and reducing death rate. These aims acquire particular urgency in pregnancy.

Ethos of care

The underlying principles of management include a pragmatic approach emphasizing rehabilitation with attention mainly paid to harm reduction; and obstetric and midwifery care focused on physical and psychological well-being in preparation for motherhood.

These aims may be defined as normalization and integration. Health-care workers need to share the same aims, and to have come to terms with the ethical issues involved (Johnstone 1994).

These aims can be achieved most effectively by management and prescribing in the community. This serves to normalize a drug user's view of herself. It is appropriate for care to take place in a way that fits in with the background and family, and where it can be delivered in a way that is acceptable, if necessary with home visits. It also means that the necessary supervision and care of the child has already been anticipated by care during pregnancy.

As part of the obligations imposed on community care staff, this means building up a detailed picture of drug habit and background, carrying out appropriate screening and antenatal care, ensuring that appropriate educational messages are conveyed, and making sure that aims are definitely planned and understood.

Another important obligation on community care staff is effective liaison and communication with other agencies. In particular, it is important to resolve the patient's anxieties about maternity unit care and to make sure that drug counsellor, social worker, obstetrician and midwife are all involved, and all giving the same message. Nothing is so guaranteed to reduce confidence as different agencies giving out different messages. For a team to be effective, people should know each other, know how to make contact quickly and easily, and be used to doing so.

Reports of contrasting responses to the needs of pregnant drug users come from north America and Europe. In the USA, coercive and even criminal justice procedures have been employed to influence management. This aggressive and punitive approach is a good ex-ample of how patients can be effectively excluded from appropriate care rather than drawn into contact with a caring service (Chaukin and Kandall 1990). The Dutch approach described in Chapter 3 attempts to provide a sympathetic environment and consequently draw all groups into a close working relationship.

Screening in pregnancy

As well as the usual pregnancy tests, there are a number of investiga-tions which may have particular importance in drug users.

Hepatitis B

This virus is spread by sharing needles or by sexual contact and, although most adults will become immune, about 5% remain as carriers of the virus. This is one of the clearest indications for screening. Without treatment, 90% of babies of women who are e-antigen positive will acquire hepatitis B infection at birth. Nearly all will remain as carriers and 25% will die by early adulthood because of liver disease. If a woman is known to be e-antigen positive, then passive and active immunization of the baby at birth will prevent at least 90% of babies from becoming infected. There is therefore a very clear gain of knowing serostatus, and testing for hepatitis B carriage should be routinely offered.

Hepatitis C

This virus is also spread by sharing and, to a much lesser extent, by sexual exposure. The benefits are not nearly so clear cut as for hepatitis B. In women who are HIV negative, only about 5% of women with hepatitis C infection will pass the virus on to their child. It is not fully understood how or when infection takes place. The 30–40% of women who are hepatitis C antibody positive but who are persistently PCR negative are at minimal risk of transmitting infection sexually, and appear to be at minimal risk of transmitting vertically. The PCR (polymerase chain reaction) test is a highly sensitive measure of the presence or absence of viral genetic material. If it is negative, it strongly suggests the absence of current viral activity. All the information at present suggests that this infection is not transmitted by breast feeding, and we currently do not advise against breast feeding. For the adult, alpha-interferon treatment has been shown to benefit some, but this should not be given in pregnancy.

HIV

This is another test where there are now clear benefits in knowing serostatus. There always were potential advantages in minimizing sexual spread but more recently combination therapy offers outstanding benefits for the individual infected. The risk of vertical transmission, usually between 15–25% in early studies from Europe and the United States, can be substantially reduced. This is mainly through use of zidovudine as shown in the ACTG076 trial which reported a 67% reduction compared with placebo (Sperling et al. 1996). The treatment shown in this trial to reduce transmission from HIV infected mother to infant has become standard therapy. It involves taking zidovudine during pregnancy, by infusion during labour and by the child for some weeks after birth. Whether it is now necessary to include a further drug, when zidovudine is so widely used is, at present, uncertain. HIV is spread through breast feeding, and this adds perhaps a 14% risk (Dunn et al. 1992). Finally caesarean section and various precautions around delivery may also have benefit (European Collaborative Study, 1994).

Because of all these benefits, it is essential not only to offer HIV testing, but to ensure that the woman is fully aware of the benefits.

Cervical intraepithelial neoplasia

It is not known whether drug use *per se* increases the risk of cervical intraepithelial neoplasia (CIN) but, because of lifestyle, there may have been greater sexual exposure to specific papilloma viruses and the woman may not have sought routine cytological screening. Women who have HIV and who are immunologically compromised are at greater risk of CIN and at greater risk of more rapid progression. Pregnancy may be an opportunity to attract the woman into cytological surveillance. Perhaps vaginal examination may not be acceptable at first contact, but this offer should be made when possible.

Cervical and vaginal infections

Drug users, particularly injecting drug users, are at higher risk of pre-term delivery. Very pre-term delivery is associated with mortality but also a higher handicap rate in survivors. Recent attention is focusing on the relationship between not only maternal infection and pre-term delivery, but also the relationship between infection and cerebral palsy in preterm survivors (Dammann and Leviton 1997). Some drug users may be at higher risk of sexually transmitted and other vaginal infections. The opportunity should be taken to screen for *Chlamydia*, gonorrhoea and also bacterial vaginosis. With all of these organisms, treatment should be followed by retest and, if necessary, repeat treatment. Group B *Streptococcus* is different in that treatment does not affect carriage rate in the long term. However, this is important information to have for treatment around labour.

Ultrasound

Ultrasound in early pregnancy is important partly to confirm gestational age, but also may provide a positive experience for the woman. In addition, women often worry more about fetal abnormality than any other problem, and feel guilt about the risk that they may have damaged the baby in early pregnancy by their drug use. In general terms, it is usually possible to be quite reassuring. However, all women should be offered fetal anomaly scanning at 18–20 weeks to exclude abnormality, with the usual explanation of implications and what is involved. This also provides a positive experience hospital and may be helpful in building a constructive relation

Pregnancy management

Pregnancy complications occur in drug using women, but not much more frequently than other women in the population. An exception to this generalization may be women using large amounts of cocaine.

Once a satisfactory relationship has been built up, it is important that there is an up-front understanding of limits, and that the principle of easy communication is established, so that when things on either side are beginning to go wrong they can be discussed and confrontation avoided. She needs to understand the hospital priority for a happy pregnancy experience for all. This does mean absolute intolerance of illicit drug use or selling in the hospital, clear limits on the number and conduct of visitors, and zero tolerance for threats of violence and abusive or threatening language. If necessary, visitors will be removed from the building and barred from returning.

It is important at an early stage to discuss neonatal abstinence syndrome. The mother should be warned that it may occur, that her dose is not a reliable predictor, that it can present after several days and can last for weeks. She needs also to know that NAS is usually easily manageable. The baby needs her support, understanding and patience. The evidence is that if properly looked after, the baby will come to no short-term developmental harm.

If the woman has to be admitted antenatally, she should have her drugs prescribed in hospital. It is best for hospital staff to check the dose of medication from the usual prescriber for all women on admission. This is safer and less confrontational since the woman regards it as routine and not something done because she is not trusted or is suspected of lying. It is important to identify the source of outside or community prescribed drugs and to notify the practitioner or prescriber that this is not necessary during the period of hospital admission.

If this is not done, the drugs may be picked up for her and sold on the street. Explanation that this is the hospital rule will always be accepted as reasonable, providing that the system for ensuring that dispensing restarts on her discharge works with the same efficiency!

There may be problems defaulting from appointments. This may mean that the antenatal visit was not a priority at that particular time but it might mean that she doesn't like the atmosphere provided and that she doesn't feel the care is geared for her. This may be helped by not giving early appointments, by the receptionists ensuring that the woman has correctly noted the appointment time, by showing some flexibility and by treating the patient with courtesy and consideration.

Repeated non-sterile injection over years destroys peripheral veins, often leaving track marks (thrombosed, fibrosed veins). Venous access may be very limited, even in women who stopped injecting years before. Usually, a small amount of blood can be obtained peripherally by taking time, asking her advice about likely sites and using the smallest needle or butterfly. Occasionally, external jugular veins have to be used.

Intrauterine growth restriction is more likely, and care should be taken to assess fetal growth carefully by clinical examination, with ultrasound if necessary and with ready recourse to antenatal fetal monitoring if required.

Antenatal fetal monitoring may sometimes be necessary. It is often difficult for drug using women to come up to a central hospital to a fetal monitoring programme and this should be started only when strictly necessary. Cardiotocography is commonly non-reactive, particularly in the first few hours after opiates, but baseline variability usually still occurs. Biophysical profile is less affected and will usually be normal even after drug ingestion. But again, fetal activity may be greatly reduced and often repeat or extended monitoring is required. Care and experience are important in interpreting biophysical monitoring. There is a risk of intervening unnecessarily because of drug induced fetal responses but also a risk of falsely attributing genuine fetal compromise to drug intake. As a general rule, effects are maximal in the first few hours after drug use, and are worse if a new drug or an excessive dosage has been taken. Drug use reduces fetal activity (and hence fetal heart rate accelerations) but will not cause oligohydramnios or fetal heart rate decelerations. Doppler studies seem unaffected and, as the concern is usually with intrauterine growth restriction and possible utero-placental problems, umbilical artery Doppler waveform should give fairly long-term prediction.

Occasionally, there may be concern about the ability of the woman to look after her child. This happens if previous children are in care, or there is a history of previous child abuse, or if she has a chaotic lifestyle, a partner with a chaotic lifestyle, or if she is socially isolated with no support network. Case discussions are important at an early stage to involve all interested parties, to forestall emergency meetings and crisis confrontation later. And equally, if there is no concern, it may be important to emphasize how the system works to the woman. It ensures that women are getting the help they need and is a framework for deciding whether a formal case conference is necessary. Many women worry that their baby may be taken away into care purely because they use drugs. This, of course, should not be true. They are very likely not to share their worries with healthcare workers and, for this reason, raising the issue only to dismiss it in a reassuring way can be important. Social work assessment involves judgement about the safety of the child. This is not directly linked to maternal drug use though chaotic drug use may affect safety, and is always a factor to be considered.

Management of labour

Women using drugs are often particularly frightened about labour, and worried they will not get adequate pain relief. Ideally, a relationship with the midwives involved in delivery will have been built up during pregnancy, and she will have seen round the labour ward.

Labour is often quite short, with women delaying coming into hospital, either because of fear or because they think they might be withdrawing or because of difficulty with transport. The babies are often not large.

Many women do still have fears that their needs will not be recognized or met, and that they will experience antagonism during their care. It is very important that the midwife makes a particular effort to be reassuring and supportive, and careful explanation at all times is appreciated.

It is very important that adequate pain relief is given. This can be with opiates although much more frequent injections are likely to be needed. Because of the high fear about pain which many drug users have, epidural anaesthesia may be very useful. Basal substitution treatment should continue. Substitution treatment with methadone does not, of course, cover pain relief. On the other hand, pethidine is not a satisfactory opiate substitute since cross-dependence is incomplete. Venous access may be limited as discussed above. Where labour is straightforward, no intravenous line is needed. However, if it does seem as if there may be complications, it is sometimes better to set up an intravenous line electively using an external jugular vein if necessary, soon after admission, rather than be faced with the task in an emergency situation.

Naloxone should not be used to reverse opioid induced respiratory depression in the new-born because of the risk of precipitating an acute opiate withdrawal crisis.

Meconium staining is common. Some babies will be growth-restricted. There must therefore be careful surveillance during labour. This should follow local hospital obstetric and neonatal guidelines for meconium staining. In a few cases, this will be a manifestation of fetal compromise but the large majority of labours and deliveries will be straightforward.

Postnatal care

Because of increased metabolism of some drugs in late pregnancy and because of the increased distribution space, plasma concentrations in late pregnancy fall. These changes correct rapidly after delivery and a woman taking the same amount of drug will, in effect, be increasing her biologically active dose. Because these changes are under-researched, and different for different drugs, it is difficult to provide guidelines for any routine changes to drug prescription. However, it is important that the woman herself understands this mechanism. If she is over-sedated, she may not be able to care for the baby properly. Reduction in dose is therefore often appropriate at this time, but has to be guided by maternal state rather than any fixed percentage rule.

The above physiological postpartum changes are one reason why over-sedation might occur. But the patient may have taken extra or different drugs, either because friends bring new drugs as a present to celebrate the birth, or to help cope with the many stresses of this time, or because she feels so 'shattered', having slept poorly. This may be a risk for childcare and episodes of loss of consciousness (described locally as 'gouching') could result in the baby falling or having other accidental injury. A small amount of damage limitation can be done by emphasizing that the woman should use a mat on the floor for feeding and changing rather than risk the baby falling off a high surface, that someone should be with her when she baths the baby, and that there are shields for fires and stoves. Ultimately however, there has to be some arrangement that the child has 'good enough' mothering 24 hours a day, and community staff need to ensure that such a strategy is satisfactorily in place.

The advice from most reviews is that women should not breast feed unless they are taking less than 20 mg of methadone daily. This is based on a US report (Committee on Drugs, 1989). However, this recommendation does not seem to be based on any good evidence. Limited local experience has not shown important short-term risk to the baby in women taking higher doses. One study in a group of women taking an average of 52 mg of methadone daily showed that breast feeding babies were exposed to a daily intake of about 0.04 mg/kg in a 3 kg infant (Blinick et al. 1975). This is a small dose. The balance is therefore between the known benefits of breast feeding against uncertain risks. My own opinion, in the light of current information and local experience, is that drug using women who are HIV negative should usually be actively encouraged to breast feed with careful surveillance of the baby. Having said this, this tends to be a population whose use of breast feeding is extremely low.

Neonatal abstinence syndrome is common (Finnegan 1985, 1986). A score is very helpful for all concerned, including the woman herself. It is also helpful if this has been explained carefully during the pregnancy. The NAS score is, of course, only one aspect of assessment and should be interpreted in the context of the individual woman's childcare skills since these vary considerably. This score is also geared for term infants, and some symptoms do not have the same severity significance in preterm babies. Several scores are described. We use a modified Finnegan score (Table 12.2). Infants are scored at 2 hours of age and then 4-hourly until 5 days of age or until symptoms abate. A score of greater than 8 merits 2-hourly scoring. All symptoms occurring with the 2–4 hour period are scored, so that the score represents the entire period, not just a single point in time. The score has a high inter-observer reliability and results in fewer infants being treated than if clinical judgement alone is used.

The onset of symptoms usually occurs within the first 24–72 hours after birth (Shaw and McIvor 1994). Timing is partly dependent on half-life of drug, e.g. methadone withdrawal tends to be later than heroin withdrawal. The acute symptoms may persist for several weeks. Seizures can occur up to 30 days later and the mean age of onset is 10 days (Finnegan, 1979).

The basis of management of NAS is to avoid additional stressors. The baby should be nursed in a quiet, soothing environment, with dim lighting, and given small feeds frequently. Pharmacologic therapy is recommended for Finnegan abstinence scores greater than 8 for an average of three scores, or for two scores greater than 12. The logical, and physiologically appropriate drug for opioid withdrawal seems to be methadone, but there are potential problems in discharging the infant of opiate abusing parents home on this drug. Our current neonatal practice is to use chlorpromazine (loading dose 3 mg/kg, maintenance 0.3–0.75 mg/kg, 4–6 hourly).

Admission to the neonatal unit should be considered if there is a Finnegan score greater than 11 or there are clear clinical indications (convulsions, marked tremors, significant respiratory distress, poor feeding with dehydration or vomiting).

This is one of the most important times for good communication and a 'seamless' transition from hospital to community care is vital. Community staff should be involved in management in hospital, and be party to decisions about discharge home. All basic arrangements, including contraceptive plans, should be in place.

Table 12.2 Neonatal Abstinence Score

Date of birth .... Name .... Time of birth							
Record 4 hourly		1	2	3	4	5	6
Date .... Time							
Sings and symptoms	Score						
Cry: high pitched:							
intermittent	2						
or continuous	3						
Sleeps after feeds for:							
< 1 hour	3						
< 2 hours	2						
< 3 hours	1						
Tremor:							
mild, when disturbed	1						
marked, when disturbed	2						
mild, when undisturbed	3						
marked, when undisturbed	4						
Increased muscle tone	2						
Generalized convulsion	5						
Frantic fist-sucking	1						
Poor feeding	2						
Regurgitation	2						
Diarrhoea	2						
Dehydration	2						
Frequent yawning	1						
Sneezing	1						
Nasal stuffiness	1						
Sweating	1						
Mottling	1						
Temperature:							
.... < 37.5°C	1						
.... < 37.5°C	2						
Repiratory rate:							
.... > 60/min	1						
> 60/min indrawing	2						
Excoriation:							
.... nose	1						
.... nose and knees	2						
.... nose, knees and toes	3						
Total score							
Signature							

Note:
If score > 8, call paediatrician and record 2 hourly.
If sore > 11, consider admission to NNU.
Modified from Finnegan (1979).

Conclusion

The principles of management of the pregnant drug user are not much different from any other problem in pregnancy. The needs and issues may just be more obvious. There is a requirement for accurate information, clear communication, mutual respect, support and a partnership of care. For most users, pregnancy is not a very high risk for mother or baby, and most pregnancies will be straightforward. Greater problems may surround the long-term background risks for mother and child. Pregnancy is a short interlude in the life of a drug user, but an important one. Most drug users have the same aspirations for family life as other women and may cope extremely well.

References

Abel, E.L., Sokol, R.J. 1986: Foetal alcohol syndrome is now leading cause of mental retardation. (Editorial). *Lancet* **i**, 222.

Abel, E.L. 1996: 'Moderate' drinking during pregnancy: Cause for concern? *Clinica Chimica Acta* **246**, 149–54.

Altshuler, L.L., Szuba, M.P. 1994: Course of psychiatric disorders in pregnancy: Dilemmas in pharmacologic management. *Neurologic Clinics* **12**, 613–35.

Ashworth, M., Gerada, C. 1997: Addiction and dependence II Alcohol. *British Medical Journal* **315**, 358–60.

Bevan, R., Kenney, A. 1996: Smoking and women's health. *The Diplomate* **3**, 274–9.

Bingol, N., Fuchs, M., Diaz, V., Stone, R.K., Gromisch, D.S. 1987: Teratogenicity of cocaine in humans. *Journal of Pediatrics* **110**, 93–6.

Blinick, G., Inturissi, C.E., Jerez, E., Wallach, R.C. 1975: Methadone assays in pregnant women and their progeny. *American Journal of Obstetrics and Gynecology* **121**, 617–21.

Buchi, K.F. 1996: Maternal substance use: A review of its prevalence in the United States. *Ambulatory Child Health* **2**, 59–68.

Chasnoff, I.J., Landress, H.J., Barrett, M.E. 1990: The prevalence of illicit-drug or alcohol use during pregnancy and discrepancies in mandatory reporting in Pinellas County, Florida. *New England Journal of Medicine* **322**, 1202–206.

Chaukin, W., Kandall, S.R. 1990: Between a 'rock' and a hard place: perinatal drug abuse. *Pediatrics* **85**, 223–5.

Cohen, M.S., Rudolph, A.M., Melmon, K.L. 1980: Antagonism of morphine by naloxone in pregnant ewes and foetal lambs. *Developmental Pharmacology and Therapeutics* **1**, 58–69.

Committee on Drugs, American Academy of Pediatrics 1989: Transfer of drugs and other chemicals into human milk. *Pediatrics* **84**, 924–36.

Cregler, L.L., Mark, H. 1986: Medical complications of cocaine abuse. *New England Journal of Medicine* **315**, 1495–500.

Czeizel, A. 1988: Lack of teratogenicity of benzodiazepine drugs in Hungary. *Reproductive Toxicology* **1**, 183.

Dahl, R.E., Scher, M.S., Williamson, D.E., Robles, N., Day, N. 1995: A longitudinal study of prenatal marijuana use: Effects on sleep and arousal at age 3 years. *Archives of Pediatrics and Adolescent Medicine* **149**, 145–50.

Dammann, O., Leviton, A. 1997: Maternal intrauterine infections, cytokines and brain damage in the preterm newborn. *Pediatric Research* **42**, 1–8.

Day, N.L., Richardson, G.A., Goldschmidt, L., Robles, N., Taylor, P.M., Stoffer, D.S., Cornelius, M.D., Geva, D. 1994: Effect of prenatal marijuana exposure on the cognitive development of offspring at age three. *Neurotoxicology and Teratology* **16**, 169–75.

Doberczak, T.M., Kandall, S.R., Friedmann, P. 1993: Relationships between maternal methadone dosage, maternal-neonatal methadone levels, and neonatal withdrawal. *Obstetrics and Gynecology* **81**, 936–40.

DolanMullen, P., Ramirez, G., Groff, J.Y. 1994: A meta-analysis of randomized trials of prenatal smoking cessation interventions. *American Journal of Obstetrics and Gynecology* **171**, 1328–34.

Drews, C.D., Murphy, C.C., Yeargin-Allsopp, M., Decoufle, P. 1996: The relationship between idiopathic mental retardation and maternal smoking during pregnancy. *Pediatrics* **97**, 547–53.

Dunn, D.T., Newell, M.N., Ades, A.E., Peckham, C.S. 1992: Risk of human immunodeficiency virus type 1 transmission through breast feeding. *Lancet* **340**, 585–8.

Ellard, G.A., Johnstone, F.D., Prescott, R.J., Ji-Xian, W., Jian-Hua, M. 1996: Smoking during pregnancy: the dose dependence of birthweight deficits. *British Journal of Obstetrics and Gynaecology* **103**, 806–13.

Ellwood, D.A., O'Connor, M.C. 1989: Maternal narcotic addiction. In: Studd, J. (ed.) *Progress in obstetrics and gynaecology.* Churchill Livingstone, Edinburgh, pp. 91–102.

Eriksson, M., Larsson, G., Zetterstrom, R. 1981: Amphetamine addiction and pregnancy. *Acta Obstetricia et Gynecologica Scandinavica* **60**, 253–9.

Esmail, A., Meyer, L., Pottier, A., Wright, S. 1993: Deaths from volatile substance abuse in those under 18 years: Results from a national epidemiological study. *Archives of Disease in Childhood* **69**, 356–60.

European Collaborative Study 1994: Caesarean section and risk of vertical transmission of HIV-1 infection. *Lancet* **343**, 1464–7.

Evans, A.T., Gillogley, K. 1991: Drug use in pregnancy: Obstetric perspectives. *Clinics in Perinatology* **18**, 23–32.

Farkas, A.G., Colbert, D.L., Erskine, K.J. 1995: Anonymous testing for drug abuse in an antenatal population. *British Journal of Obstetrics and Gynaecology* **102**, 563–5.

Farrell, M., Ward, J., Mattick, R., Hall, W., Stimson, G.V., Des Jarlais, D., Gossop, M., Strang, J. 1994: Methadone maintenance treatment in opiate dependence: A review. *British Medical Journal* **309**, 997–1001.

Finnegan, L.P. 1979: Pathophysiological and behavioural effects of the transplacental transfer of narcotic drugs to the foetuses and neonates of narcotic-dependent mothers. *Bulletin Narcotics* 1–58.

Finnegan, L.P. 1985: Effects of maternal opiate abuse on the newborn. *Federal Proceedings* **44**, 2314–17.

Finnegan, L.P. 1986: Neonatal abstinence syndrome: assessment and pharmacotherapy. In: Rubaltelli, F.F., Granati, B. (eds). *Neonatal therapy: an update*. Elsevier, Amsterdam, pp. 122–47.

Finnegan, L.P., Kandall, S.R. 1997: Maternal and neonatal effects of alcohol and drugs. In: Lowinson, J.H. *et al.* (eds). *Substance abuse: a comprehensive textbook*. Willams and Wilkins, Baltimore, pp. 513–34.

Forman, R., Klein, J., Barks, J., Mehta, D., Greenwald, M., Einarson, T., Koren, G. 1994: Prevalence of foetal exposure to cocaine in Toronto, 1990–1991. *Clinical and Investigative Medicine* **17**, 206–11.

Fredricsson, B., Gilljam, H. 1992: Smoking and reproduction: Short and long term effects and benefits of smoking cessation. *Acta Obstetricia et Gynecologica Scandinavica* **71**, 580–92.

Fried, P.A. 1989: Cigarettes and marijuana: Are there measurable long-term neurobehavioural effects? *Neurotoxicology* **10**, 577–84.

Fried, P.A. 1991: Marijuana use during pregnancy: Consequences for the offspring. *Seminars in Perinatology* **15**, 280–87.

Fried, P.A., Watkinson, B., Siegel, I.S. 1997: Reading and language in 9–12 year-olds prenatally exposed to cigarettes and marijuana. *Neurotoxicology and Teratology* **19**, 171–83.

Gillogley, K.M., Evans, A.T., Hansen, R.L., Samuels, S.J., Batra, K.K. 1990: The perinatal impact of cocaine, amphetamine, and opiate use detected by universal intrapartum screening. *American Journal of Obstetrics and Gynecology* **163**, 1535–42.

Goldschmidt, L., Richardson, G.A., Stoffer, D.S., Geva, D., Day, N.L. 1996: Prenatal alcohol exposure and academic achievement at age six: A non-linear fit. *Alcoholism: Clinical and Experimental Research* **20**, 763–70.

Hall, W., Solowij, N., Lemon, J. 1994: The health and psychological consequences of cannabis use. In: *Monograph Series No 25. National Drug Strategy*. Australian Government Publishing Service, Canberra, pp. 77–91.

Hartmann, K.E., Thorp, J.M., Pahel Short, L., Koch, M.A. 1996: A randomized trial of smoking cessation intervention in pregnancy in an academic clinic. *American Journal of Obstetrics and Gynecology* **87**, 621–6.

Holzman, C., Paneth, N. 1994: Maternal cocaine use during pregnancy and perinatal outcomes. *Epidemiologic Reviews* **16**, 315–34.

Johnstone, F.D. 1990: Drug abuse in pregnancy. *Contemporary Review in Obstetrics and Gynaecology* **2**, 96–103.

Johnstone, F.D. 1994: Drug addiction and obstetric practice. In: Bewley, S., Ward, H. (eds). *Ethics in Obstetrics and Gynaecology*. RCOG Press, London, pp. 237–49.

Johnstone, F.D., Raab, G.M., Hamilton, B.A. 1996: The effect of human immunodeficiency virus infection and drug use on birth characteristics. *Obstetrics and Gynecology* **88**, 321–6.

Jones, H.E., Kunko, P.M, Robinson, S.E., Balster, R.L. 1996: Developmental consequences of intermittent and continuous prenatal exposure to 1,1,1-trichloroethane in mice. *Pharmacology Biochemistry and Behaviour* **55**, 635–46.

Kaltenbach, K., Finnegan, L.P. 1984: Developmental outcome of children born to methadone maintained women – A review of longitudinal studies. *Neurobehavioural Toxicology and Teratology* **6**, 271–5.

Kaltenbach, K., Finnegan, L.P. 1987: Perinatal and developmental outcome of infants exposed to methadone *in utero*. *Neurotoxicology and Teratology* **9**, 311–13.

Kaltenbach, K., Finnegan, L.P. 1988: The influence of the neonatal abstinence syndrome on mother-infant interaction. In: Anthony, E.J., Chiland, C. (eds). *The Child in this Family: Perilous Development: Child Raising and Identify Formation under Stress*. Wiley-Interscience, Chichester, pp. 223–30.

Kandall, S.R., Gaines, J., Habel, L., Davidson, G., Jessop, D. 1993: Relationship of maternal substance abuse to subsequent sudden infant death syndrome in offspring. *Journal of Pediatrics* **123**, 120–26.

Kendrick, J.S., Merritt, R.K. 1996: Women and smoking: an update for the 1990s. *American Journal of Obstetrics and Gynecology* **175**, 528–35.

Kline, J., Levin, B., Kinney, A., Stein, Z., Susser, M., Warburton, D. 1995: Cigarette smoking and spontaneous abortion of known karyotype: Precise data but uncertain inferences. *American Journal of Epidemiology* **5**, 417–27.

Konovalov, H.V., Kovetsky, N.S., Bobryshev, Y.V., Ashwell, K.W.S. 1997: Disorders of brain development in the progeny of mothers who used alcohol during pregnancy. *Early Human Development* **48**, 153–66.

Koren, G., Shear, H., Graham, K., Einarson, T. 1989: Bias against the null hypothesis: The reproductive hazards of cocaine. *Lancet* **ii**, 1440–42.

Laegreid, L. 1990: Clinical observations in children after prenatal benzodiazepine exposure. *Developmental Pharmacology and Therapeutics* **15**, 186–8.

Laegreid, L., Conradi, N., Hagberg, G., Hedner, T. 1992a: Psychotropic drug use in pregnancy and perinatal death. *Acta Obstetricia et Gynecologica Scandinavica* **71**, 451–7.

Laegreid, L., Hagberg, G., Lundberg, A. 1992b: Neurodevelopment in late infancy after prenatal exposure to benzodiazepines – a prospective study. *Neuropediatrics* **23**, 60–67.

Langa, A. 1993: Volatile substance abuse: A brief report. *British Journal of Clinical Practice* **47**, 94–6.

Linn, S., Schoenbaum, S.C, Monson, R., Rosner, R., Stubblefield, P.C., Ryan, K.J. 1983: The association of marijuana use with outcome of pregnancy. *American Journal of Public Health* **73**, 1161–4.

MMWR 1990: Statewide prevalence of illicit drug use by pregnant women – Rhode Island. *MMWR* **39**.

Mack, G., Thomas, D., Giles, W., Buchanan, N. 1991: Methadone levels and neonatal withdrawal. *Journal of Paediatrics and Child Health* **27**, 96–100.

Malpas, T.J., Darlow, B.A., Lennox, R., Horwood, L.J. 1995: Maternal methadone dosage and neonatal withdrawal. *Australian and New Zealand Journal of Obstetrics and Gynaecology* **35**, 175–7.

Marzuk, P.M., Tardiff, K., Leon, A.C., Hirsch, C.S., Stajic, M., Portera, L., Hartwell, N. 1995: Fatal injuries after cocaine use as a leading cause of death among young adults in New York City. *New England Journal of Medicine* **332**, 1753–7.

Marzuk, P.M., Tardiff, K., Leon, A.C., Hirsch, C.S., Stajic, M., Portera, L., Hartwell, N. 1997: Poverty and fatal accidental drug overdoses of cocaine and opiates in New York City: An ecological study. *American Journal of Drug and Alcohol Abuse* **23**, 221–8.

Mattick, R.P., Hall, W. 1996: Are detoxification programmes effective? *Lancet* **347**, 97–100.

Medrano, M.A. 1996: Does a discrete foetal solvent syndrome exist? *Alcoholism Treatment Quarterly* **14**, 59–76.

Mendelson, J.H., Mello, N.K. 1996: Management of cocaine abuse and dependence . *New England Journal of Medicine* **334**, 965–72.

Morris, P., Binienda, Z., Gillam, M.P., Klein, J., McMartin, K., Koren, G., Duhart, H.M., Slikker, W.Jr., Paule, M.G. 1997: The effect of chronic cocaine exposure throughout pregnancy on maternal and infant outcomes in the rhesus monkey. *Neurotoxicology and Teratology* **19**, 47–57.

Morrison, C.L. 1995: The medical problems of illicit drug misuse in pregnancy and harm minimization. In: Siney, C. (ed.) *The pregnant drug addict*. Books for Midwives, pp. 15–23.

Neerhof, M.G., Macgregor, S.N., Retzky, S.S., Sullivan, T.P. 1989: Cocaine abuse during pregnancy: Peripartum prevalence and perinatal outcome. *American Journal of Obstetrics and Gynecology* **161**, 633–8.

Noble, A., Vega, W.A., Kolody, B., Porter, P., Hwang, J., Merk II, G.A., Bole, A. 1997: Prenatal substance abuse in California: Findings from the perinatal substance exposure study. *Journal of Psychoactive Drugs* **29**, 43–53.

Nulman, I., Rovet, J., Altmann, D., Bradley, C., Einarson, T., Koren, G. 1994: Neurodevelopment of adopted children exposed *in utero* to cocaine. *Canadian Medical Association Journal* **151**, 1591–7.

O'Campo, P., Davis, M.V., Gielen, A.C. 1995: Smoking cessation interventions for pregnant women: Review and future directions. *Seminars in Perinatology* **4**, 279–85.

Okacha, C.I. 1995: Treating the patient with benzodiazepine addictions. *Hospital Update*, 396–401.

Ostrea, E.M., Ostrea, A.R., Simpson, P.M. 1997: Mortality within the first 2 years in infants exposed to cocaine, opiate or cannaboid during gestation. *Pediatrics* **100**, 79–83.

Oulellette, E.M., Rosett, H.L., Rosman, N.P., Weiner, L. 1977: Adverse effects in offspring of maternal alcohol abuse during pregnancy. *New England Journal of Medicine* **297**, 528–30.

Passaro, K.T., Little, R.E., Savitz, D.A., Noss, J. 1996: The effect of maternal drinking before conception and in early pregnancy on infant birthweight. *Epidemiology* **7**, 377–83.

Pastuszak, A., Milich, V., Chan, S., Chu, J., Koren, G. 1996: Prospective assessment of pregnancy outcome following first trimester exposure to benzodiazepines. *Canadian Journal of Clinical Pharmacology* **3**, 167–71.

Pegues, D.A., Engelgau, M.M., Woernle, C.H. 1994: Prevalence of illicit drugs detected in the urine of women of childbearing age in Alabama public health clinics. *Public Health Reports* **109**, 530–38.

Pietrantoni, M., Knuppel, R.A. 1991: Alcohol use in pregnancy. *Clinics in Perinatology* **18**, 93–111.

Richardson, G.A., Day, N.L., Goldschmidt, L. 1995: Prenatal alcohol, marijuana, and tobacco use: Infant mental and motor development. *Neurotoxicology and Teratology* **17**, 479–87.

Richardson, G.A., Conroy, M.L., Day, N.L. 1996: Prenatal cocaine exposure: Effects on the development of school-age children. *Neurotoxicology and Teratology* **18**, 627–34.

Robertson, J.R., Ronald, P.J.M., Raab, G.M., Ross, A.J., Parpia, T. 1994: Deaths, HIV infection, abstinence, and other outcomes in a cohort of injecting drug users followed up for 10 years. *British Medical Journal* **309**, 369–72.

Schuckit, M.A. 1997: Substance use disorders. *British Medical Journal* **314**, 1605–608.

Seivewright, N.A., Greenwood, J. 1996: What is important in drug misuse treatment? *Lancet* **347**, 373–6.

Sell, L., Finch, E., Farrell, M., Strang, J. 1996: Addictions. *British Journal of Hospital Medicine* **56**, 136–40.

Shaw, N.J., Mcivor, L. 1994: Neonatal abstinence syndrome after maternal methadone treatment. *Archives of Disease in Childhood* **71**, F203–F205.

Sperling, R.S., Shapiro, D.E., Coombs, R.W., Todd, J.A., Herman, S.A., McSherry, G.D., O'Sullivan, M.J., Van Dyke, R.B., Jimemez, E., Rouzioux, C., Flynn, P.M., Sullivan, J.L. 1996: Maternal viral load, zidovudine treatment and the risk of human immunodeficiency virus type 1 from mother to infant for the Paediatric AIDS Clinical Trials Group Protocol 076 Study Group. *New England Journal of Medicine* **335**, 1621–9.

Stewart, D.E., Streiner, D.L. 1995: Cigarette smoking during pregnancy. *Canadian Journal of Psychiatry* **40**, 603–607.

Tardiff, K., Marzuk, P.M., Leon, A.C., Portera, L., Hartwell, N., Hirsch, C.S., Stajic, M. 1996: Accidental fatal drug overdoses in New York City: 1990–1992. *American Journal of Drug and Alcohol Abuse* **22**, 135–46.

Tenenbein, M., Casiro, O.G., Seshia, M.M.K., Debooy, V.D. 1996: Neonatal withdrawal from maternal volatile substance abuse. *Archives of Disease in Childhood* **74**, F204–F207.

Wakschlag, L.S., Lahey, B.B., Loeber, R., Green, S.M., Gordon, R.A., Leventhal, B.L. 1997: Maternal smoking during pregnancy and the risk of conduct disorder in boys. *Archives of General Psychiatry* **54**, 670–76.

Walsh, R.A., Redman, S., Brinsmead, M.W., Byrne, J.M., Melmeth, A. 1997: A smoking cessation programme at a public antenatal clinic. *American Journal of Public Health* **87**, 1201–204.

Windham, G.C., Fenster, L., Hopkins, B., Swan, S.H. 1995: The association of moderate maternal and paternal alcohol consumption with birthweight and gestational age. *Epidemiology* **6**, 591–7.

Wong, P.P.L., Bauman, A. 1997: How well does epidemiological evidence hold for the relationship between smoking and adverse obstetric outcomes in New South Wales? *Australian and New Zealand Journal of Obstetrics and Gynaecology* **37**, 168–73.

Woodburn, K.R., Murie, J.A. 1996: Vascular complications of injecting drug misuse. *British Journal of Surgery* **83**, 1329–34.

Woods, J.R., Jr. 1996: Adverse consequences of prenatal illicit drug exposure. *Current Opinion in Obstetrics and Gynecology* **8**, 403–11.

Zaren, B., Cnattingius, S., Lindmark, G. 1997: Foetal growth impairment from smoking – is it influenced by maternal anthropometry? *Acta Obstetricia et Gynecologica Scandinavica* **76**, 30–33.

Zuckerman, B., Frank, D.A., Hingson, R., Amaro, H., Levenson, S.M., Kayne, H., Parker, S., Vinci, R., Aboagye, K., Fried, L.E., Cabral, H., Timperi, R., Bauchner, H. 1989: Effects of maternal marijuana and cocaine use on foetal growth. *New England Journal of Medicine* **320**, 762–8.

Zuspan, F.P., Gumpel, J.A., Mejia-zelaya, A., Madden, J., Davis, R. 1975: Foetal stress from methadone withdrawal. *American Journal of Obstetrics and Gynecology* **122**, 43–6.

13 Shared care

Claire Gerada and Michael Farrell

Introduction

Within the United Kingdom (UK) and most of Europe all indications are that the rate of rise of illicit drug use shows no abatement. Until its recent abolition, the number of users notified to the Home Office Addicts Index in the UK had steadily increased. Women and people under 21 years old show the largest increase in notifications. Similar high levels of drug use were found in a UK population survey of psychiatric morbidity (Meltzer *et al.* 1995) where an overall rate of alcohol and drug dependence of 4.7% and 2.2% respectively was elicited. Men were three times more likely than women to be alcohol dependent, and twice as likely to be drug dependent. Alcohol and drug-dependence was especially prevalent in young men aged between 16 and 24 years, with a yearly prevalence for drug dependence of 111/1000 being found. Other indicators of drug use include drug-related deaths, drug-related offences and numbers of prisoners serving sentences for drug-related crimes. All these continue to rise. Despite this rise there has been considerable success in containing rates of infection amongst injecting drug users in the UK, although in many developing countries this is different (Des Jarlais *et al.* 1997). Co-incidental with increasing numbers of drug users, access to specialist drug services has become more difficult with long waiting times for first appointment This has necessitated the continued need to find new avenues of care for these patients. General Practitioners (GPs) and the primary healthcare team (PHCT) are being encouraged to include the care of drug users as part of their every day remit, with shared care the vehicle for this. Policy makers argue that GPs are best placed to see and care for drug users early on in their drug using careers. From a cautious start primary care services have responded to the challenge of treating this frequently disenfranchised group of patients. The chapter will review shared care as it currently stands in the UK and how to best involve GPs in the care of drug using patients.

Definition of primary care

Primary care implies a readily available service, accessed by self-referral and provided in a community or home setting. It involves first contact care, which can be delivered by a variety of professionals such as a doctor, nurse, probation officer or community pharmacist. Many countries have developed primary care although there are national differences in the structure and organization of general practice. These variations include the mode of payment of GPs, the gate-keeper function of general practice, and its relationship to secondary specialist services and practice characteristics such as work load, length of consultation and access to investigations. Where primary care is developed, such as in the Netherlands, Denmark, UK and members of the Commonwealth like Canada, Australia and New Zealand, the GP forms the core and focal point of primary healthcare. He or she is the point of first contact for most patients (including drug users) and provides generalist and, increasingly, specialist care. In these countries the GP provides general medical care to a relatively stable list of patients united in households, composed of both sexes, and of all age categories. Primary care, however it is delivered, should have four attributes: longitudinality (person focused care over

Table 13.1   What do we mean by primary care?

- It is first contact care
- It s readily accessible by self referral
- It is provided in a home or community setting
- It is led by professionals who have trained for a generalist role
- It is continuing and personal and the fixed point for referrals to secondary care
- It is capable of providing acute care, high technology' care and specialist care according to the training needs of the individual/s

(Adapted from *Primary Care development. Future options for General Practice* (Meads, 1996)).

time); comprehensiveness; coordination of care for patients requiring secondary specialist services and accessibility for first contact care. The concept of 'primary care for all' is an international one seen as fundamental by the WHO (Horder 1983).

Primary care involvement in the UK – a brief history

The 1960s and 1970s

In the 1960s the growth of opiate addiction in the UK was in part attributed to over-liberal prescribing by a handful of doctors (Stimson and Oppenheimer 1982) many of whom were involved in private practice. Specialist clinics (drug dependency units), run by consultant psychiatrists, were established for the treatment of opiate dependency. These together with attached in-patient facilities were the mainstay of treatment of drug addiction in the 1970s. The role of the GP was largely ignored (Edwards 1981). The number of drug users continued to rise and surged in the late 1970s. Waiting times for treatment of several weeks or months was not uncommon. The delay between seeking and receiving help was a significant obstacle to engaging in treatment (ISDD 1988). It became apparent that to reach a greater number of users and to successfully engage them in treatment a different approach to the traditional outpatient/inpatient one needed to be found (Department of Health and Social Security 1985).

The 1980s and 1990s

Throughout the 1980s GPs had been encouraged to help and treat patients with drug related problems (ACMD 1982, 1988, 1989), particularly as a means of reducing the then burgeoning HIV and AIDS problem. However few GPs were willing or able to offer their services other than (at best) providing general medical services. The 1980s saw the rise of community drug teams (CDTs) as the vehicle for specialist services to deliver community treatment to drug users. Though some CDTs employed a GP as part of the team there was little extension into mainstream general practice; in many cases the workers and the attached GP took over the primary care function for drug users. Parallel with this was the expansion of the primary care 'liaison' role of the voluntary street agencies. A common practice was for the agency to act as the advocate for the patient, attempt to find them a GP who would prescribe substitute medication and then to provide the GP with the primary care support necessary to do this.

With regard to primary care, both models had problems. The former did not transfer skills to GPs, and left them isolated and ignorant of the care that their patients may be receiving from an outside source. This model reinforced the status quo, not encouraging GP involvement, instead continuing the expert–generalist split. Patients were not encouraged to register with a GP leaving this vulnerable group without proper access to primary care services. Patients were encouraged to access the specialist service directly by-passing the normal primary care referral system. Community drug teams failed therefore to effect liaison between primary and second-ary care and this instead resulted in poor collaboration with GPs (Strang *et al.* 1992). With the later model 'street agency' involvement, the GP was left vulnerable to over enthusiastic referrals. As a doctor was seen to be sympathetic to the needs of drug users and took them on for care, so the practice became overwhelmed with referrals. The GP was frequently unaware that the staff recommending dosage regimes did not have a medical or nursing qualification that entitled them to do so. Injudicious prescribing was sometimes advised, such as high doses of methadone linctus, injectable prescribing or con-comitant benzodiazepines. Naively the GP felt comfortable that he or she was being advised by an 'expert' and prescribed accordingly.

Both these models propagated the continuance of negative atti-tudes. GPs that did become involved quickly became overwhelmed and disillusioned and the rest were able to remain prejudiced and ignorant. This uneven distribution of care contributed to the rise of the 'maverick' GP, that is a doctor prescribing large amounts of substitute medication but without adequate time, training or support to monitor patients who were abusing their treatment regimen.

During this time many practices were overwhelmed with drug users asking for help. This was especially problematic in areas of high prevalence of drug use. For example in one London Health authority, with five times the national average for Home Office notifications, 5%

Table 13.2 Barriers to GP involvement

- Difficulty in establishing rapport, fears of being taken advantage of and deceit
- Negative attitudes to drug users (Glanz and Friendship 1990)
- Disgust at injecting practices
- Lack of skills
- Concern about legal status and potential litigation
- Fear of contracting HIV
- Fear of censure from colleagues for substitute prescribing
- Possible effect on other practice patients
- Disillusionment at patient's relapses
- Costs of prescribing

of the 400 GPs were treating 50% of drug users known to be current primary care patients.

The 1990s onwards

In the UK payments for managing drug users additional to those for general medical services were ruled out by the health authorities in the mid-1980s. This is now beginning to change (Wilson *et al.* 1994). Not surprisingly, those GPs with large numbers of drug users as patients became concerned about the increased workload these patients brought to them and in some areas obtained additional financial and staff remuneration for the 'non-core' (i.e. deemed to fall outside general medical services) work. Clinics run by General Practitioners are being established, especially in areas with poor specialist provision. There is now a growing number of GPs prepared to take on a significant role in responding to drug users if they are adequately resourced. For most patients, management in a general practice setting with close association with outside agencies seems to be the ideal. On the whole drug users will seek out doctors who they feel understand and are sympathetic to their problems and will care for them competently (Hindler *et al.* 1996). In a study of users' views General Practitioners were identified as one of drug users most frequent points of first contact with services, 70% of respondents who had ever contacted a service had sought help from a GP (Stimson *et al.* 1995). Treatment for substance use is effective and individuals can demonstrate the capacity for change despite severe problems. There is no single treatment approach, though the provision of methadone, counselling and on-site medical and psychological services has been shown to reduce injecting drug use (Department of Health 1997). General practice offers an appropriate setting for these interventions in close association with other agencies which provide more extensive counselling, group work, social activities and psychological interventions.

Definition of shared care

Shared care is a complex term frequently used but poorly defined and with various interpretations. In the UK it is promoted as a way of integrating primary and secondary services and many shared care schemes exist, usually for the management of chronic diseases. It can broadly be classified and constructed in five different ways, based on the mode of information exchange between the participants (Hickman *et al.* 1994). These are:

- Community clinic/'mini-clinic'/shifted out-patient – Here a specialist undertakes a clinic in a primary care setting, The specialist may use this opportunity to train the GP and practice staff to become more independent of his or her advice.
- Liaison and consultancy – Here the community or hospital team and GP meet fact to face to discuss and agree the management of patients under shared care. This usually involves a period of initial training program. The hospital specialist, either in a routine out-patient clinic or in a community clinic sees new patients. When stable the patient is referred back to general practice.
- Shared care record cards, where the exchange of information is made through a booklet or 'cooperation' card, commonly carried by the patient. Most commonly used with ante-natal and child health surveillance.
- Computer-assisted shared care, where a circuit of information is established between the GP and specialist on data collected at each patient visit and mediated through computer generated summaries.
- Electronic mail, where hospital specialist and GP both have access to the same data on patients shared between them. The use of e-mail has been described in a positive manner within a medical context (Singarella *et al.* 1993). It is particularly well-developed in The Netherlands where in some case discharge letters are transmitted from hospital to primary care with an hour of the patient being seen (Branger *et al.* 1992).

Most research involving the first two has been carried out on the delivery of integrated diabetic care, which accounts for half of all shared care schemes in operation in the UK. The liaison model being met with enthusiasm from patients and doctors alike (Worth *et al.* 1990), with no loss or reduction in diabetic control. Shared care should be seen as part of a range of treatment options which can be offered. Health and allied professionals do not work in a vacuum and

Table 13.3   Examples of good practice in the care of drug users

Professional	Role
1. GP	Treatment of acute episode of illness
	Immunization
	HIV testing
	Cervical sreening
	Family planning advice
	Identiy a problem drug user*
	Assessment of illicit drug use*
	Referral to secondary drug service*
2. Pharmacist	Daily dispensing of methadone
3. Practice nurse	Abscess dressing, skin care
4. Social worker	Welfare rights, legal advice
5. Drug agency	Provision of injecting paraphernalia
	Safer sex advice
	Benefit advice
	Referral for rehabilitation treatment

*General practitioners may require additional training to develop these skills.

most care of patients involves different professional skills coming together. However shared care should imply care that goes beyond that provided as part of normal good clinical practice. Whilst many of the activities listed in Table 13.3 could be part of a shared care regimen they should and can be provided by the professional involved irrespective of others involved in the care of that patient.

Shared care for drug users must involve joint participation of specialist (usually consultant psychiatrist) and generalist (General Practitioner) in planned delivery of care, informed by enhanced information exchange, beyond the routine discharge and referral letters. Professionals involved in delivering shared care must be readily accessible and able to respond quickly. In most instances the GP maintains a central coordinating role for the patient.

Development of shared care

Shared care, between the specialist and the generalist is seen as the ideal model to be used to facilitate primary care involvement. The challenge of shared care for substance users has been explored now for over three decades. A public health perspective has driven much of this on the tackling of alcohol and other drug problems. The sheer scale of the problems made it clear that whatever the expansion of specialist services they would not be able to tackle all alcohol and other drug problems in the community. A prototype for shared care, that of the community alcohol team, developed the multidisciplinary team in the early 1970s. In many parts of the world problems associated with non-prescribed drugs have increased. In general statutory agencies (health or otherwise) were slow in responding to new drug subcultures and often the response was from a small network of specialist agencies with a focus on in-patient and residential therapeutic community support. Over time as the size of the problem grew, increasing emphasis was put on the need to develop a broader community-based response to grapple with the growing problem. Such community-based agencies tended at first to be specialist in orientation, but as they expanded they developed better links and working relationships with other generic community agencies. Community based teams aimed to provide shared care, with the key identifiable tasks of the team being:

- Direct work with clients
- Provision of advice, support and training to others involved with the client
- Service coordination or liaison
- Service development.

A number of factors account for the continued development of shared care and these are driving the momentum for closer integration of primary and secondary care services. They include:

- The general shifts towards a better balance of primary and secondary health care provision.
- The improvement in addiction training given to GPs enabling them to care for substance users.
- Patient preference to be treated where possible in the community – GP treatment rated as better for ease of access and confidentiality (Telfer and Cludlow 1990).
- The increasing levels of problem drug use and extended waiting lists for assessment and treatment.
- The increasing numbers of patients presenting to primary care in crises (for example homeless, chaotic state) or with complex drug problems.
- Concerns about the different standards of clinical care.
- The evolution of primary care which in many cases includes a range of specialist personnel, including community psychiatric nurses, clinical psychologists and specialist alcohol workers.
- The nature of drug dependency, a chronic disorder likely to continue over many years.
- Economic considerations. The emergence of managed care for alcohol and drug misuse such as in the USA (Armstrong 1997).

Why is shared care important?

A review of services in England (Department of Health 1997) found that treatment works when directed toward reduction of the immense harm caused by drug misuse. However, to be effective, treatment must embrace care in its widest sense. As the primary health care team is a frequent point of contact for drug users they are vital in providing continuity of care to improve general health and sustain improvements. By facilitating GP care access to specialist services for those patients requiring specialist interventions and support can be enhanced. Only with shared care can more patients be enabled to begin treatment and hence begin the process of change. This later point is especially pertinent to younger drug users. Many opiate users in London and other centres are under 25 years, yet this age group is under-represented in treatment agencies (Gillam *et al.* 1992).

Aims of shared care

Where care is shared, the GP with whom the patient is registered or attending, should in most circumstances maintain overall clinical responsibility. The GP and specialist should agree who is clinically responsible for providing different aspects of the care programme, such as hepatitis B immunization, substitute prescribing and other components. Shared care is not solely limited to prescribing issues. It can include agreements about interventions to support drug users whom wish to give up without a need for prescribing and structured interventions, for example counselling and non-pharmacological therapies.

The aims and objectives of shared care should be closely related to the aims and objectives of the local drugs strategy. Ideally, the skills of the PHCT supported by shared care can be used to retain the drug users in treatment and therefore enable the patient to make changes along a harm reduction spectrum and to facilitate a non-drug using lifestyle. Drug services in primary care could help promote better

Table 13.4   Aims of shared care

- Reduce referrals to the specialist service for patients with less severe problems, including patients requiring long term prescribing
- Selectively encourage referrals for patients with more complex problems
- Mutually enhance the skills of the general practice team and those involved in providing shared care
- Improve drug users access to primary care services
- Develop locally agreed guidelines for treatment

health among drug users who, despite their increased health needs, have limited access to primary care services. Of 112 attendees to a health clinic based at a non-statutory 'street agency' only 38% were registered with a GP and many of those who were registered were reluctant to attend their GP. Shared care aims to redress this balance (Gerada *et al.* 1992).

Shared care – a UK review

A recent survey of shared care provision across the UK (Gerada and Tighe in press) shows there to be great diversity across the country. A total of 120 health authorities were contacted and asked to furnish details of their shared care provision. The responses were examined to ascertain the following:

- Needs assessment: audit of existing care
- Shared care protocol (e.g. suitability for shared care)
- Non-prescribing treatment options
- Prescribing treatment options.

Eighty-nine authorities responded to the request for details of their shared care arrangements. Thirty had carried out a local need assessment, identifying training and support from secondary services as the main pre-requisites for successful GP involvement. Twenty-six of the 89 responding health authorities had designed a shared care policy. In some areas the provision was a planned response to needs (patient, GP and financial) and in others *ad hoc* arrangements developed in the absence of a well coordinated policy. Provision varied from sophisticated models with agreed protocols for referral, liaison and treatment to less formalized arrangements.

It is apparent from the review that shared care arrangements across the country were very varied, with most health authorities not having any formal arrangements in place. Services seemed to develop on an *ad hoc* basis, with poorly defined lines of responsibility and an array of local protocols and policies in place. The more the secondary

Table 13.5   Shared care provision

Result of 89/146 responses of Health Authority Review	
No GP provision	13%
Ad hoc provision only	44%
Advocate General Medical Services only	6%
Direct supervision (e.g. shifted outpatient)	11%
Specialist support (Consultant-liaison)	7%
Specialist GP	7%
Unknown/unstated	12%

services meet local needs, the less so the shared care arrangements. Elsewhere, for example in areas with a large geographical spread, shared care formed an important part of a comprehensive range of service provision.

No single model of shared care can be advocated; different arrangements must be developed depending on local drug service organization, prevalence and type of drug use, availability of specialists and the organization of primary care.

A joint working group the Royal College of Psychiatrists and GPs concluded that effective shared care could be achieved if some or all of the following measures are in place: close contact between GP and specialist, integrated training, audit, locally agreed management protocols and well defined responsibility for control and monitoring of prescribing (Anon 1993).

Shared care – examples of good practice

As stated before there is no single model of shared care. It may be an integral part of secondary specialist service coordinated by specialist GPs or Professionals Allied to Medicine (PAM) such as psychologists or psychiatric nurses, part of the voluntary sector drug misuse treatment service or combinations of all of these.

In the shared treatment of drug users the following are practical examples currently in operation:

- Consultant-led specialist service with full-time medical facilitator and nursing support (Greenwood 1992). Patients assessed and stabilized at a clinic and then referred to participating GPs for opiate and benzodiazipene prescribing with a treatment plan that involves regular contact with a named key worker. Random urine testing and sanctions for continued illicit drug use. Changes in medication negotiated with community drug worker and case conferences called to address complications that arise. The specialist service manages only a small number of patients with complex needs.
- Staged care with consultant- (psychiatrist or specialist GP or PAM) led drug team assessing and commencing treatment with central prescribing for an agreed limited period followed by GP taking over prescribing with support of a key worker attached to the practice or from specialist service (King 1997). In some instances GP clinical assistants are involved in the assessments.
- Liaison team (led by consultant psychiatrist or specialist GP or PAM) with a team suitable qualified staff (alcohol and drug specialist) employed by specialist provider. The team is based in primary care and facilitates and supports GPs to manage the

treatment of drug users. The team is peripatetic and aims to enable the GPs to treat the users rather than members of the team taking over care themselves. One such example is the Consultancy Addiction Liaison Service based in southeast London, a team of four, (specialist GP, drug and alcohol worker and team leader) supporting GPs treating patients in the community.

- A 'one-stop' clinic led by specialist general practitioner and employing a range of additional services, such as psychologist, social worker, drug and alcohol workers (Cohen and Schamroth 1990, Ronald *et al.* 1992). In some cases the GP see referrals and carries out assessments on behalf of other GPs within a locality (Wilson *et al.* 1994). In this later example methadone maintenance clinics are run jointly by GPs and drug counsellors in two Glasgow practices. The patients are seen in separate clinics within general practice rather than during normal surgeries – which could run into problems of stigmatization and congregation of drug users. The GP is mainly involved in initial assessment of patients, stabilization on methadone and then with intercurrent illness and serological testing.
- In the USA there is a strong desire to move some treatment into office-based settings. To date the regulations of methadone treatment prevent this. The concept of multidisciplinary clinics, which include various services, including general medical, has been growing (Smith and Frawley 1993).

Working within a multidisciplinary team

For shared care to be successful it must be underpinned by multi-disciplinary working which itself must have a good management structure. Overtreit (1980) wrote on the particular problems of management within multidisciplinary teams as being due to:

- Poor line management
- Poor case coordination and case liaison
- Difficulty in formulating and agreeing priorities for workload
- Uneven distribution of workload within the team
- Poor review of long-term cases
- Uncertainty about the role of the team in relation to general services and how the team fits into the overall service and strategy.

The Task Force review (McKeith 1997) highlighted similar problems in multidisciplinary team working, with a particular emphasis on weak management and poor resource utilization within community drug agencies.

Shared care pitfalls

Dual diagnosis

Not all patients can be managed within a shared care model as not all patients are suitable for general practice treatment. Some very chaotic patients, using large amounts, with more than one diagnosis or physically very unwell may be better managed by a specialist unit. The recent National Treatment Outcome Research Study reinforces this view finding that a quarter of those accessing specialist treatment services over a 2 year period had experienced seriously troublesome suicidal thoughts, one sixth had been an in-patient in a general psychiatric ward, a tenth on a general medical ward. Eleven per cent of the patients had been a patient of a community psychiatric team and half of the whole study group had attended accident and emergency. Over half of drug dependent individuals in the community have current mental health problems and the rates of mental illness are significantly higher among those entering treatment services. Patients with substance abuse problems had spent twice as many days in hospital in the previous 2 years as those without. In a study carried out by Weiss *et al.* (1992) to review the problems inherent in assessing rates of psychiatric disorder in substance misuse, rates for current major depression ranged from 2 to 100%, rates of life-time depression ranged from 24–38%, rates for anxiety between 16 and 19%. Looking at the issue the other way, a study of 121 psychotic patients in south east London (Menezes *et al.* 1996) showed the one-year prevalence rate for any substance problem to be 36.3%, for alcohol problems to be 31.6% and for drug problems to be 15.8%. With regards to serious physical illness, population studies estimates that between 60–70% of injectors are hepatitis C positive. Alcohol dependence is very common amongst dependent drug users and it is important to take this into account when assessing a patient for primary care treatment. Duel diagnosis is further discussed in Chapter 5 which deals with psychiatric comorbidity and Chapters 6 and 7 which deal with medical complications and HIV and AIDS.

Medical cost

Treatment of drug users in primary care, with or without shared care, has real costs to general practice. Reports of outcome among drug users do not take into account any impact on other areas of GPs' work, but studies of consultation rates and prescribing patterns appear to show that opiate users make greater demands on GPs' time and resources than other patients. In one Edinburgh survey attendances for patients increased more than five-fold after starting to use heroin (Bucknall *et al.* 1986). In another survey the mean annual consultation rate was 19.5 compared with 4.4 for the practice population as a whole, with HIV positive patients consulting 25 times per year compared with 16 for those that were negative (Ronald *et al.* 1992). In London, Leaver *et al.* (1992) compared 29 heroin users with 58 non-drug-using patients registered at the same practice and matched them for age, sex and GP. The heroin users made significantly more routine consultations than the control group over a six month period, though in keeping with another similar study (Neville *et al.* 1988) most of the increase in consultations was directly related to heroin use, consultation for general medical care being lower in heroin users. This leaves a window of opportunity in that good shared care should mean that these areas of care can be delegated, leaving the GP free to attend to the vast medical needs of his or her patients.

Financial cost

Cohen and Schamroth (1990) estimated that the costs of prescribing methadone in general practice was £663 per patient per year for GP time and £500 per patient per year for methadone prescribing costs. This contrast with a figure double that calculated by Wilson *et al.* (1994), who estimated cost per patient a few years later to be £2030. This latter figure includes the cost of laboratory monitoring. These figures represent, however, maximum costs and are comparable to

Table 13.6 Estimated annual costs of methadone maintenance in general practice

	Cost per patient
General Practitioner and Practice time*	208
Counsellor time[†]	173
Dispensing fees	806
Methadone	323
Toxicology[‡]	520
Total	2030

Figures based on average dose of methadone of 60 g dispensed daily.
*Three minutes weekly at £80/hour.
[†]Twenty minutes weekly at £10 per hour.
[‡]Analysis of urine every fortnight.
Source: Wilson *et al.* (1994)

specialist service costs at £1000–£2000 per patient per year. All these figures pale into insignificance when compared with the cost of maintaining a habit through stealing. It is estimated that £70 000 worth of goods needs to be stolen by a heroin addict to support a habit of half a gram per day.

Criminal justice system: prisons and the probation service

It is clear that a significant minority of people in prison and in other parts of the criminal justice system have drug problems. An estimated quarter of all offenders may have serious problems with illicit substances. Only a small proportion of these individuals will currently be in contact with treatment services. There has been increasing pressure to improve the process of identification and to create incentives for drug users to self-declare theft problems whilst in custody. Availability of skilled and competent responses is an important element once these problems have been revealed. There is also a desperate need for increased and more comprehensive treatment within the prison system and probation service. The challenge is to develop methods which enhance the links between the community-based treatment services and the criminal justice system. This may be particularly important for individuals who have received substantial treatment within prison and require ongoing management after release from prison. Clear plans for continuity of care between prison and the community are rational but very sparingly delivered. Primary care practitioners have an important role in assessment after release and where possible promoting continuity of care with previous treatment in custody.

This whole area poses one of the greatest challenges to models of multidisciplinary working, but may also possibly be one of the areas where such multiagency working markedly enhances the effectiveness of overall response.

Requirements for shared care

Whatever the shared care arrangements, all the professionals involved must be suitably qualified for the work/advice that they deliver. In most circumstances those involved in shared care should be able to offer the GP the following:

- initial assessment of drug misuser
- treatment planning for drug misuser
- setting up practice policies and guidelines in relation to treating drug misusers

- training to primary health care team on aspects of drug misuse relevant to that member of the team
- establish systems to evaluate number of drug users in treatment, their retention and compliance rates
- draw up continuing care arrangements, for example review dates, outcome criteria, and referral criteria to secondary care.

Good practice in shared care should include regular, ideally, face to face communication between the carers.

Shared care guidelines

The development of shared care guidelines should take into account the national policy but be locally determined taking into account local services. The guidelines should involve all providers including GPs, pharmacists and other professionals involved in the care of drug users.

Guidelines might specifically include

- Standardized assessment, treatment and referral protocols, including maximum substitute prescribing doses, acceptable formulations, and frequency of urine testing, criteria for review and termination of treatment
- Roles and responsibilities of shared care professionals
- Mechanism for support, e.g. key worker, liaison worker, shared care team
- Identification of skills, knowledge and training needs and a strategy how to address these needs
- Agreed monitoring and evaluation arrangements
- Arrangements to keep abreast of new developments
- Arrangements to provide a strategic overview on the development of local drug misuse services and patterns of drug misuse

Shared care can only work in the context of well-resourced secondary services is they in the statutory or voluntary sector. The expertise of specialist services would be expected in the following situations.

- Patients with serious risk to physical or mental health with co-morbidity for example. schizophrenia, or physical disease such as liver problems, or complex needs, frequent relapse, multiple drug use, concurrent alcohol use, and other complications of drug use
- Patients requiring injectable prescriptions
- Patients with serious forensic history

- Patients requiring in patient or day care
- Patients requiring a large element of psychosocial therapy or support
- Patient serving rehabilitation services.

Treatments that work using shared care model

At the present time the importance of evidence based interventions is increasing and there is a need to ensure that services are fashioned and delivered using the skills that have been demonstrated to have the greatest impact. Severe alcohol and drug dependence is a very serious condition that increases mortality rate between 15 and 30-fold when untreated (Shaw 1978).

The traditional sceptical view on the value of treatment for the drug dependent patient is often based on personal anecdotal experience and negative clinical experiences. The large treatment studies indicate very significant impact on actual consumption and reduction in related physical, psychological and social problems to such an extent that there are grounds for substantial therapeutic optimism and hope even in the face of some of the most intractable problems (McLellan et al. 1993). Treatment for drug abuse does bring about improvement in about 30% of cases (Department of Health 1997). Over the last few years there has been an emphasis on the value of less intensive interventions, particularly for alcohol users. In the drugs field the overriding emphasis has been to attract and retain patients in treatment so as to stabilize an often chaotic lifestyle, reduce criminality, morbidity from HIV and hepatitis and ultimately reduce mortality in conditions where it is higher than the general population (Ward et al. 1992). Treatment is often categorized as being pharmacological, psychological or combination of both.

The following interventions can be carried out in primary care with shared care support:

Detoxification

This is the process of coming off drugs, usually by giving gradually decreasing doses. The final goal could be abstinence or, more realistically, low dose maintenance. Detoxification can be carried out over days, weeks or months and it usually involves the prescribing of substitute medication. There are well-established regimens for most substances producing withdrawal syndromes. Chlordiazepoxide is the treatment of choice for alcohol dependence and lofexidine, clonidine or methadone linctus for opiates. The choice of detoxification programme depends on what has been found during the assessment period, the severity of physical dependence, the nature of drug-related problems, and previous experience of detoxification. Detoxification may need to be repeated; some patients resume illicit use whilst undergoing detoxification and others afterwards. Rather than treating a relapse as a failure, any worthwhile period of abstinence should be encouraged and praised. Detoxification may involve the use of symptomatic medication rather than substitute treatment. For example, with opiate detoxification symptomatic relief with antispasmodics (dicyclomine hydrochloride, hyoscine) to relieve abdominal pain, loperamide for diarrhoea, or neuroleptics such as chlorpromazine can be used. Further issues relating to detoxification are considered in Chapter 10.

Pharmacological treatment to prevent relapse

Disulfiram is the drug of choice for abstinent alcohol patients and naltrexone for those abstinent from opiates. It is most suitable for people who have decided to abstain and need extra support beyond will power to remain so. Naltrexone is an opiate antagonist. It is taken orally and blocks the effect of opiates for up to 72 hours (it therefore needs to be taken at least three times a week). It should be administered to an individual 7 days after achieving abstinence from heroin and 10 days after last methadone dose. The use of pharmacological relapse prevention methods requires a high degree of motivation on the part of the patient. They should be ideally administered under close supervision from a close family member or the General Practitioner with shared care support.

Maintenance or substitution treatment

The most commonly prescribed drug for opiate dependence is methadone mixture. If the patient adheres to the treatment regime then it should remove the need to obtain drugs illicitly and eliminates the need to inject with all the potential dangers this poses. Maintenance involves providing the patient with an adequately prescribed dose to prevent the onset of the abstinence syndrome. Having achieved stabilization, the patient is subsequently maintained on base-line daily dose of opiate for a prolonged time, perhaps indefinitely.

There is firm evidence that the provision of methadone to opiate misusers through well-managed and structured maintenance and or reduction programmes results in improvements in several aspects of lifestyle and behaviour.

Treatment of additional psychiatric morbidity

This includes management of depression and anxiety. Counselling is a central part of all drug use treatment, including methadone maintenance and reduction programmes. Counselling can be part of general information giving or more structured form treatment such as cognitive therapy, relapse prevention, motivational interviewing. A detailed account of diagnosis and treatment of psychiatric disorders in and associated with drug use is the topic of Chapter 5.

Drug counselling

At its simplest level this constitutes an advisory service. It is usually provided by professions other than the general practitioner, in parallel with GP treatment. Sessions should occur regularly by appointment rather than on an *ad hoc* drop in basis. The frequency of sessions should be determined jointly by the patient, the counsellor and the GP and not be part of a consultation linked to the issuing of a prescription. Many kinds of problem can be dealt with in the sessions. Where appropriate, specific treatments can be discussed, such as specific psychological techniques, drug-free therapeutic communities, and in-patient or out-patient treatment. Other areas that can be discussed are ways of avoiding encounters with drug using friends or acquaintances and how too avoid high-risk situations. Practical solutions for dealing with boredom can also be discussed. Drug counsellors usually liaise with others in order to help with practical areas of daily living. Counselling is usually a supportive relationship and should not become a specific analytical psychotherapeutic intervention.

Relapse prevention

This behavioural treatment requires additional training and is usually delivered by trained drug counsellors as part of a shared care programme. It involves identifying high-risk situations where there is an increased likelihood of drug taking. These may be negative emotional states, such as interpersonal conflicts and social pressure. The patient is encouraged to record their use of drugs and identity factors that trigger relapse. With the help of the therapist, coping strategies can be looked at to deal with these situations in the future. A structured approach has defined objectives and requires additional training for the clinician.

Role of professions allied to medicine

Shared care necessitates the involvement of multiprofessional groups. Some of these are attached to primary care, others separate from them. The multidisciplinary response to drug use necessarily involves a variety of professionals who must collaborate and cooperate. Shared care should be seen as a partnership between medical and non-medical practitioners.

Professions allied to medicine include:

- Practice nurses
- Health visitors
- Clinical psychologists
- Counsellors
- Social workers
- Nurse practitioners.

The future

The future, certainly in the UK and other European countries, points to increasing involvement of General Practitioners who will increasingly drive decisions in commissioning and purchasing of healthcare. The danger is that as the pendulum swings towards non-specialist doctors being the provider of care to drug users, that the role of the specialist will be diminished. One area of concern is that GPs will work in isolation and that there will be an increase in non-specialist involvement. Increasing numbers of patients merely collect prescriptions from reception staff without contact with medical or nursing staff; this is likely to be less effective. It may lead to lack of urine analysis or appropriate history-taking or any discussion around harm reduction, immunization, sharing injecting equipment, offers of hepatitis immunization or indeed any basic health checks. In order to prevent these problems evaluation of best practice and the success or failure of different approaches is essential. As stated often in various chapters in this book, research funding is vital.

Summary

The development of continuing evolution of shared care and the increasing involvement of the primary healthcare team is evidently the way forward in the UK. Similar developments in many western countries are being driven by increasing numbers of drug users and the recognition of the range of conditions they suffer from. Financial constraints make similar developments the likely model in developing countries. Early contact is essential if prevention of blood-borne

Table 13.7 Roles of professionals allied to medicine

Practice Nurse (ENB 1996a)

Assessment of:
- The individuals level and pattern of drug misuse
- The needs of particular groups service users affected by substance abuse

Identification of:
- Range of short-term goals and interventions
- Ethical, legal, political and cultural issues relevant to the nursing care of people affected by substance misuse
- The role of the registered nurse in contributing to a multi-disciplinary and multiagency response to prevention and treatment of drug misuse

Provision of:
- Access and referral to health care and treatment and rehabilitation services for people affected by substance misuse
- Education on health lifestyles and harm reduction interventions
- Information on generic and specialist sources of advice, help and treatment
- Care and management of critical incidents, including withdrawal, overdose and accidental ingestion of substances (ENB 1996a)

Promotion of:
- Sexual and reproductive health for substance misusers

Health Visitors (ENB 1996b)

All of above and

Assessment of:
- The impact of substance use and misuse and related lifestyles on the care of children and identification of relevant legal issues
- The health issues of women during pre-conception, pregnancy and the puerperium in relation to the issue of substances.

Social Workers (CCETSW 1992)

Identification of:
- Substance misuse problems at an early stage

Ability to:
- Use existing social work skills when working with substance misusers
- Employ minimal interventions
- Employ risk reduction strategies
- Engage in preventive action

Knowledge of:
- The nature and range of substance misuse problems
- At least two conceptual models of substance dependence
- Principal UK legislation relating to child care

Table 13.7 Continued

Drug Practitioners

Ability to provide:
- Expert knowledge of the impact of substance misuse and related harm on the health, well being and functioning of the individual, family, community and society
- Comprehensive assessment of people with substance misuse problems and prioritise interventions
- Expert care planning and management of people with substance misuse problems within a multidisciplinary and multiagency framework
- Expert clinical management of physical, psychological and behavioural problems associated with substance misuse and related lifestyles
- An expert resource to colleagues in the care and management of people who misuse drugs
- Management of challenging behaviour associated with drug use and their impact on others

Identification of:
- Health education and specialist substance misuse treatment needs of under services population groups, e.g. people from ethnic minority groups, women
- The needs of elderly, homeless, young people, women and offenders and ex-offenders

viruses is going to be effective and access to a wide variety of specialist help over a number of years makes the primary care physician an ideal coordinator of treatments. Economic constraints in most countries are likely to demand the most cost-effective models of care for drug users as they do for other conditions, and evidence of effective clinical practice will be expected. Ensuring that multidisciplinary community-based agencies in partnership with primary care deliver the most effective treatment possible for these serious conditions presents a major challenge for practitioners, policy makers and researchers for the coming decade. The identification of particular interventions that have been demonstrated to be more effective will then need further studies to determine the different settings in which these interventions can be delivered. Such careful study will help to articulate and define the interface between specialist and generic community-based interventions.

References

Advisory Council on the Misuse of Drugs 1982: *Treatment and rehabilitation.* HMSO, London.

Advisory Council on the Misuse of Drugs 1988: *Aids and drug misuse, Part 1.* HMSO, London.

Advisory Council on the Misuse of Drugs 1989: *Aids and drug misuse, Part 2.* HMSO, London.

Anon. 1993: *Shared care of patients with mental health problems*. Report of a Joint Royal College Working Group. Occasional Paper 60. Royal College of General Practitioners London, pp. 1–10

Armstrong, G., 1997: Managed Care. In: Lowinson J.H., Ruiz P., Miliman R.B., Langrod J.G. (eds). *Substance abuse. A comprehensive textbook*, 3rd edn. Williams & Wilkins, Baltimore, pp. 911–21.

Branger P.J., van der Wouden J.C., Schudel B.R., Verboog, E., Dulsterhout, J.S., van der Lei, J., van Bemmel, J.H. 1992: Electronic communication between providers of primary and secondary care. *British Medical Journal*, **305**, 1068–70

Bucknall, A., Roberston, J., Foster, K. 1986. Medical facilities used by heroin users. *British Medical Journal* **293**, 1215–16.

Cohen, J., Schamroth, A. 1989. General Practice management of drug misusers. *The Practitioner* 1471–4.

CCETSW 1992: *Substance misuse: guidance notes for diploma in social work*. ENB, London.

Des Jarlais, D.C., Freidman S.R., Hagan, H., Paone, D., Vlahov, D. 1997: Drug use. Vancouver conference review. *AIDS Care* **9**, 53–7.

Department of Health and Social Security. 1985: *Misuse of drugs. Government response to the 4th report of the social services committee session 1984–1985.* HMSO, London.

Department of Health. 1997: *The Task Force to review services for drug misusers.* Report of an independent review of drug treatment services in England. DOH, London.

Edwards, G. 1981: The background. In: Edwards, G., Busch, C. (eds). *Drug problems in Britain: a review of ten years experience.* Academic Press, London.

English National Board 1996a: *Curriculum guidelines for substance misuse.* ENB, London.

English National Board 1996b: *Substance use and misuse: Guidelines for good practice in education and training of nurses, midwives and health visitors.* ENB, London.

Gerada, C., Orgel, M., Strang, J. 1992: Health clinics for problem drug users. *Health Trends*, **24**, 68–9.

Gerada, C., Tighe, J., in press. A review of shared care protocols for the treatment of problem drug users in England, Scotland and Wales. *British Journal of General Practice.*

Gillam, S., Dubois-Arber, F., Stirzacker, L., Croft, A., Das Gupta, N. 1992: Evaluating the drug dependency unit. *Public Health*, **106**, 209–15.

Glanz, A ., Friendship, C. 1990: *The role of GPs in the treatment of drug misuse. Findings from a survey of GPs in England and Wales.* Report prepared for the Department of Health, London.

Greenwood, J. 1992: Persuading general practitioners to prescribe – good husbandry or recipe for chaos? *British Journal of Addiction* **87**, 567–74.

Hickman, M., Drummond, N., Grimshaw, J. 1994: Shared care for chronic disease. *Journal of Public Health Medicine* **16** (4), 447–54.

Hindler, C., King, M., Nazareth, I., Cohen, J., Farmer, R., Gerada, C., 1996 Characteristics of drug misusers and their perceptions of general practice care. *British Journal of General Practitioners* **46**, 149–52.

Horder, J. 1983: General Practice in 2000: Alma Ata Declaration. *British Medical Journal* **286**, 191–4.

Institute for the Study of Drug Dependence 1988: Drug indicators project: study of help-seeking and service utilization by problem drug takers. ISDD, London.

King, L. 1997: Structured GP liaison for substance misuse. *Nursing Times* **93** (4), 30–31.

Leaver, E., Elford, J., Morris, J., Cohen, J. 1992: Use of general practice by intravenous heroin users on a methadone programme. *British Journal of General Practice* **42**, 465–8.

McLellan, A,T., Arndt, I.O., Metzger D.S., Woody G.E., O'Brien C.P. 1993: The effects of psychosocial services in substance abuse treatment. *Journal of the American Medical Association* **269**, 1953–9.

McKeith, J. 1997: *The organization and management of Community Drug Agencies.* Policy Press, London.

Meads, G. (ed.) 1996: Primary care development. In: *Future options for General Practice*: Radcliffe Medical Press. The British Dilemma.

Meltzer, H., Baljit, G., Petticrew, M., Hinds, K. 1995: OPCS surveys of psychiatric morbidity in Great Britain. Report 2. Physical complaints, service use and treatment of adults with psychiatric disorders. HMSO, London.

Menezes, P.R., Johnson, S., Thornicroft G., Marshall, J., Prosser, D., Bebbington, P., Kuipers, E. 1996: Drug and alcohol problems among individuals with severe mental illness in South London. *British Journal of Psychiatry* **168**, 612–19.

Neville, R., McKellican, J., Foster J. 1988: Heroin users in general practice Ascertainment features. *British Medical Journal* **296**, 755–8.

Overtreit, J. 1986: *Organization of multidisciplinary community teams.* BIOSS working paper. Brunel University, Uxbridge.

Ronald, P., Witcome, J., Robertson, J.R., Roberts, K., Shishodia, P., Whittaker, A. 1992: Problems of drug abuse, HIV and AIDS: the burden of care in one general practice. *British Journal of General Practice* **42** 232–5.

Shaw, N. et al. 1978: *Responding to drinking problems.* Croom Helm, London.

Singarella, T., Baxter, J., Sanefur, R.R., Emery, C.C. 1993 The effects of electronic mall on communication in two health sciences institutions. *Journal of Medical Systems* **17**, 69–86.

Smith, J.W., Frawley, P.J. 1993: Treatment outcomes of 600 chemically dependent patients in a multimodal inpatient program including aversion therapy and Pentothal interviews. *Journal of Substance Abuse Treatment* **10**, 359–69.

Stimson, G., Oppenheimer, E. 1982: *Heroin addiction: Treatment control in Britain.* Tavistock, London.

Stimson, G., Hayden, D., Hunter G., Metrebian, N., Rhodes, T., Turnbull, P., Ward, J. 1995: *Drug users' help seeking and views of services.* A report prepared for the Task Force. DOH, London.

Strang, J., Smith, M., Spurrell, S. 1992: The community drug team. *British Journal of Addiction* **87**, 169–78.

Telfer, I., Cludlow, C. 1990: Heroin misusers: what they think of their general practitioners. *British Journal of Addiction* **85**: 137–40.

Ward, J., Darke, S., Hall, W., Mattick, R. 1992: Methadone maintenance and the human immunodeficiency virus: current issues in treatment and research. *British Journal of Addiction* **87**, 447–53.

Weiss, R.D., Mirin, S.M., Griffin, M.L. 1992: Methodological considerations in the diagnosis of coexisting psychiatric disorders in substance abusers. *British Journal of Addiction* **87**, 179–87.

Wilson, P., Watson, R., Ralston, G.E. 1994: Methadone maintenance in general practices patients, workload, and outcomes. *British Medical Journal* **309**, 6414.

Worth, R., Nicolson, A., Bradley, P. 1990: Shared care for diabetes in Chester: Preliminary experience with a 'clinic-wide' scheme. *Practical Diabetes* **7**, 266–8.

Care in the community

Anne Whittaker and John MacLeod

Introduction

The use of psychoactive drugs is widespread throughout most societies and appears to be increasing (ISDD 1997). The clandestine nature of illegal drug use means that all of the many surveys into its extent are subject to considerable bias and their results must be treated with caution (Home Office 1995; Miller and Plant 1996). Within this they show a consistent picture, a large number of people use drugs and most of them never encounter the sort of problems seen amongst clients of drug services. Problems can be associated with the use of any drug. In general their severity depends on the legal status of the drug involved and the pattern of its use. For moderate, non-dependent users of any drug, legal status is extremely important in determining whether or not problems are likely. For heavy dependent use the distinction becomes less important. Similar issues arise around neglect of self, disintegration of social functioning, inability to meet responsibilities and a general narrowing of life focus till it includes nothing but the drug and issues around its acquisition and consumption. For illegal drugs, problems of personal criminality, criminal control of production and distribution and its consequences to the consumer and membership by default of a criminal subculture are simply added to the previous list. Injecting drugs, particularly illegal drugs, brings its own set of special problems. It has been estimated that 2% of adults in UK urban centres regularly inject drugs (Frischer *et al.* 1993).

The following Chapter concerns care in the community as it relates to *problem* drug users, in simple terms clients of drug services, proportionately a small subgroup of drug users but one which attracts a disproportionate (though not necessarily unjustified) amount of attention and concern.

Perhaps the most useful paradigm of problem drug use was provided by Zinberg (1984) who suggested that whether or not a persons' drug use became problematic was a product of the interplay between the triad of drug (the pharmacology of the substance used), set (the personal characteristics of the drug user) and setting (the environment in which the use occurred). Pearson (1987) has described how in the UK an over-supply of cheap high quality heroin in the 1970s in conjunction with many aspects of the social setting of urban poverty combined to create the picture of problem drug use and problem drug user that is typically seen today.

Of course not all problem drug users come from socially disadvantaged urban backgrounds. Many rural communities are now experiencing what was initially an almost exclusively urban phenomenon. Drug problems can also be associated with affluence and privilege. The extent of this association is difficult to assess. Affluent drug users' problems are less likely to become visible if they have money, family support and access to private care and this group are less visible to the average drug worker or General Practitioner.

The consequences of problem drug use to the individual, their immediate family, their community and 'society' generally are considerable if difficult to quantify. Problem drug use is a chronic relapsing condition associated with a number of physical, psychological and social problems. A variety of services may be required in order to address these.

'Care in the Community' can have two related meanings in this context. Services that are designed to maintain clients in the community (in their homes or in 'homely' surroundings) and more specifically in the UK, services which are covered by the 1990 NHS and Community Care Act.

The development of community-based medical care

Glanz (1994) described the development of UK general practice and the changing relationship between General Practitioners (primary care doctors) and problem drug users. There is little to add to his account other than to confirm that, as predicted, primary care services in most developed countries are once again coming to the fore of the therapeutic response to problem drug use. Of all the community based agencies in the UK, general practice has a unique relationship with problem drug users based on its relative accessibility and the power to prescribe. Within this General Practitioners have recognized the generic primary care physician often has less specific training about drug problems than other non-medical practitioners (Martin 1996).

As Glanz described, UK general practice originated in the early 19th century as a means of meeting middle-class demands for a family doctor. As such it was in origin firmly individually based and curative (rather than preventive) in orientation. In the UK the prestige of general practice fell as the prestige of hospital specialists rose. By the 1960s morale and direction of British general practice was at its lowest ebb (Hart 1988). In 1967 the Dangerous Drugs Act took away the right of General Practitioners to prescribe heroin or cocaine to drug addicts. This role was thereafter restricted to addiction specialists, generally psychiatrists.

In contrast, primary care was about to undergo something of a renaissance internationally. Though high technology medicine was aspired to and revered in most of the world its shortcomings were becoming apparent. It was very expensive, whole health budgets of a country could be spent on one teaching hospital in the capital city. It gave little return in terms of improved population health (McKeown 1979), it was curative and reactive rather than preventive and proactive. Its priorities often reflected medical fashion rather than objective importance. Conversely, primary care had several advantages. It was community-based, so theoretically closer to the people and their real problems. It was the only medical service regularly in contact with a significant proportion of the population and hence the only viable setting for primary prevention. It was based in minimal technology at a time when the dangers of technological medicine were being discussed (Illich 1977). It seemed to offer the potential for community participation which was seen as being essential to *healthy* healthcare. Above all where resources were finite, primary care was relatively cheap. Thus throughout the world primary care rose to prominence combining as it did the attractions of both economy and political correctness. In 1978 this prominence was underlined in the declaration of Alma Ata, when the WHO announced its target of

'Health For All' by the year 2000 to be achieved through the mechanism of primary healthcare (Horder 1983).

British general practice was also picking up from its mid-1960s low. A Royal College was founded and compulsory vocational training was introduced. Then came the 1990 NHS reforms. The 'new contract' was generally seen as a bad thing by most GPs in terms of its likely consequence of increasing their workload. However, antipathy to this stick was tempered by enthusiasm for the carrot of the promised 'Primary Care-led NHS' and a significant minority (perhaps as much as a third) of GPs were excited at the prospect of fundholding, a system they saw as being financially advantageous for them and providing improved care for their patients. Unfortunately fundholding has probably only resulted in these advantages for certain types of patient at certain types of practice. Generally these are patients who made little demands of health services in practices serving relatively affluent areas. Clearly problem drug users are poor candidates for reaping the benefits of this system of allocating funds.

From all the above it may seem an unlikely scenario that care for drug users has become such a prominent part of the work of GPs in most parts of the UK. Yet by 1997 a survey of around 300 GPs in Manchester showed virtually all were working with drug users and that twice as many had predominantly positive as opposed to negative feelings about this work (Davies and Huxley 1997). Indeed their main 'negative' feeling was that they had less training than they would have liked to do the job properly! Two things hastened these changes. Firstly, as mentioned, the late 1970s and early 1980s saw a coincidence of oversupply and suitable socioeconomic setting that led to a genuine explosion of injection heroin use amongst the urban poor. This phenomenon happened in many European cities. From being viewed as largely irrelevant deviancy drug use began to be seen as a significant social threat. Secondly by tragic coincidence this same period saw the emergence of a new and deadly blood-borne pathogen – HIV.

The influence of HIV

It is impossible to look meaningfully at current service provision outside of the HIV context. Following reports of epidemics of infection amongst injectors in North America a similar situation was discovered in the Scottish cities of Edinburgh and Dundee (Robertson et al. 1986, Des Jarlais et al. 1989). The UK Advisory Council on the Misuse of Drugs (ACMD 1988) concluded that HIV represented a greater threat to public health than drug misuse. Drug services

throughout the UK were expanded to meet this threat. The ACMD
envisaged a significant role for GPs within these new AIDS prevention services. Specialist services were hardly likely to cope. They were
too small and they generally met users far too late in their 'career' of
drug use for effective prevention. The ACMD suggested that all GPs
should be prepared to work with drug users. Apocalyptic scenarios
were painted as to the potential devastating effect of a generalized
HIV epidemic. The message to primary care workers was clear. Even
if they were not particularly concerned with the problems of individual drug users they should be concerned with the public health
implications of 'the drug problem'.

As a postscript and with the benefit of some hindsight one can
critically examine the fears that shaped policy 10 years ago and the
consequences of the policy they shaped. A generalized UK epidemic
of HIV has never materialized, and most people now seem to agree
that it is unlikely that it ever will. It is difficult to know if it was ever
really on the cards. Hepatitis B is a blood-borne virus which by the
early 1980s was virtually endemic amongst UK injectors, yet has
never generalized far beyond this community (probably as a result of
fairly fixed assortative sexual mixing patterns in a society characterized by little mobility between social strata). However to say based
on this that HIV was never a real population threat would probably
be foolish. It is also true that heterosexual spread is occurring, mainly
in the communities originally most blighted by problem drug use, if
at a lesser level than originally predicted (Robertson *et al.* 1998).

The other epidemic that has failed to materialize is that of HIV
amongst UK drug injectors themselves. In 1997 Edinburgh and
Dundee are still the only UK cities to experience very high seroprevalence. If this were the consequence of preventive efforts then it
would represent a real and significant benefit to drug injectors of a
policy that as stated was not actually devised with their benefit in
mind. Problem drug users can die of many things but in the aging
Edinburgh cohort AIDS is now the principal cause of mortality
(Shishodia *et al.* 1998). Again it is difficult to know if low seroprevalence is a consequence of successful prevention. Glasgow, a city
only 40 miles from both Edinburgh and Dundee offers little clarification. There are more Glaswegian injectors than in the other two cities
combined and 'harm reduction' policies were adopted later than in
most UK settings. Equipment sharing is still acknowledged to be
widespread, Hepatitis C seroprevalence is very high yet HIV seroprevalence remains very low (Bloor *et al.* 1994, McKeganey *et al.*
1995). Hepatitis C may of course have spread prior to harm reduction
campaigns though this is unclear, the current consensus appears to be
that the continuing low prevalence of HIV amongst UK injectors does
represent a success of prevention campaigns (Stimson 1996).

The philosophy and development of 'Care in the Community'

In most developed countries the perceived need to reform health care has gone along with changes in the service approach to drug users. The imperative to provide economic value has driven policy. A result has been the merging of services and the concentration on primary medical care and community social care as the main focus of development for the care of drug users. The financial attractions of this are self-evident, the saving of resources by using generic services to provide additional areas of care. These new responsibilities for non-specialists however created new demands on already over-stretched agencies. There is no unifying philosophy underpinning 'care in the community'. Rather it represents a concept which has developed in the latter half of this century in Europe and North America informed by various ideological and economic considerations.

The stated ideals behind 'community care' as we know it today include: 'deinstitutionalization', 'normalization', 'independent living', 'decentralization', and 'case management'. 'Deinstitutionalization' supports the idea that more people who need long-term care should be supported to live at home or in a 'homely' environment rather than stay in residential or institutional settings. 'Normalization' (Wolfensberger 1972), argues for the integration of people with chronic and severe disabilities into the wider community. 'Independent living' advocates and supports people to achieve their maximum potential and independence within the community. 'Decentralization' emphasizes a change in the planning, delivery and organization of services to people in need from a centralized base to a local community base. 'Case management' is an approach to caring for people with multiple needs in the community by assessing, planning, implementing and evaluating their care on a continuous basis.

Community care policy

The implementation of 'community care' has been a process of social and cultural change.

In the UK, the NHS and Community Care Act (1990) relates to the care needs of older people, people with learning disabilities, people with physical disabilities, people with mental health problems, people who are homeless and vulnerable, people with alcohol-related problems, people with drug-related problems, and people with HIV/AIDS. The national policy framework encourages Local Authorities to look at services to vulnerable adults as a whole and community care guidance also requires authorities to consider specifically the needs of carers.

Policy has been stimulated by the increasing elderly population and the implications for costs. The need to transfer adults with severe learning disabilities and mental health problems who need long-term care from institutional settings (healthcare) into the community (social care) was also a driving force. The main policy objectives in 'Caring for People' (Department of Health 1989) were based on the recommendations in the Griffiths report (Griffiths 1988).

The stated central aim of community care in 'Caring for People' (para 1.8) is to enable people

- to live as independently as possible in their own homes, or in 'homely' settings in the local community.
- to provide the right amount of care and support to help people achieve maximum possible independence ... and to ... achieve their full potential.
- to give people a greater individual say in how they live their lives and the services they need to help them to do so.

The six key objectives for service delivery in 'Caring for People' (para 1.11) are:

- to make proper assessment of need and good case management the cornerstone of high quality care.
- to clarify the responsibilities of agencies, and so make it easier to hold them to account for their performance.
- to promote the development of domiciliary, day and respite services to enable people to live in their own homes wherever feasible and sensible.
- to ensure that service providers make practical support for carers a high priority.
- to promote the development of a flourishing independent sector alongside good quality public services.
- to secure better value for taxpayers money by introducing new funding structure for social care.

The main changes proposed were that social service authorities should become the main agencies responsible for assessing individual need, deciding whether 'publicly-funded care can and should be arranged', designing care arrangements and securing their delivery 'within available resources'.

The practice of 'care management' is central to community care policy. Care management is considered appropriate 'where an individual's needs are complex or significant levels of resources are involved'. In these circumstances a nominated 'care manager' takes responsibility for ensuring the care plan is implemented, monitored and reviewed.

The NHS and Community Care Act also had financial implications. The new funding system introduced 'a single unified budget to cover the costs of social care' for which local authorities had responsibility. Funds were transferred from the Department of Social Security (the 'care component') to social service departments (the 'community care budget'). Financial assistance since 1993 is dependent on an 'assessment of need' by a local authority. Residential care is paid by local authorities, depending on their 'pricing policy', and users are required to undertake a financial assessment to assess whether or not they can help pay for their care. Community care assessments include this financial assessment.

The Community Care Act has led to a number of changes in the way services operate in the UK. It has meant a split in the purchaser/provider role, joint planning and purchasing, the development of a 'contract culture' and 'service agreements' for agencies providing care. It has also meant the creation of NHS Trusts and 'fund-holding' GPs (budgets held by GPs), the closure of long-stay hospitals and changes in hospital discharge arrangements. These arrangements continue to evolve with new legislation increasing the trend to community centred medical agencies.

Community care legislation emphasizes a 'needs-led' rather than a 'service-led' approach. The concept of 'need', however, has been left ambiguous. The Social Work Services Group (SSI and SWSG 1991) guidance defines 'need' as shorthand for 'the requirements of individuals to enable them to achieve, maintain, or restore an acceptable level of social independence or quality of life as defined by the particular care agency or authority'.

Concurrent policy

In addition to the legislation surrounding 'community care' which is essentially a social policy, practitioners need to take account of the more specific guidelines on drug policy.

In the UK, the Advisory Council on the Misuse of Drugs (ACMD) has issued guidance on drug policy and practice over a number of years. The AIDS and Drug Misuse (1989) report recommends that for the most part, care for drug users 'will and should be provided in the community'. ACMD guidance suggests that local Community Care Plans take into account the needs of couples, families and support for the 'informal' carers of drug misusers. They also suggest that local authorities, health authorities, housing and the voluntary sector should look for 'imaginative solutions' in the provision of accommodation for drug users. They recommend that community nursing services should be expanded and all General Practitioners and dentists should be prepared to treat drug misusers, including those with

HIV infection. The ACMD emphasizes the role of planning, coordination and liaison in providing services to drug misusers in the community.

Similar changes have occurred in the United States where an acceptance of drug misuse as a medical problem and inclusion of treatment in Medicaid and federal funding programmes has been curtailed by the need to contain costs. The emergence of 'Managed Care' for both insured and uninsured patients has changed the way in which drug users will receive care. A fundamental element of this new approach to healthcare delivery is prevention and community care. The three essential elements of managed care are improved access to primary care, cost containment and quality assurance (Armstrong 1997). Difficulties arise in the inclusion of substance abuse care due to its various manifestations of an acute illness or a chronic long-standing disorder. As the new approach takes hold patients and care providers will notice new rules.

Community care and drug users

A number of difficulties immediately arise when we attempt to translate and integrate the care and treatment of drug users into the philosophy and ideals of community care.

'Normalization' of illicit drug use is not considered a desired goal of most societies despite the fact that drug use is widespread. Most legal systems support this view and social and drug policy aims to reduce the incidence of drug use and drug related problems. The current climate of an international 'war on drugs' emphasizes that society appears to have little intention of accepting or integrating drug use into normal life.

The philosophy of 'deinstitutionalization' is not particularly relevant for drug users as most live in the community, although not necessarily in a 'homely' environment. 'Institution' for drug users generally means prison. Community care policy also emphasizes a move from healthcare to social care for people who require long-term support. Since the advent of HIV drug users have been encouraged to make more contact with health services. Social care alone is inadequate for most drug users who may also need services such as substitute prescribing, needles and syringes, psychiatric and psychological care, HIV treatment and general medical care.

The idea of 'independent living' is also not easily applicable to drug users. Drug use is normally seen as a problem, not a disability with drug use portrayed as being abnormal and unacceptable behaviour. Problems associated with drug use are often seen as being 'self-inflicted' and drug users as undeserving of compassion. Societies do not want to see people reaching their maximum drug using 'potential'. Drug policies emphasize strategies which tend to organize (segregate), control (limit) and monitor (label) people who use drugs. Society seems likely to continue to characterize drug users as a homogeneous group of people which they will stigmatize, label, reject, and punish. Realistically, not many 'communities' are willing to provide help and support to their local drug users. Organized community groups often actively discriminate against their drug using members, advocating action which is designed to exclude them from their area.

The 'care management' approach advocated in community care policy was really not developed with drug users in mind or on top of the agenda. The shift from a service-led, controlling approach to a person-centred, enabling approach is still rhetoric rather than reality in relation to the management of most drug users. It has also been difficult to get practitioners to leave their agency setting and their passive role of waiting for clients to come to them and be assertive in going out to deliver treatment and support to drug users in the community. This is a difficult barrier to overcome as there is often a great fear of drug users, a perception of more physical risk and an underlying feeling that clients should show that they are 'motivated'. In the UK, local authorities and health boards have had to give priority to securing services to those client groups who are seen as 'most in need'. For most local authorities services for drug users are considered low priority in comparison with their other responsibilities. Drug users are probably viewed as the most undeserving of all people entitled to community care services.

The role of different agencies in community care

Social Services

Social service departments are responsible for meeting the social care needs of vulnerable people in the community and have the lead role in ensuring that community care policy and practice is implemented. Social care includes the provision of residential, day and domiciliary care services and respite care. Social services are able to charge for these services after they take into account the users ability to pay. The key responsibilities for social services in community care are: assessing individual need; designing packages of care; securing the delivery of services; monitoring the quality of services; financially assessing the client's ability to pay for services; and appointing a 'care manager' to facilitate these tasks. Social services are to act as an 'enabling authority', developing a 'mixed economy of care' by making use of services in the independent sector. They must also 'plan, purchase and commission' community care services, making community care plans available to the public.

Health

Healthcare is considered an essential component of community care and 'will help people to continue to live in their own homes for as long as possible'. Health Authorities and healthcare workers are expected to make some specific contributions to community care. These are: to take part in the assessment process for community care for individuals; to collaborate with local authorities in planning and providing services; and to prepare and produce plans for community care. The role of the General Practitioner described in 'Caring for People' (paras 4.11–4.13) points out that they will often be the first point of contact for people requiring community care. It recognizes the 'key role' played by GPs in caring for people in the community. GPs assessing drug users will initiate referral on to other services and, through linkage with substitute prescribing, can make attendance more likely. GPs are especially important in recognizing the needs of carers and other family members affected by a person's drug use. They are increasingly more involved in community care and government policy states that locally agreed arrangements should be developed to enable them to make their 'full contribution to community care'. Guidance suggests that 'complex and bureaucratic procedures should be avoided' and the policy on community care assessment states that 'where advice is needed by the local authority in the course of assessment, this should be obtained from the GP orally (e.g. by phone) as far as possible' and 'a record should be kept of the advice given'. Many health authorities have offered financial and other incentives to GPs for treating drug users. ACMD recommendations state that GP involvement with drug users should increase and training is essential. They also advocate that 'shared care' systems are developed so that GPs and specialists can combine to monitor the treatment provided to drug users and in particular, drug users with HIV infection. This is considered in more detail in Chapter 13.

Housing

Housing is essential in community care. It is a basic requirement in ensuring that people are able to remain in the community. Assessment of housing needs is part of a 'comprehensive assessment' and is critical for drug users who typically have difficulty in securing and maintaining suitable housing. Rehousing from prison and following on from residential detoxification and rehabilitation placements is also an important part of community care. The role of housing is also essential when providing services such as supported accommodation, housing adaptations and furnished tenancies which can help drug users maintain independent living in the community.

The independent sector

Community care policy gives high priority to the development of a flourishing independent sector by advising local authorities to shift the balance of service provision towards the non-statutory sector. Drug services have traditionally been provided by the voluntary sector as many statutory services have been reluctant to provide the kind of service that drug users were willing to access. The voluntary sector has undergone considerable change since the implementation of community care. Community care policy has emphasized cost-effectiveness, so many drug services have had to conform to the specific requirements of purchasing bodies and their HIV prevention agenda. Unfortunately, this may have led to a lack of innovation in service provision, reducing the likelihood that more unorthodox user-centred approaches to service provision are offered and generating a general mainstreaming of services for drug users.

The private sector, in comparison, have traditionally not been active players in the drugs field reflecting a lack of demand and financial incentives throughout most of the UK apart from London. Substitute prescribing of injectables is more widespread in private clinics compared with NHS facilities raising issues of equity. Private detoxification, respite and rehabilitation units are few. Some private residential treatment units offer detoxification (funded by health authority agreement) followed by a period of rehabilitation (funded by social services).

Volunteers

The role of volunteers in community care is considerable as they contribute to service provision in virtually every setting. Examples of these are day care, domiciliary care (meals on wheels, sitter services, home visiting), supported accommodation, peer education projects, residential accommodation, driving services, befriending, advocacy, and advice and information services. Most projects of this nature employ some paid staff and many 'volunteers' receive some remuneration for example travel or child-care expenses. The management of most non-statutory services is predominantly undertaken by volunteers usually in the form of management committees.

User involvement

Community care policy states that it is a statutory responsibility to consult users in the planning process. Users and carers should be made aware of their rights in relation to community care. They should be encouraged to make suggestions and complaints about assessment arrangements and service provision. Support should be offered, including training where necessary, in order to promote the development of user groups, forums, carers support groups and other self-help groups. Drug users can be difficult to consult and organize into reliable user groups which offer a balanced view on local community care services. Views on the needs of drug users tend to be polarized and the special stigma attached to certain subgroups of drug users (e.g. those who are HIV positive, those who work in prostitution) tends to prohibit open and public consultation. Service satisfaction questionnaires and other methods of anonymous information gathering are sometimes required in order to gain a more extensive picture of drug service acceptability and quality.

The whole question of participation of people in receipt of care in the defining of their problems and the discovery of appropriate solutions to them is one which preoccupied international community health in the aftermath of Alma Ata (Rifkin and Walt 1986, Newell 1988). Individual or community participation is also presented as being central to both the 'New Public Health' and the 'New General Practice'. Participation has never featured prominently in UK medicine which came from the tradition of expert service for a fee. McDermott (1992) recently provided a sceptical overview of user participation in UK drug projects. He concluded that 'participation' usually involved tokenism, cheap labour, intellectual and creative 'asset stripping' and the legitimization of an establishment agenda through creation of the illusion that it originated outside the establishment.

Service provision for drug users in the community

Different approaches to the care and treatment of drug users are applied in many different types of service provision. No one service delivery type has been shown to be universally effective with all drug users so it is important to consider all available methods. In this section the main types of service provision for drug users are outlined. It is important to remember that these are not necessarily mutually exclusive. Many drug users access multiple services at any one time.

Substitute prescribing services

The line between 'substitute prescribing' (Dole and Nyswander 1965) and simply giving drug users legal drugs, thus decriminalizing that part of their drug use, is indistinct. 'Substitute' implies that in some way the drug prescribed is different from the drug users customary illegal drug of choice. In some cases (for example substitution of methadone for heroin) the prescribed drug may be taken in a 'healthier' manner, orally rather than intravenously and generally it will have been subject to more rigorous standards of quality control during its preparation. In some cases (for example in opiate users whose drug of choice was oral methadone anyway) the only difference is it is free and legal. 'Substitute' also implies that the prescribed drug is taken instead of illicit drugs. Many drug users on substitute prescriptions acknowledge that they use illicit drugs in addition to their prescription though generally in lesser quantities than before. Research has, perhaps unsurprisingly, shown that the substitute prescriptions most successful at reducing their recipient's illicit drug intake are those involving the higher daily doses of the substitute drug.

The argument as to whether a methadone prescription achieves it effect primarily through social rather than pharmacological mechanisms is likely to run for some time. Most 'drugs of abuse' have at some time been prescribed to drug users as part of a therapeutic intervention. In most instances it has been explicitly recognized that any associated therapeutic benefit derives from a social mechanism.

The delivery system of substitute prescribing programmes varies considerably throughout the UK and the world. Some programmes are managed and controlled by psychiatrists working within the mental health field, some by public health department services, some by doctors within primary care services. Drug users are sometimes required to attend prescribing clinics on a daily basis, or to attend their local chemist for daily dispensing, or to self-administer their supply on a daily basis. Some substitute prescribing services are mobile.

Ward *et al.* (1992) concludes that the available evidence on methadone maintenance prescribing suggests that it is more effective than no treatment in retaining drug users in treatment, in reducing the use of illicit drugs, in reducing drug-related criminal activity and imprisonment. Ward also flags up the general lack of high quality research in this area. It does seem disappointing that we do not seem to have progressed much further than the conclusion that providing free legal drugs is popular with drug users and sometimes reduces their recourse to expensive illegal drugs with all the consequences that may have. Further discussion of these issues and of the practicalities of substitute prescribing can be found in Chapter 9.

Needle exchange services

Needle exchange services supply clean needles and syringes, impart information on safer injecting practices and collect used needles and syringes. Many also offer safer sex advice and condoms and some also offer ancillary services (e.g. HIV testing, substitute prescribing, pregnancy testing etc.) on site. Pharmacy-based needle exchanges are also found in most major towns and cities throughout Europe and increasingly in North America.

Practitioners should ensure that all drug injectors know:

- how to inject as safely as possible
- how to clean used injecting equipment if necessary
- where the nearest needle exchange service is located
- where the nearest pharmacy supply is located
- what options they have if they wish to stop injecting drugs.

Out-patient services

Most specialist drug dependency units are attached to mental health services and offer out-patient appointments for assessment and follow-up with a staff member from the team. Drug teams are often multidisciplinary and follow a 'key worker' system whereby each drug user is allocated a named member of staff who is their main contact and counsellor. A number of drug teams are staffed by community psychiatric nurses who offer home visiting and appointments in satellite clinics based in the community or in GP surgeries.

Out-patient detoxification is also offered by drug dependency units, prescribing GPs and other specialist drug agencies. 'Outreach' clinics are sometimes located in agencies that work with sex industry workers.

Community health services can provide needle exchanges, community psychiatric nursing service, maternity and other child care services. District nurses, health visitors and clinical psychologists also offer services specifically to drug users in some health authorities.

Residential services/in-patient care

Limited beds are available within the NHS for the purposes of drug detoxification and tend to be located within mental health services or, less often, acute services. Admissions are normally planned following referral from the GP and an assessment by the Consultant. Other medically staffed private clinics and some voluntary sector drug rehabilitation units also offer supervised drug detoxification. Typically most drug users who wish to undertake a planned and supervised detoxification enter into one of these establishments.

Crisis centres

Drug crisis centres follow a harm reduction approach and offer the goal of stabilization to the chaotic and vulnerable drug user. They are usually direct access, offering emergency admission and have a short-stay (1 to 4 week) programme of care. Services offered include crisis intervention work, individual and group counselling, harm reduction information and advice, practical help and support, and referral on to community agencies for follow-up on discharge. They are found in most major cities and are normally (in the UK) joint funded by Health and Social Services.

Rehabilitation units and therapeutic communities

Residential rehabilitation care for drug users tends to be solely provided by the independent sector. Drug rehabilitation units follow an abstinence model and offer the goal of drug-free living for those who wish to come off drugs. Most units accept people once they have completed their drug detoxification and offer a comprehensive range of support. Residential services vary in the services they offer. Therapeutic approaches vary between those informed by one or more psychotherapeutic theories to religious or quasi-religious philosophies. Programme length varies but is normally either short stay (4–8 weeks), medium stay (2–6 months), or long stay (6–18 months). Number of available places can be anything from 5 to 45. Staffing levels and types of interventions range from 24 hour support to a 1 hour-a-week individual session and no weekend staff cover. Services typically offered include individual, family and group counselling; relapse prevention; training in social skills and independent living skills; employment, training and leisure activities and other alternatives to drug using behaviour. Many also focus on offending behaviour as drug users who enter into residential care often have an extensive forensic history. Most residential rehabilitation units accept single people only and do not accommodate children. Special units which admit families, couples, or women with their children are limited. Fees can range enormously. Therapeutic communities in the USA encompass all aspects of substance misuse. They are responding to changes in funding arrangements by offering a treatment model which allows an allocation of residential stay per year (O'Brien and Devlin 1997).

Day care services

Day care services for drug users can include counselling and support services, drop-in centres, group work programmes, social skills training, relapse prevention training, leisure activities and other alternatives to drug use as well as structured day programmes up to 5 days a week. Day care is normally provided in the agency setting, although many services offer outreach and home visiting. A range of service providers including health service drug dependency units, voluntary sector drug agencies, self-help groups and social work drug agencies provide day care.

Support and counselling services

Most services offering support and counselling are 'day care' providers. Support can include offering drop-in sessions, welfare rights advice, practical help with independent living tasks, advocacy, and user involvement. Individual, couple, family and group counselling is also offered by a number of drug agencies. Ideally 'counsellors' should have relevant approved training and supervision. Counselling approaches can vary depending on the training of the counsellor, but most personal issues of significance can be addressed by most counsellors. Most often issues such as low self-esteem, loss and bereavement, sexual abuse, relationship difficulties, anxiety and depression are explored. Counselling and support services are likely to have a limited impact if practical problems are not addressed, i.e. housing, welfare benefits, evening activities, social contact, child care etc. Many drug services which offer support and counselling therefore also offer help with these practical problems and will liaise with other agencies for additional services.

Preventative and educational services

Drug prevention and drug educational services attempt to address a wide range of issues relating to drug use and include a number of service providers. Information, advice and skills development training are provided by health service teams, voluntary sector drug agencies, youth services, peer education projects, educational establishments, community education departments, social services (especially the criminal justice service) and the police. Drug education, taken in its widest sense, is incorporated into most services in contact with drug users.

Peer led services

Many successful and innovative services have been provided using a peer led approach. Preventative, educational, care and support type services are all provided by ex-drug users and current drug users in a number of settings. The use of indigenous workers to provide services to drug users has been strongly advocated (ACMD 1993) in order to maximize contact with drug users (particularly in detached and outreach services) and to increase the 'street credibility' of the information and advice giving in harm reduction services. Work with young people and 'hard-to-reach' drug using populations has often incorporated this approach.

Detached/outreach services

The fact that, historically only a limited proportion of drug users made contact with drug agencies, as well as the concern over HIV/AIDS, prompted a number of agencies to employ 'outreach' strategies to recruit clients. Outreach work usually means working with drug users in the community setting and encouraging them to attend the agency for more in-depth work. Detached work usually involves workers making contact with drug users in the community (often in their own home), with no expectation that they should attend agency premises. Most outreach and detached drug services are provided by the voluntary sector because of the informal nature of the work. Many use indigenous workers who do not necessarily have formal qualifications. Workers target places and communities where drug users can be contacted, then use 'snowballing' techniques (drug users introducing the worker to other drug users) to meet more and more drug users who are out of contact with services. Most workers offer information, advice and support through a mixture of brief or minimal interventions, facilitation, education and training, and casework. The emphasis is on taking the service to the user rather than the user taking themselves to the service.

Vocational service initiatives

Some drug services offer leisure, training, education and employment opportunities as part of a day care programme to encourage drug users to develop alternative activities to drug use. This type of service is normally provided by the voluntary sector and self-help groups. It is also incorporated into most residential rehabilitation programmes. Few health service drug dependency units offer this kind of service as part of their programme.

Complementary therapies

Many drug service providers are now encouraging and offering a range of complementary therapies as part of their care programme for drug users. Many different types of complementary therapies are now available from a wide range of disciplines. Most take a holistic view of the person and complement orthodox or conventional medicine and counselling. Many focus on the use of 'bodywork' or hands-on techniques such as aromatherapy, osteopathy, shen, therapeutic massage, acupuncture, cranial sacral therapy, Alexander technique and chiropractic treatment. Others such as homeopathy, hypnotherapy and herbalism involve no touch at all.

The benefits for drug users are their palliative and relaxing effects on the mind and body, relieving sleeplessness, anxiety and stress. A number of voluntary sector services for HIV positive people offer complementary therapies as a way of reducing the effects of stress and influencing the immune system.

Assessment

Assessment in community care is a key task and will determine whether or not the drug user will require a formal care plan and care management service. The NHS and Community Care Act (1990) states specific guidance on assessment procedures for people entitled to community care services.

The assessment process can be broken down into three distinct components:

- the initial referral
- the initial or preliminary assessment
- the comprehensive or in-depth assessment.

Assessment systems should be needs-led not service-led; they should have an initial assessment or screening process to help determine the type of assessment required; they should ensure the full participation of the user and his or her carer; they should take into account all aspects of a person's physical, psychological and social functioning; they should include the involvement of all other relevant agencies; they should be non-discriminatory; they should have a flexible response system; and the outcome should be recorded in a systematic way.

Assessment is a continuous process following entry into the system. It should be kept as simple as possible, avoiding duplication.

Initial referral and 'screening'

The demand for community care services in general is high so a process of screening is undertaken to focus services on those who need them most and to decide whose needs are complex and who require a full assessment. Many drug users will have needs that are fairly straightforward and can be readily addressed by existing services. Drug agencies undertaking assessments will receive referrals from other agencies as well as self-referrals. Basic referral forms should be used in order to gain a minimum of information at referral which includes: personal details; minimal information about drug use; basic information about medical, psychological and social factors; and reason for referral.

Initial or preliminary assessment

At the initial interview, practitioners will make a judgment as to whether or not the drug user requires a more comprehensive assessment or a formal care plan. Most Local Authorities and drug services have criteria and priority levels which they use to determine the type of response required. At this stage the drug user should be given an indication of what is involved in the assessment, the policy on confidentiality, and whether or not the participation of others is expected. During the initial assessment information should be made available to the drug user about what to do if they wish to use the complaints procedure or appeal against the decisions made at or after assessment. The initial assessment should be used to establish the level of need and the severity of the problem.

The initial assessment should cover the following areas:

- personal information
- current and previous drug use
- physical and mental health details
- criminal and legal factors
- social information (e.g. accommodation, benefits, employment)
- family circumstances
- user expectations and wishes
- other agency involvement
- the outcome of the initial contact.

The outcome of the assessment should be recorded in a systematic way and the drug user should be informed so that they clearly understand what this means for them. Carers should also be informed of the conclusions of the assessment.

Comprehensive or 'in-depth' assessment

Many drug users have complex needs and will require a more formal assessment so that a care plan can de devised.

The information required in a comprehensive assessment should include the following:

- personal details
- family and relationship details (including interviews with partners and carers)
- child care and parenting information (including child protection matters)
- social details (including housing, employment, training, leisure activities)
- significant life events (in childhood, adolescence and adulthood)
- social supports and networks (including psychosocial behaviour)
- comprehensive history of drug use and associated problems
- drug treatment history
- risk behaviour (including injecting practices and sexual practices)
- criminal history and current offending behaviour
- financial status and budgeting skills
- physical health problems and medical care
- past and present mental health problems (including current emotional maturity and coping strategies)
- self-concepts (including problem perception, self-esteem and self-efficacy)
- perceived needs and motivation to address needs
- personal resources and abilities
- resources and abilities of partners and carers
- other agency assessments
- specialist assessments
- the conclusions and suggested interventions of the assessment.

Carers' needs assessment

The drug users perception of need is the starting point in assessment but there will be circumstances where this is at odds with the carer's view, or where it is detrimental to the carer's needs. A separate assessment for the carer may be required as many carers of drug users and drug users with HIV infection have significant support needs of their own. Carers will sometimes require support, counselling, home care, respite and other forms of service provision to enable them to continue their task.

Specialist assessments

Specialist assessments may be required to investigate a particular problem, to gain more specific information about a problem and to establish underlying causes and/or possible solutions. These assessments might be clinical, for instance in the case of HIV positive drug users who are attending a specialist medical clinic, or technical, as is the case for drug users with disabilities who need housing adaptations. Independent living skills might also need to be assessed to find out what people can do for themselves and occupational therapists may undertake these particularly for drug users with a physical disability or cognitive impairment.

Assessing drug users for residential care

Under community care legislation all local authorities are responsible for assessing drug users who may require residential rehabilitation care. Funding for the placement is financed from the community care residential budget.

Service eligibility criteria for access to residential care where the local authority is responsible can vary but generally includes the following guidelines:

- The client is motivated to accept help with their drug problem and a period of treatment and/or rehabilitation is required because:
  - there is an immediate risk to self or others, and/or
  - there is an urgent need to reduce the harm associated with the drug use, and/or
  - there is a high risk to the successful and appropriate maintenance of current living circumstances

  and

- this required period of treatment and/or rehabilitation is not available from community-based services or if available is not effective because:
  - accommodation is required which provides a model of care which cannot be provided in current living circumstances, and/or

- there is a need to leave the existing social environment, and/ or
- the required intervention is only available in a residential setting, and/or
- the use of community services is unlikely to work or has failed because: the living situation is unsuitable
- the individual is unable to access community services due to a chaotic lifestyle community services are insufficient or inappropriate to meet the individual's assessed needs.

Multidisciplinary and multiagency assessments

Gathering together a number of assessments from different agencies and professionals can be very time consuming. It can also mean overcoming a number of problems. Some of the issues that arise include: duplication and overlaps in professional concern, knowledge and skill; understanding and appreciating different roles and responsibilities; recognizing particular areas of expertize; accepting differences in opinions; acknowledging the range of approaches to treatment and care; understanding differences in the language used; and policies on confidentiality and access to records. Assessors need to use considerable discretion when sharing information about drug users as much of the information gained will be 'sensitive' and possibly compromising from a purely legal standpoint.

Practitioners who are undertaking an assessment of a drug user should follow these guidelines:

- Use an checklist when undertaking an assessment
- Record your assessment in a systematic way
- Consider the possible financial implications
- Listen to the drug user, be willing to take their advice on what they need and respect their choice of lifestyle
- Keep a sense of proportion – keep the needs of the client in context
- Maintain a positive approach, be inquisitive and use your imagination
- Know about available resources and services
- Value the drug user's experience – it is probably a lot more than you have or will ever have!
- Try to be objective and recognize your own prejudices
- Realize that rather than malicious deceit, some dishonesty on the part of the client may simply reflect that they are telling you what they think you want to hear.

Care planning

Care planning involves developing a 'package of care' which will meet the clients' needs. It is a systematic approach and includes what care and treatment will be provided, as well as the desired outcome. Care plans need to be realistic and achievable. They should describe not only what input will be provided, but by whom, when, how and at what cost. They should empower the drug user not disempower them. A care plan should be a plan of action which can be monitored, measured and reviewed as necessary. Its creation will involve the client, other service providers (both informal and formal) as well as the assessor and 'care manager' if a care management service is required. The care plan should be clearly agreed by all parties in advance of its implementation. The drug user should know who is responsible for implementing, monitoring and reviewing the plan.

A model care plan

Care plan structures and formats are diverse as different assessment agencies and service providers use different practices depending on their organization.

A model care plan for a drug user would include:

- a format that allows for easy monitoring of specific aspects of the plan
- a format which breaks down the information gathered at assessment into specific objectives
  For example:
  - drug using behaviour
  - sexual behaviour
  - offending behaviour
  - alternatives to drug use
  - health care
  - employment and training
  - leisure activities
  - personal relationships
  - child care
  - social contacts
  - financial affairs
  - accommodation
  - attendance at service providers including counselling
- a format that includes a separate section for identifying the need or problem, a section which clearly states the objective or goal to be achieved, a section for the description of the intervention or service required in order to achieve the goal, and a section to identify the review date (Fig. 14.1).

Care Plan

Client/Patient's Name:

Care Manager/Key Worker's Name:

Date:

Identified need/problem	Goals to be achieved	Interventions/service provision required	Review date

Figure 14.1 Care Plan

'Aftercare' planning

Planning 'aftercare', or discharge planning as it is also known, is important since the ultimate goal of any residential or inpatient treatment programme should be successful reintegration of the client into the community. The care manager is the key person to support the client to achieve this and should develop the aftercare plan well in advance of the drug user returning to the community. Many drug users, however, leave residential care on an unplanned basis and make aftercare planning difficult. Drug users are often most at risk in the period immediately following residential care so intensive follow-up support is particularly important at this stage.

Developing a care plan

Developing a care plan involves using skills that ensure all the different parts of the care plan are linked together. Liaison is crucial in ensuring that all parties are clear about the overall plan. In particular, each party needs to be aware of their role and responsibility. If there are potential difficulties or dilemmas anticipated in the implementation of the care plan then these need to be aired in advance. Coordination and negotiating skills are essential in order to ensure the smooth progress of the care plan. Care plans should also recognize, acknowledge and record unmet need. Most drug users will have multiple problems and the resources available will realistically only go so far in meeting those needs. If the client is homeless and on the waiting list for a tenancy they may remain homeless for some time. Having no place to live or even temporary accommodation is a serious unmet need! The best made care plan in the world is difficult to follow through in these circumstances.

Implementing a care plan

Contracting and purchasing skills are often required to negotiate the right kind of service provision. Care managers in local authorities often have to go 'shopping' for the best price, particularly for 'care at home' services, supported accommodation and residential drug re-habilitation services. Individual 'service contracts' sometimes need to be devised. An informal approach is best used where openness and honesty encourage the development of a care plan which is viable. Implementing a care plan means collaborative working and being willing to act as an advocate for the drug user in order to secure appropriate services. Care should be taken to integrate formal care with informal care so that they complement each other.

Monitoring care plans

Monitoring a care plan is an ongoing process which involves regular communication with the client, carer and service providers in order to keep the progress of the care plan in check. It is important that all parties inform each other if something isn't going according to plan so that changes can be made. Continuous feedback and sometimes 'hard evidence' (e.g. attendance information) is required in order to proceed with the plan. Often the client's multiple needs are dependent and interrelated with each other. If one part of the care plan is missing or interrupted, then this will have an effect on all the other parts.

Reviewing care plans

A review date should be agreed when the care plan is first written. Care plans should then be reviewed at regular intervals. All parties involved in the care plan should be encouraged to attend the review. Verbal or written reports should be received from those who cannot attend. The review should be an opportunity to 'fine tune' the plan, to scrap any unrealistic goals, to agree new goals, as well as to evaluate the existing goals that have or have not been achieved.

Practitioners who devise care plans for drug users should follow these guidelines:

- Develop a systematic approach to developing, writing, implementing, monitoring and reviewing care plans.
- Distribute copies of the care plan to the client, the carer and all the service providers involved. Re-read the care plan regularly.
- Encourage clients to take responsibility for achieving planned objectives. Recognize clients may try to avoid this responsibility for various reasons.

Care management

Community care policy emphasizes that assessment and care management should be the 'cornerstone of good quality care'. Care management, however, is an ambiguous term applied to a number of activities and functions. There is no single, acceptable definition of care management. The Social Services Inspectorate of the Department of Health (SIS and SSI 1991) define care management as: 'any strategy for managing, coordinating and reviewing services for the individual client in a way that provides for continuity of care and accountability to both the client and the managing agency'.

Table 14.1 Care management: key tasks and process

Initial assessment →	Comprehensive assessment →	Care planning →	Service delivery →	Monitoring/review
Engagement	Detailed assessment of:	Identifying:	Coordinating the delivery of services including:	Liaison
Develop initial rapport	• drug use	• need	• health care	Evaluation
Encourage client to share needs/problems and at-risk behaviour	• physical health	• goals to be achieved	• social care	Review meetings
Use of inclusion/exclusion criteria	• mental health	• interventions required	• independent sector care	Gaps in services
Prioritize level of need	• legal	Negotiating services	• family care	Reassessment
	• financial	Costing package of care	• home care	Feedback
	• housing	Securing finance	• housing	Report writing
	• daily living skills	Advocacy	• voluntary services	Case closure
	• occupation/day time activity	Set review date		
	• relationships			
	• social network			
	• current supports			
	• history of service use			

Care management should be a continuous process which includes assessment of needs, planning care, implementing care packages, monitoring care plans and reviewing needs (Table 14.1). It is a separate process from service provision. An important feature of care management is the gathering together of relevant knowledge and skills from a variety of disciplines i.e. 'multidisciplinary' and 'multi-agency' working. Care management has brought a much higher emphasis to this as standard practice. Roles, responsibilities and accountability of all participating agencies needs to be clearly defined. Collaborative practice ensures a coherent delivery of care. Coordinating packages of care means maintaining links with other agencies, negotiating boundaries, locating gaps in service provision, accountability to the user, coordination of the work of different professionals, and cost-effectiveness in the allocation of resources. The care management model, as a process, should ensure coordinated services that facilitate a person functioning as normally as possible in the community.

Care management models exist along a continuum. Different models have different constructs ranging from the 'care manager' who is purely a purchaser of services and who has little contact with the client to the 'care manager' who, after assessing the client, is also the provider of services. Social service departments throughout the UK have implemented very different styles of care management.

Care management and drug users

The 'care management' model has been described (Bokos *et al.* 1993) as wholly appropriate for many drug users and several characteristics of drug users lend themselves to a care management approach. Drug users often require long-term treatment and a comprehensive network of support in order to remain stabilized in the community. Care management focuses on improving and coordinating service delivery to clients with chronic problems and multiple needs. The size of practitioners' caseloads and the lack of resources in most drug agencies prohibits coordination of health and social services in order to comprehensively meet clients' needs. A care management approach emphasizes the integration and coordination of these services thereby enhancing the effectiveness of care programmes to drug users. In a climate of increasingly limited resources and an increase in drug use throughout the world the effective utilization of existing services is crucial. Bokos *et al.* (1993) describe the results from an evaluation study of a care management model for intravenous drug users in Chicago which showed that through its ability to identify available services, to purchase services, and to reduce barriers to treatment and care, the care management model is highly effective in helping injecting drug users access drug treatment.

Undertaking care management tasks with drug users

Practitioners who undertake a 'care management' role when working with drug users need to fulfil a variety of functions and possess a number of skills. Managing care for a drug user is normally a challenge. Drug users have special characteristics that affect practitioners and consequently affect their ability to be effective care managers.

Drug users who come into contact with services have often been abusing drugs for many years and are part of the drug culture. In this culture drug use is an integral part of their life and they often perceive no way out, no other lifestyle. They tend to be unemployed, from a socially disadvantaged background and have low self-esteem. The person's low self-worth is often reinforced by society's stigmatization, discriminization and rejection. Frequent unsuccessful attempts at changing their lifestyle after repeated treatment episodes also leads to a sense of failure – and repeated failures breed low self-esteem. Care management with drug users needs to place a high degree of priority on relapse prevention work and aggressive interventions with service providers (i.e. housing, welfare benefits, medical and social support services) in order to ensure the most effective care and treatment is received. Drug users are often discouraged from accessing generic services because they are viewed as an undeserving and undesirable client group. The care manager must deal with these attitudes and concerns and attempt to negotiate their cooperation and participation.

Drug users also cause problems for a number of caring agencies (particularly statutory services) as they often present in crisis and are orientated towards immediate gratification. Care management is considered a long-term planning process and most services are accessed on a voluntary basis. Care management practice has been developed in response to people who require long-term care and have complex needs. The client needs to understand this. The care management process involves a series of tasks designed to stabilize, support and maintain the client living in the community. These goals take time to achieve and, in fact, may never be fully realized.

The greatest challenge for the care manager in working with drug users is in developing and maintaining a therapeutic working relationship with the client. Trust, openness, honesty, reliability and cooperation may be difficult to establish. Drug users also tend to hold little respect for practitioners and their organizations that they come into contact with. They are often openly disparaging about services that they have received or are receiving and may attempt to 'split' service providers involved in their care. In an attempt to maintain control over their situation and to maximize the benefits of their chosen lifestyle their behaviour can be manipulative and seductive. For a care manager, attempting to implement a coordinated care package, this can be a problem and will undermine the very core of care management.

Drug users sometimes lead unconventional and unstable lifestyles so it takes a unique care manager with an open mind and good counselling skills to develop and maintain a relationship with them. It is important to show a genuine interest in your client's life in all its complexity and to avoid being obviously judgemental. Don't be frightened to admit your ignorance and allow your curiosity and naiveté. Most clients can immediately recognize inexperience but will not necessarily be contemptuous of it as long as it is allied to a willingness to learn.

It is important to be familiar with community care policy and current practice and to know what the agreed procedures are for referrals, screening, assessments and care management. Having a clear understanding of the role and responsibilities of agencies in community care is essential and developing ways of utilizing these policies and practices when working with drug users. Finally the practitioner must take into account the special characteristics and behaviour of drug users when managing their care.

The management of drug users with special needs

The following section covers the particular issues that may arise in relation to care for members of particular social groups. The groups covered reflect the authors' practical experience rather than the belief that only these following groups have special needs. The wider issues of care provision for socially marginalized groups generally is covered in Chapter 15.

HIV infected drug users

Many of the people who contracted HIV infection through injection drug use had left their drug use behind before they discovered they were infected and of these most never return to it. Many, however, have current unresolved drug problems and are also HIV infected. Practitioners need to be aware that HIV infected problem drug users can provoke a range of negative and unhelpful responses, both in the practitioner themselves and in others. Fear is a common response. It may be presumed that the drug user (often a young man with a history of violence and criminality) now has 'nothing to lose' and is consequently likely to be particularly aggressive and unpredictably volatile. The belief that the drug user may be 'better off dead' can also feature and can be reinforced by the users own apparently nihilistic attitude to life.

HIV infection has still not quite been normalized into 'just another chronic illness' but real improvements in care have occurred in the past 2 years (these and specific clinical issues are described in Chapters 5, 6 and 7) and problem drug users have as much potential and right to benefit from these as any other infected individual. People will generally only use a service if they feel it has something to offer them. A common approach of many services is to exploit the fact that drug users generally will attend to pick up a substitute prescription, and to tie this attendance in as an opportunity to review their health generally and to discuss other therapeutic options in the areas of antiviral therapy and prophylaxis against opportunistic infection. It is often the case that the only 'therapy' the drug user is inclined to discuss is their substitutes. This situation is not helped by the fact that many antivirals and prophylactics have genuine and unpleasant side effects, and that some of the newer antivirals, particularly the protease inhibitors, have to be taken in fairly inflexible regimens involving dietary restrictions that many drug users find difficult to incorporate into their lifestyles. Generally the best approach is one of persistence in reminding clients what the latest position on therapeutic options is, whilst remembering that as with any therapy they should at all times be free to decline to avail themselves of it. Many problems are manageable in primary care without the need for hospital admission.

Prevention of further viral transmission is another important issue. 'Safer sex' messages may not meet with much enthusiasm. A difficulty can arise in that a practitioner who has access to privileged information may know that a sexual partner of an HIV positive drug user is at a risk of infection the person themselves is unaware of. In such a situation, some practitioners would be prepared to break confidentiality as a last resort. Generally this approach is only advisable if every other option has truly been exhausted, and in practice it is likely to make any subsequent trusting relationship with the drug user difficult. It is often more useful to present this issue in selfish rather than altruistic terms. That is to stress the infected persons need to protect themselves from reinfection or from exposure to other infections which might cause them particular problems in their immunocompromised state. Many drug users are genuinely concerned about transmitting infection to a partner, but require support and advice about ways of discussing this sensibly.

Terminal care is the other main area of potential challenge. in a young person is something that both the community practitioners find difficult to deal with. This difficulty may be compounded when the process of dying is occurring in less than ideal physical circumstances, sometimes with a lack of social support. There may be the additional problems of living with young children, people with their own unresolved drug problems or frail elderly parents. Chronic pain is commonly a feature of the terminal phases of AIDS. The principles of maintaining people in as comfortable a state as possible whilst preserving as much of their pre-morbid functioning as is feasible are no different from those in general terminal care. Practitioners can be prone to inappropriate reticence in prescribing increasing doses of a substance of abuse to a person whose main lifetime health problem was substance abuse. There may also be more legitimate concerns that in the some 'home' situations it may be difficult to be sure that psychoactive drugs prescribed are being consumed by the person they were prescribed for. As ever, flexible pragmatism is the order of the day.

Drug use and child care

Many drug users will have children. Practitioners working closely with drug users will be aware of the parenting and child care abilities of the drug user. The effects of parental drug use on the children will be evident to a greater or lesser extent. Drug use and its associated problems may or may not have consequences for the children. Help and support for the drug user to care of their children is normally offered by most practitioners in specialist drug services. Practitioners working with drug users are expected to intervene when concerns over child care become evident. This action and responsibility can be uncomfortable and difficult for the practitioner to manage. Some drug users will already be in contact with social services departments and practitioners will work collaboratively with the agency to promote the welfare of the child as well as the drug user. Drug users typically report experiencing difficulties in caring for their children when their drug use results in them either being intoxicated on a regular basis or in a state of drug withdrawals on a regular basis. Both extremes result in an unusual mental state that prohibits normal functioning. The ability adequately to supervise and care for a child in these circumstances is seriously compromised. Drug users should ensure that there is another responsible adult available to care for their children at these times. Practitioners should sensitively address child care matters with drug using parents and support them to provide the best possible care for their children.

The Children Act (1989) and the Children (Scotland) Act 1995 defines a 'child' as a person under 18 years of age and regards parental responsibilities towards children as follows:

- to safeguard and provide the child's health, development and welfare
- to provide direction and guidance
- to maintain personal relations and direct contact on regular basis
- to act as child's legal representative.

The Act defines Local Authority duty to 'children in need' as:

- to promote the welfare of children in need
- to provide services to promote upbringing by parent.

Practitioners working with drug users who have children should keep in mind the spirit of the Children's Act.

Drug users who work in the 'sex industry'

Of all sub-groups of drug users the one probably most multiply stigmatized and most challenging to work with is that of prostitute women who are also problem drug users. A prostitute is stigmatized firstly for simply being a prostitute. Often she is also a mother. She may be HIV infected, and is then likely to attract special public outrage and condemnation. Within the community of sex workers itself prostitutes with drug problems are marginalized and liable to find themselves working in the most dangerous and unhealthy situations. Internationally prostitute women were at one time the focus of fear as the group with the greatest potential to propagate HIV throughout the community generally. Whether this potential is actually realized seems to depend on many other factors. It is generally agreed now that in the UK prostitutes have not played, and are not likely to play in the future, a significant part in the dynamics of HIV transmission.

However, this has only become apparent in retrospect and consequently from the late 1980s UK prostitutes, along with their international counterparts, became the focus of a massive disease surveillance and HIV preventive effort. Of necessity this effort was channelled through the few existing contact points that there were at that time. Principally these were genitourinary medicine services, projects promoting the political legitimacy of prostitution, charitable organizations, some with a religious focus, and a few 'self-help' groups. With some exceptions these projects were generally not orientated towards drug users or their problems. Nor was the funding that they were now able to access motivated by concern to address these problems, rather projects were paid to quantify and contain a disease threat. This lead to more problems. Projects who perceived their funding to be in jeopardy generally responded by overstating this disease threat thus increasing public paranoia and the marginalization of prostitutes – particularly those with drug problems.

The relationship between illicit drugs and prostitution is long-standing, partly because the 'industries' of illicit sex and illegal drugs are often controlled and organized by the same people. The popular explanatory model that characterizes this link as a simple economic one; the prostitute only 'works' to earn money to buy drugs, but this is an oversimplification. Many economic factors (not least the need to pay expensive fines) make it hard for women to stop prostitution once they have started. However it is more the case that both prostitution and problem drug use have the same 'risk factors', most importantly childhood sexual abuse (Widom and Kuhns, 1996). A woman can enter prostitution and subsequently develop problematic use of drugs which are generally freely available. Her drug problem can escalate as she attempts to use intoxication as a coping strategy against the realities of 'business'.

Unfortunately women may find that 'prostitute projects' with their disease surveillance agenda may not be equipped to offer much help with drug problems and conversely that 'drug projects' may have little understanding of the complex issues around prostitution. Thankfully most drug services seem to now be recognizing the significance of sexual abuse and its many sequelae. Prostitutes' self-organizations seem more reluctant to embrace problem drug use as an issue for them. This is understandable as an association between prostitution and problematic behaviour is contrary to the picture of 'a job like any other' they are often trying to promote.

Work with drug using prostitutes can occur in a variety of settings and should be guided by a few basic principles. The first is that sexual health is important but not so important that it should dominate the agenda. In most recent UK-based surveys, sexually transmitted disease prevalence amongst prostitutes is lower than amongst people attending genitourinary medicine clinics and only slightly higher than estimated prevalence in the population generally (Scott *et al.* 1995). This almost certainly reflects the level of condom use amongst prostitutes. In most situations with clients condom use is the rule rather than the exception. Most disease surveillance projects have found that new sexually transmitted infections in prostitutes are more likely to originate from a partner (based on presumptive evidence) rather than a commercial client. The fact that many clients are prepared to pay extra for unprotected sex both confirms the preference of prostitutes for protection, and suggests where responsibility for any consequent STD transmission should lie.

Symptomatic infections can be treated if they arise; screening for asymptomatic chlamydial, gonococcal or HIV infection can be carried out at 6-monthly intervals using simple 'near patient' tests. Hepatitis B vaccination can be offered to the non-immune. In a UK setting it is sufficient to check syphilis serology once, unless clinically indicated (most women will have had it checked during pregnancy in any case). The importance of regular cervical cytology and reliable contraception is the same as it is with any sexually active young woman.

Substitute prescribing for drug using prostitutes is essentially no different to substitute prescribing in any other context. Practitioners must be wary of making the assumption that by giving a prostitute free drugs one will remove her need for involvement in prostitution. Certainly substitute prescribing in this context can be useful in reducing the economic pressure on a prostitute and may help her exit prostitution (if this is what she wishes). Conversely given the complexity of the situation even 'scripted' prostitutes often continue to work in prostitution. Practitioners need to be aware of this and to guard against unrealistic expectations or setting people up to fail.

Drug use and mental health problems

Two different types of serious mental health problems can arise for drug users. The first, and in some ways less serious type, is drug-induced psychosis. This is normally a temporary condition that is resolved after the cessation of the causal drug. Some drug-induced psychoses, however, are precipitated by the sudden or dramatic cessation of a drug of dependence. Drugs types which are most commonly associated with drug-induced psychosis are stimulants, hallucinogens and solvents.

The second type, which has long-term consequences for the drug user, is major psychiatric illness (typically psychoses). Clients with a 'dual diagnosis' of drug dependency and a psychiatric disorder are often difficult to manage. They will often have disturbances in affect, thoughts and behaviour. Many will show a serious deterioration in their personality over time, exacerbated by continued drug use. Their social functioning can be very poor with limited independent living skills. Health and community care authorities have a duty under the Mental Health Act to cooperate and provide care for people with mental health problems. This is often difficult to achieve with drug users who are not particularly welcomed in generic mental health services. Drug services may not want to treat people with severe mental health problems and generic mental health services may be reluctant to treat drug users.

Ideally, individual care plans for drug users with long-term mental health problems should include the following:

- assessment and review by a psychiatrist on a regular basis
- assessment and review by a social worker for social care needs
- provision of social care needs
- provision of housing
- provision of daytime activities
- provision of information and support to carers to enable them to continue to provide care.

Sometimes drug users with mental health problems will decline to cooperate with the agreed care plan and treatment regime. People who are 'informal patients' are free to do this.

Homeless drug users

Many drug users will report problems with accommodation and may end up homeless. Many homeless people will develop drug-related problems. The two appear to go hand in hand. Depending on the reason for their homelessness depends on the type of intervention required to help them address this need. Reasons might include: the effects of their drug use, disruption in the family, violence and abuse, poor independent living skills, mental health problems, not managing their finances to pay rent fees, and eviction. Drug users can also be quite a transient population, moving frequently. They may present for assessment and treatment with no fixed abode. Procedures and protocols need to ensure that individuals are not excluded because of eligibility criteria which requires a duration of residence or a permanent address. Contact with housing departments and associations is necessary. Medical statements, letters of support, financial assistance, advocacy and representation may all need to be offered.

Drug users and the criminal justice system

The use of illicit drugs, in itself, involves criminal activity and most drug users will encounter the criminal justice system at some point in their 'drug using career'. Some will have spent considerable time in prison as a result of their drug-related offending behaviour. Alternatives to custody include fines, probation and community service orders as well as bail conditions which stipulate participation in drug treatment programmes. Conditions of residence may also be the subject of criminal justice orders. Close liaison with practitioners in the criminal justice field is often normal practice for drug service workers. Joint care plans need to be sensitively devised to allow both services to work with the drug user in a constructive and collaborative way. Criminal justice practitioners are expected to work with offenders to achieve specific objectives and these are not always compatible with drug service objectives (i.e. reducing drug-related offending behaviour rather than eliminating it altogether!).

Community care for drug users internationally

Care in the community for drug users outside the UK can be usefully divided into care projects in other parts of the developed world and those throughout the less developed world.

In other parts of the developed world, community care for drug users is essentially the same, in terms of its components and motivating agendas as that in the UK. Differences exist but these are generally minor. Australia has had for some years a well organized, pragmatic harm reduction approach in which the supervised substitute prescribing of methadone to heroin users has featured prominently. Probably more therapeutic approaches to problem drug use have been developed in North America than in any other country, in part reflecting the extent and long history of drug problems in the USA. The North American approach has placed more emphasis on a role for the criminal justice system and less on harm reduction. Needle exchange schemes have been particularly difficult to establish however recent fairly unequivocal evidence of their usefulness in numerous settings looks likely to change this. Throughout Europe the approach has been more or less similar to that in the UK. In some countries, Spain and the Netherlands for example, the decriminalization of possession of softer drugs – basically cannabis – has been incorporated into the community response to drug problems. This has generally been a success in reducing cannabis use itself and reducing policing costs; it may also have reduced the likelihood of cannabis users graduating to more problematic drug use though the dynamics of this relationship are not at all clear. It has probably not reduced the prevalence of problem drug use generally. There are several reasons for this but the main ones are probably that cannabis use is not intimately linked to problem drug use and that decriminalization of one drug in several small areas is only likely to have a minimal impact on international drug trade and the problems that result from it.

In the less developed world, problem drug use is a phenomenon that arose relatively recently. Opium smoking has long been a feature of some countries in Asia and the use of mild plant-based stimulants and hallucinogens has also long been recognized in Africa and Latin America. In general though, use of these substances was not associated with a significant public health problem.

Many countries of the less developed world had found that in economic terms, drugs were the most lucrative cash crop that subsistence farmers could grow. Even given the pittance paid to tenant farmers by landlords generally, a Colombian peasant in the 1970s could make at least three times as much growing coca as growing coffee. The same was true of opium production. Initially the raw product was exported for refining in or close to the consumer countries. This had several drawbacks. Transport of the unrefined drug was less efficient, increasingly vigorous law enforcement was making home refining less feasible and from the perspective of the increasingly confident (and affluent) producer country criminals who controlled production it made more economic sense if they could offer a finished product.

As a result, from the 1970s onwards large amounts of high purity immediately usable illicit drugs were produced throughout much of the less developed world. Supply soon exceeded demand and prices consequently fell. Rather than over-saturate the market in this way, producer and transit countries expanded into new home markets. Traditionally few people in drug-producing countries actually used the drugs they produced for a number of cultural and economic reasons. This situation has changed dramatically in the past 20 years. In the setting of endemic social deprivation that exists in most of the less developed world, problem drug use has become epidemic.

The service response to this epidemic was at first slow, after all it was only one of many public health problems in the less developed world and was not generally considered to be at the 'top of the list'. Recognition of the potential threat of HIV changed this perspective as it had done throughout the developed world. In some places this change happened too late for effective prevention and the new focus on drug users simply allowed the description of an epidemic of HIV, levels of seroprevalence typically going from below 5% to over 50% in the space of a year. In some countries, Brazil for example, there also appears to be a growing generalized heterosexual epidemic. Whether this represents an initial epidemic amongst drug users that then spread outwith this community is not clear, possibly the two epidemics developed in parallel, certainly experience in Africa suggests that a significant level of injection drug use is not essential to the establishment of a general population epidemic. In Brazil, attempts to introduce harm reduction measures met with significant opposition. The impetus for them has subsequently reduced as there is some perception that they would now represent closing the stable door after the horse has bolted. Again the over-riding concern is not helping drug users but containment of the threat they are perceived to pose.

In many countries where this threat is still thought to exist (those where HIV infection is high in drug injectors but low in the population generally and those with a growing injecting 'scene' where HIV seroprevalence is either still low or not known) harm reduction initiatives have been implemented. These are generally based around syringe exchange, peer education and the provision of oral substitutes and can now be found throughout most of Asia, and much of Latin America. Initiatives are currently underway to introduce similar schemes in parts of the former Soviet Union. Within these projects, methadone still predominates as the substitute used but there have also been limited experiments using buprenorphine (in India), tincture of opium (in south east Asia) and coca preparations (in Peru, whereas in most of Latin America cocaine rather than heroin is the injectors main drug of choice) (Ball, 1996).

The service response to a growing phenomenon of problematic injection drug use in Africa will be interesting to observe. Such a situation is likely as new drug transit routes through Africa seem to be associated with the precipitation of local use as they have elsewhere. So far injecting does not seem to be the predominant method of use, but experience suggests it eventually will be. Since many parts of Africa already have an established HIV epidemic services aimed at preventing transmission from drug users may be less evident, and funding to work with drug users may be less available than in other settings. Despite this a community response motivated by concerns at growing levels of problem drug use rather than potential HIV transmission has been seen in some parts of Africa, notably Kenya (Beckerleg et al. 1996). One suspects that more of these community level mutual aid schemes exist throughout many parts of the world, but remain hidden as generally they do not involve academics and are thus unlikely to be described in the international literature.

The future

There are several possible futures for the community-based response to problem drug use. We have already noted how the service agenda of the last 10 years has been dominated by concerns about HIV transmission. This is likely to remain the case throughout most of the less developed world, though possibly will be less evident in areas where HIV is already endemic. In the developed world the agenda is likely to become less HIV orientated and more driven by concerns around protection of the community from drug-related crime (Home Office 1995). What this change in orientation will actually mean for services or for drug users is unclear (Strang et al. 1997).

Drug problems arise for a variety of reasons the most important probably being a fertile social setting. Trends in social inequality in the UK do not give any reason for belief that less rather than more problematic drug use will be a feature of the future (Wilkinson 1996). The case is often made for alternatives to the current policy of drug prohibition in terms of the benefits this could lead to for care providers, drug users and society generally (Wodak and Owen 1996). So far, policy makers internationally seem to have little enthusiasm for this approach. Interesting experiments in social policy and drugs legislation are evident in many European countries (Dorn *et al.* 1996). Unlikely changes may be less remote than expected.

One thing that is certain is that ending prohibition would not eliminate problem drug use; legalization of alcohol has not eliminated alcohol problems. However it would allow meaningful research both on the longer term consequences of the use of drugs and on the extent of 'recreational' drug use. Currently this is not possible due to the clandestine nature of drug use and the consequences of honest reporting to the individual, consequently one can only guess at possible future health and social problems and the number of people likely to experience them.

References

Advisory Council on the Misuse of Drugs 1988: *AIDS and drug misuse, Part 1.* HMSO, London.

Advisory Council on the Misuse of Drugs 1989: *AIDS and drug misuse, Part 2.* HMSO, London.

Advisory Council on the Misuse of Drugs 1993: *AIDS and drug misuse, update.* HMSO, London.

Armstrong, G. 1997: Managed care. In: Lowinson, J.H., Ruiz, P., Millman, R.B., Langrod, J.G. (eds). *Substance abuse. A comprehensive textbook*, 3rd edn. Williams & Wilkins, Baltimore.

Ball, A. 1996: Averting a global epidemic. Commentary on editorial by Stimson. *Addiction* **91**, 1095–8.

Beckerleg, S., Telfer, M., Kibwana Sizi, A. 1996: Private struggles, public support: rehabilitating heroin users in Kenya. *Drugs: Education, Prevention and Policy* **3** (2),159–69.

Bloor, M., Frischer, M., Taylor, A., Covell, R., Goldberg, B., Green, S., McKeganey, N., Platt, S. 1994: Tideline and turn? Possible reasons for the continuing low HIV prevalence among Glasgow's injecting drug users. *Sociology Review* **42**, 738–57.

Bokos, P.J., Mejta, C.L., Monks, R.L., Mickenberg, J. 1993: A case management model for intravenous drug users. In: Inciardi, J.A., Tims, F.M., Fletcher, B.W. (eds). *Innovative approaches in the treatment of drug abuse: programme models and strategies.* Greenwood Press, London.

The Children Act 1989: HMSO, London.

The Children (Scotland) Act 1995: HMSO, London.

Davies, A., Huxley, P. 1997: Survey of general practitioners' opinions on treatment of opiate users. *British Medical Journal* **314**, 1173–4.

Department of Health 1989: Caring for people: community care in the next decade and beyond. Cm 849. HMSO, London.

Des Jarlais, D.C., Friedman, S.R., Novick, D.M., Sotheran, J.L., Thomas, P., Yaucovitz, S.R., Mildvan, D., Weber, J., Creek, M.J., Malansky, R. 1989: HIV-1 infection among intravenous drug users in Manhattan, New York City, from 1977 through 1987. *Journal of the American Medical Association* **261**, (7), 1008–12.

Dole, V.P., Nyswander, M. 1965: A medical treatment for diactyl-morphine (heroin) addiction. *Journal of the American Medical Association* **193**, 80–4.

Dorn, N., Jepsen, J., Savona, E. (eds). 1996: *European drug policies and enforcement.* Macmillan, London.

Frischer, M., Leyland, A., Cormack, R., Goldberg, D., Bloor, M., Green, S. 1993: Estimating the population prevalence of injecting drug use and infection with human immunodeficiency virus among injecting drug users in Glasgow, Scotland. *American Journal of Epidemiology* **138**, 170–81.

Glanz, A. 1994: The fall and rise of the general practitioner. In: Strang J., Gossop M. (eds). *Heroin addiction and drug policy. The British system.* Oxford University Press, London.

Griffiths Sir R. 1988: *Community care: agenda for action.* A report to the Secretary of State. HMSO, London.

Hart, J.T. 1988: *A new kind of doctor.* Merlin Press, London.

Home Office 1995: *Self-Reported Drug Misuse in England and Wales: Findings from the 1992 British Crime Survey.* Home Office Research and Planning Unit Paper 89.

Horder, J. 1983: Alma Ata Declaration. General practice in 2000. *British Medical Journal* **286**, 191–4.

Illich, I. 1977: *Medical nemesis.* Calder and Boyars, London.

The Institute for the Study of Drug Dependence. 1997: *Drug use in Britain 1996.* ISDD, London.

Martin, E. 1996: Training in substance abuse is lacking for GPs (Letter). *British Medical Journal* **312**, 186.

McDermott, P. 1992: User friendly, User run. *Druglink* November/December, 11.

McKeganey, N., Abel, M., Taylor, A., Frischer, M., Goldberg, D., Green, S. 1995: The preparedness to share injecting equipment: an analysis using vignettes. *Addiction* **90**, 1253–60.

McKeown, T. 1979: *The role of medicine, dream, mirage or nemesis?* Blackwell, Oxford.

Miller, P.M., Plant, M. 1996: Drinking, smoking and illicit drug use among 15–16 year olds in the UK. *British Medical Journal* **313**, 394–7.

Newell, K.W. 1988: Selective primary health care: the counter revolution. *Social Science and Medicine* **26** (9), 891–8.

NHS 1990: *The NHS and Community Care Act 1990.* HMSO, London.

O'Brien, P., Devlin, C.J. 1997: The therapeutic community. In: Lowinson, J.H., Ruiz, P., Millman, R.B., Langrod, J.G. (eds). *Substance abuse. A comprehensive textbook.* Williams & Wilkins, Baltimore, pp. 400–405.

Pearson, G. 1987: Social deprivation, unemployment and patterns of heroin use. In: Dorn, N., South, N. (eds). *A land fit for heroin?* Macmillan, London.

Rifkin, S.B., Walt, G. 1986: Why health improves: defining the issues concerning comprehensive primary health care and selective primary health care. *Social Science and Medicine* **23** (6), 559–66.

Robertson, J.R. , Bucknall, A.B.V., Welsby, P.D., Roberts, J.J.K., Inglis, J.M., Brettle, R.P. 1986: Epidemic of AIDS related virus (HTLV-III/LAV) among intravenous drug abusers. *British Medical Journal* **292**, 527–9.

Robertson, J.R., Wyld, R., Elton, R., Brettle, R.P. 1998: Heterosexual transmission of human immunodeficiency virus in men and women in a Scottish cohort. *AIDS* (in press).

Scott, G.R., Peacock W, Cameron S. 1995. Outreach STD clinics for prostitutes in Edinburgh. *International Journal of STD and AIDS* **6** (3), 197–200.

Shishodia, P., Robertson, J.R. Milne, A. 1998: Deaths in a cohort of drug injectors in an Edinburgh general practice 1981–1997. *Health Bulletin. Scottish Office* **56** (2), 553–6.

SIS and SSI 1991: *Assessment and community care.* Department of Health, London.

Stimson, G.V. 1996: Has the United Kingdom averted an epidemic of HIV-1 infection among drug injectors? (editorial plus commentaries). *Addiction* **91**, 1085–99.

SSI and SWSG 1991: *Care management and assessment: manager's guide.* HMSO, London.

Strang, J., Clee, W.B., Gruer, L. , Raistrick, D. 1997: Why Britain's drug czar mustn't wage war on drugs. *British Medical Journal* **315**, 325–6.

Ward, J., Mattick R., Hall, W. 1992: *Methadone maintenance treatment.* University Press, Sydney, NSW.

Widom, C.S., Kuhns, J.B. 1996 Childhood victimization and subsequent risk for promiscuity, prostitution and teenage pregnancy, a prospective study. *American Journal of Public Health* **86** (11), 1607–12.

Wilkinson, R. 1996: *Unhealthy societies: the afflictions of inequality.* Routledge, London.

Wodak, A., Owen, R. 1996: *Drug prohibition, a call for change.* NSW University Press, Sydney.

Wolfensberger, R. 1972: *The principle of normalization in human services.* NIMR, Toronto.

Zinberg, N. 1984: *Drug, set and setting, the basis for controlled intoxicant use.* Yale University Press, New Haven.

15 Marginalized groups

Richard Starmans

Introduction

Individuals or groups of individuals may be marginalized from what is otherwise mainstream society for a variety of reasons. They may be differentiated by virtue of one characteristic, i.e. being female or being of a different ethnic origin, but otherwise be part of the culture they inhabit by virtue of being employed, enjoying social status or conforming to social norms. They may suffer from stigmatization due to a disapproval of behaviour such as drug use, prostitution or alcohol abuse. When these characteristics are multiplied in the same individual he or she is likely to suffer increasing marginalization, if not rejection, by society.

Such isolation can be counteracted by being in a supportive group or organization, the enlargement of which may become an organized subculture with a status of its own. Association may be lifelong and unchangeable, or may be for a period in the life of the individual. At any point in time conflicting needs may encourage conformity to the subculture or generate the initiative to move out of it into another stream of society. Multiple problems will make movement less likely and more difficult. A situation has arisen in US society as well as others in which individuals are socialized into a cycle of deviant behaviour. This helps to perpetuate hopelessness and maintains the disenfranchisement of poor people and their communities within the larger society (Johnson and Muffler 1997).

Drug use comes in many shapes and forms. Infrequent, recreational cannabis use in college students may be necessary to be part of the majority as is more dependent drug-taking in areas of social and economic deprivation. Drug use in these circumstances may be sustained or encouraged by a requirement to be in the majority. For drug users, friends appear to be a more important source of social support than relatives (Stowe *et al.* 1993). Treatment or management of drug use has to consider this carefully when one is attempting to change behaviour. Movement away from drug use may only be possible when the peer group normal behaviour changes, as students move into employment or drug users grow older, have families or achieve employment.

For many drug users, however, drugs remain a part of the culture within which they exist and other characteristics or membership of other minority groups continue to encourage or support drug use. There is a clear link between unemployment and drug use (Peck and Plant 1987).

This chapter is about the provision and design of services for drug users who have additional reasons for being in minority groups. It overlaps with previous chapters about care in the community and has reverberations with chapters on AIDS care and descriptions of other services for drug users. Despite being the last chapter in the book, an understanding of issues in it are essential to those involved with the management of drug users. Without sympathy for the traps inherent in being poor, being deprived or being outside mainstream society, working with drug users is likely to be difficult. This may be why health and social care workers find this area of their jobs problematic. Equally important, the provision of adequate and effective services at a local or national level depends upon an understanding of how societies and minorities within societies sustain themselves. Drug users are in general a censored group although many successful and apparently healthy individuals use some kind of drugs. There are reasons why some individuals use drugs and minimize the damaging effects whilst others do not. This chapter will examine problems causing drug users to be on the edge of society. These problems are to do with the place of drugs in the approval of the public and politicians, but also the problems which bring individuals into contact with drugs and sustain the dependency upon drugs. It will also consider why some drug users live in double or multiple jeopardy, having one or several additional stigmata or problems to contend with.

Within any group of drug users some can be considered as (extra) marginalized. These include:

- homeless people
- the unemployed

- those under 25 who are neither students nor living with their parents
- those in ethnic minority groups
- people without legal residence status (e.g. illegal immigrants)
- those in sexual minorities
- people in temporary housing (a hotel, a homeless shelter, friends)
- those working in the sex industry

These characteristics are not mutually exclusive. The general characteristics are that the needs of these people are not usually addressed by the existing healthcare organization (Bleach and Ryan 1995). Even in countries in which there is an ample supply of care for drug users in general, the accessibility remains poor. AIDS care and care focusing on drug use should be coordinated and integrated (Woerkom and Tiemeijer 1997). Language barriers may frustrate the advice and treatment (Hoeksema 1997). Continuous training of medical personal for the specific problems is essential (Bury *et al.* 1997, Junod *et al.* 1997).

Young people living in the streets have been identified as being very vulnerable to HIV in both developing and developed countries because of being beyond the reach of social and health services (Aggleton 1997). American research showed that 'trading sex' for drugs is closely related to poverty and homelessness (Elwood *et al.* 1997).

The marginalization of sex workers has been deliberate, but efforts to eradicate their industry have failed. Sex industry workers operate outside regulations and are the subject of much stigmatization. Society regarding itself as respectable, decent and normal excludes sex workers. They are associated with the spread of sexually transmitted diseases and AIDS and are considered to be incapable of raising children. Criminal acts of physical violence by police on sex workers are often considered to be expected. Trying to escape from this often leads to adopting a double lifestyle and hiding their profession. Attending social and healthcare agencies may be frustrated by the fear of repercussions (Thomas 1992).

Politicians seem to show no interest in these groups (De Clercq 1997). In North American inner cities, it appeared that people marginalized by low economic status die more frequently in hospital than at home and report unrelieved pain more frequently during the last week of their stay at home (Dancault *et al.* 1997). They are often unaware of their rights or are in the process of claiming them, because of their lack of education or the complexity of the social security bureaucracy.

Additional to the problems related to drug use and obtaining them, day-to-day life is determined by meeting other basic needs like housing, food and finance. Setting realistic targets is essential in caring for drug users and, for the subgroups described in this chapter, limited goal-setting is important. Many drug users live in unfortunate and stressful circumstances and their needs have to be carefully prioritized. For those with HIV infection, immediate needs may not include addressing their drug problem. Essential issues such as treatment of infection such as tuberculosis may prevail over longer term issues.

Existing mental health problems often complicate the stay in shelters and drop-in centres and require specific skills (Cote *et al.* 1997). Active coping strategies in HIV positive drug users seem to be inversely related to depressive symptoms, and avoidance coping seems to be directly associated to greater mood disturbances (Guidetti *et al.* 1997). It is unclear whether HIV infection has specific mental health consequences for drug users. In a review of this area, rather contrasting differences were found in studies comparing seropositive and seronegative drug users, although psychological adjustment in general to HIV infection seems to be poorer (Catalan 1995).

Drug users from marginalized groups have hardly been investigated. Research in this field designed to look at their specific problems, the way specific needs can be met and the efficiency of existing services and new initiatives in meeting these needs seems rather difficult, if not impossible, because of the nature of the people involved. In this chapter we can only present a descriptive approach of some initiatives which attempt to address the needs of this group of people and to provide an overview of efforts to address the healthcare needs of these marginalized groups. Most of these were presented at the Third International Conference on Home and Community Care for Persons living with HIV/AIDS which was held in Amsterdam in May 1997. It offers a wide spectrum of initiatives which show how people are trying to address the needs of these particular groups that fall outside the usual scope of our healthcare systems.

Some models of care in the community

Specialized – general

Healthcare for drug users may be delivered within general core services or as a separate specific service. Both approaches have strong and weak aspects. General services are, usually, easily accessible. The most obvious example is provided by general practice in those countries where these and associated primary care workers provide basic and generalized services in the community. They provide the broad spectrum of healthcare not only related to drug use. Additional care can be organized within the system. Examples in the UK of how a wide range of services for drug users can be provided in the community are reported from several centres where general practice has been the main service involved but is supported and enhanced by specialist nurses and psychiatrists (Greenwood 1990, 1992, Beamont 1997).

Drug users, however, often find it difficult to fit into the structured way in which services are organized and are often not able to show up at appointments with General Practitioners and at hospitals. This creates the need for additional support and resources in those agencies offering help for drug users and particularly for those with multiple problems. Individuals from marginalized groups may have a passive indifference to their health care needs and require encouragement and support (Chauvin *et al.* 1997).

In parallel to this, interest and motivation of the staff of the general services to address the needs of this particular group is lacking. The latter may be based on prejudices, unrealistic targets, lack of knowledge and capabilities, poor organization and excessive workload. Specialized services may be more capable of an active and outreaching approach. The staff in such services have usually been given special training and have been recruited because of an interest in working in the field. The relative advantages and disadvantages of generalist and specialist models of care have been discussed in detail in Chapter 13 and referred to in several others.

Outreach services for drug users

Since the emergence of HIV and AIDS among drug using communities in the USA, Europe and Australia the need for extended services has been recognized (Jose *et al.* 1996). Various models of outreach and extended provision of treatments include the Amsterdam bus providing specific drug therapies and needle and syringe exchange (Buning 1992), the street education and intervention in San Francisco (Watters *et al.* 1990) and the peer-based drug using education in parts of New York, Australia and elsewhere (Friedman *et al.* 1987, Crofts and Herkt 1995).

Drug user involvement in the services

Although involvement of current or ex-drug users has often been mentioned as a target in healthcare including mental healthcare, for marginalized groups the implementation of this policy-target seems extremely difficult. The 'classical' way of a more or less structured representative group like users- or patient-organizations is lacking and initiatives to get feedback on the services provided should be made by the services themselves. In the Netherlands drug users were interviewed to get feedback on the services provided (Woerkom and Tiemeijer 1997).

Examples of health services targeting people from marginalized groups

The examples presented here are selected to demonstrate several approaches to the delivering of care to difficult to reach groups. Most are only described as there are no details on their effectiveness and the initiatives are grouped around some themes.

General awareness

In Vancouver a graffiti project aims at reaching a community strongly affected by AIDS, poverty, drug use and mental health issues. Through discussions with young graffiti artists, a large outdoor highly visible mural was produced in a high-risk area. This promotes HIV education and awareness to the community (Prussick and Moth 1997).

In Kampala, Uganda marginalized groups especially women and young people are made aware of AIDS through drama derived from people's daily experience (Tibamanya and Nuwagaba 1997).

Outreaching/remodelling existing primary health care

In Thailand a project was directed from suburban health centres in slums. It attempts to integrate the care of persons living with HIV and AIDS into the work of community workers. Based on interviews with key persons in the community, community workers and healthcare personnel, training of the healthcare staff was set up to provide them with more specific medical knowledge. This included the treatment of tuberculosis, assistance in counselling for patients living with HIV and AIDS and collaboration with community groups. Difficulties encountered were due to lack of resources to do home calls in the slums and ineffective organization (Metzger *et al*. 1991).

In Lusaka, Zambia, regular home visits to patients living with HIV and AIDS with their family tried to meet spiritual, psychological, material and drug support depending on the patient's condition (Mwondela 1997).

For the treatment of tuberculosis, a system of 'directly observed treatment' (DOT) has been developed in Barcelona, Spain. The DOT team provides patients living with HIV and AIDS from marginalized groups with treatment for tuberculosis whether they are at home, in a shelter or hotel or even in the street. They move around by public transport and on motorbikes. The project aims at high rates of adherence to the anti-tuberculosis treatment reducing the number of contagious people out in the streets reducing hospital admissions and readmissions, and preventing the spread of multidrug-resistant strains (Pascual 1997).

A young person-led service attached to general practices can provide confidential, non-judgmental HIV prevention and sexual health service among young people who would not otherwise feel that they have access to help and support. These young people's drop-in centres attached to GP practices seem to have become successful in rural England (MacKenzie 1997).

New services

In Bologna, Italy, a residential house for homeless people with AIDS offers medical care and leisure activities. During their stay individuals may benefit from support and knowledge from other patients living with HIV and AIDS who may be benefiting from newer antiviral drugs. Other empowerment strategies such as counselling to increase self-esteem, self-care and seeking support coping styles helps these homeless people in regaining a social network for support and strengthening them emotionally and cognitively (Pictrantoni and Malaguti 1997).

Drop-in centres

Drop-in centres can often meet the need of persons with drug problems and/or HIV/AIDS for support and a safe social environment. This is especially useful for people who are poor. Such centres may offer complementary therapies, referral to community resources, food and nutritional advice, peer counselling, and educational and social activities and unstructured time to meet with other patients living with HIV and AIDS.

In Ottawa, Canada, a manual for setting up such centres and addressing the diversity of patients living with HIV and AIDS including drug use and mental illness has been published. They advocate active roles for patients living with HIV and AIDS in the planning and in decision making in the centre (Young 1997).

Refugees, asylum seekers migrants and ethnic minorities can be considered to marginalized as well (even without having a drug-problem). In Norway these people are targeted when they attend language (Norwegian) schools by providing them information on sexually transmitted diseases, HIV and AIDS (Omar Saho 1997).

In Glasgow, a new service for female prostitutes was set up to address their needs. It appeared in the setting up process that none of the women wanted a service designed to 'save them from prostitution'. A drop-in centre was developed which offered coffee, food and a chat, direct access to condoms and social support. The social support identified several areas where problems were prevalent. These included fines, court, welfare rights, housing, violent partners, child care, medical care and the need for a refuge when attacked. Hundreds of female prostitutes started to use the service the majority of whom were also drug users. There were strict rules like 'no drug use on the premises', but these were difficult to enforce. The non-drug users seemed to have less tolerance of the drug users and consequently started to use less of the services on offer. From discussions with the women it was then decided to split up the premises, creating space for both groups. Drug users were segregated in that, although they were offered shelter, they were unable to participate in other activities because of their drug use. Apparently, within the sex industry, drug users were further marginalized (MacIver 1992).

In Sri Lanka, workshops have been organized in order to disseminate information and guidelines. This has been specifically targeted at migrant workers and those returning to the locality (Ganasinghe 1997).

In other chapters, various other ways of approaching the problems of drug users who have special problems are discussed. As in the examples above, these strategies often depend upon the individual circumstances in the locality and the presence or absence of other infrastructural health and social services.

Strategies and policies to help marginalized groups

In recent decades it has been recognized that some individuals or groups of individuals require special attention or protection, (Ovretveit 1993). This has resulted in national and international legislation to protect, for example, the rights of women and ethnic minorities. Drug policy has consistently failed to adopt such sensitive concerns for groups within its remit and has considered drug users as a homogeneous group and has often taken a punitive and controlling approach to control rather than trying to separate components of the problem. Policy by committee or, worse still, policy by default has characterized the UK experience (Strang and Gossop 1994) and those who recognize drug use as a symptom of other problems are unfortunately in a minority (Heather *et al.* 1993).

Without stated aims to address all the requirements of those using illegal substances, it is unlikely that significant improvement can be made. A comprehensive assessment of drug users case by case has been identified in several chapters of this book as an essential prerequisite to effective treatment. A mandate and resources to deal with the complicated minority issues often identified in drug users, or brought to light by their own drug use, is an essential part of an effective service. Such a comprehensive approach to drug services is likely to bring serious long-term benefits to the individual, but also to prove cost-effective in preventing or diverting longer term problems.

Conclusions

Marginalized groups are by definition difficult to reach. This requires workers to cross the boundaries of the usual way of working. The examples provided here give exceptional indicators of ways of approaching particularly marginalized groups. These in summary are:

- promoting health education with graffiti and drama
- using key persons in the community to train the health care personnel addressing the specific needs in the community
- regular home visits (including moving around on motorbikes) to ensure medical treatment and other support
- attaching youngsters to existing services to facilitate same age people to be recognized
- activities with a low threshold, firstly to offer a safe place, but also aiming at regaining a social network and meeting peers including knowledge on (new) therapies.

From observing this wide range of examples of approaching marginalized groups it can be concluded that that there is no universal best way to target such individuals. The aims of these innovative activities presented show a wide but consistently limited scope. Each one sets out to achieve a limited range of objectives and highlights the specific difficulties which need to be addressed in the locality. None are expected to provide comprehensive care but often respond to an emergency situation in some cases with a sense of desperation.

Economic marginalization threatens to become the dominant determinant of problems for those individuals living in poorer areas of growing urban centres. Unemployment contributes heavily to the difficulties of those with poor health, mental illness, incomplete education, criminal records and other problems. Several members of families who have used drugs through several generations and waves of varying drug types have left a sector of the population in inner cities in a position of hopelessness. Improvements documented in the USA in terms of reduction in drug use have largely been outside those inner city populations (Johnston *et al.* 1995).

In the general consideration and assessment of the needs of individuals with a drug problem, the problems outlined in this chapter are essential. The management of the drug problem is often dependent on such inhibitory factors. All patients, however, have individual situations which may prevent resolution of their problems. The special situations of elderly drug users, health professionals with drug problems and the children of drug-dependent individuals are beyond the scope of this chapter, but are recognized in other sections of this book.

Although attitudes to drugs are constantly changing it is likely for the foreseeable future that as well as being an independent problem for many sectors of society, it will increasingly be a burden for the already disadvantaged. This is true for developed Western nations and for the developing world.

References

Aggleton, P. 1995: Young people and AIDS. *AIDS Care* **7**, 77–80.

Beamont, B. (ed.) 1997: *Care of drug users in general practice, a harm-minimization approach.* Radcliffe Medical Press, Abingdon.

Bleach, A., Ryan, P. 1995: *Community support or mental health.* Pavilion Publishing, Brighton.

Book of Abstracts 1997: Third International Conference on Home and Community Care for Persons Living with HIV/AIDS, Amsterdam, May 1997. Open University Press, Buckingham.

Buning, E.C., van Brussel, G., van Santen, G. 1992: The impact of harm reduction drug policy on AIDS prevention in Amsterdam. In: O'Hare, P.A., Newcombe, R., Matthews, A., Buning, E.C., Drucker, E. (eds). *The reduction of drug related harm.* Routledge, London.

Bury, J., Simmonte, M., Jaquet, C. 1997: *Training primary care staff about HIV prevention.* Presentation number 63. Third International Conference on Home and Community Care for Persons Living with HIV/AIDS, Amsterdam.

Catalan, J., Burgess, A., Kilmes, I. 1995: *Psychological medicine of HIV infection.* Oxford University Press, Oxford.

Chauvin, P., Mortier, E., Carrat, F., Imbert, J.C., Valleron, A.J., Lebas, J. 1997: A new outpatient care facility for HIV-infected destitute populations in Paris, France. *AIDS Care* **9** (4), 451–9.

Cote, P., Rochette, P., Junod, P. 1997: *IDU HIV-positive homeless with a mental health problem: a challenge for street workers in Montreal.* Presentation number 46. Third International Conference on Home and Community Care for Persons Living with HIV/AIDS, Amsterdam.

Crofts, N., Herkt, D. 1995: A history of peer-based drug user groups in Australia. *Journal of Drug Issues* **25**, 599–616.

Dancault, S., Fortin, J. 1997: *Services to highly disadvantaged persons living with for homeless people with AIDS*. Presentation number 13. Third International Conference on Home and Community Care for Persons Living with HIV/AIDS, Amsterdam.

De Clercq, K. 1997: *Migrants living with HIV/AIDS, a non-existing or not-seen problem?* Abstract number 34. Third International Conference on Home and Community Care for Persons Living with HIV/AIDS, Amsterdam.

Elwood, W.N., Williams, M.L., Bell, D.C., Richard, A.J. 1997: Powerlessness and HIV prevention among people who trade sex for drugs ('strawberries'). *AIDS Care* **9**, 273–84.

Friedman, S.R., Des Jarlais, D.C., Southeran, J.L., Garber, J., Cohen, H., Smith, D. 1987: AIDS and self-organization among intravenous drug users. *International Journal of the Addictions* **22**, 201–20.

Ganasinghe, M.R. 1997: *Aids prevention and care for migrant workers*. Presentation number 36. Third International Conference on Home and Community Care for Persons Living with HIV/AIDS, Amsterdam.

Greenwood, J. 1990: Creating a new drug service in Edinburgh. *British Medical Journal* **300**, 587–9.

Greenwood, J. 1992: Services for problem drug users in Scotland. In: Plant, P., Ritson, B., Robertson, R. (eds). *Alcohol and drugs: the Scottish experience*. Edinburgh University Press.

Guidetti, F., Starace, F., Gargiulo, M., Venuto, O., Sangiovanni, V., Chirianni, A. 1997: *Relationship of coping strategies to affective state in HIV seropositive injecting drug users*. Presentation number 5. Third International Conference on Home and Community Care for Persons Living with HIV/AIDS, Amsterdam.

Heather, N., Wodak, A., Nadelmann, E.A., O'Hare, P. (eds). 1993: *Psychoactive drugs and harm reduction: from faith to science*. Whurr Publishers, London.

Hoeksema, K. 1997: *'Do I want to speak your language?'* Presentation 067. Third International Conference on Home and Community Care for Persons Living with HIV/AIDS, Amsterdam.

Johnson, B.D., Muffler, J. 1997: Determinants and perpetuations of substance abuse, sociocultural. In: Lowinson, J.H., Ruiz, P., Millman, R.B., Langrod, J.G. (eds). *Substance abuse. A comprehensive textbook*, 3rd edn. Williams & Wilkins, Baltimore, MD.

Johnston, L.D., O'Mally, P.M., Backman, J.G. 1995: *National survey results on drug use from the Monitoring the Future Study. Volume II. Secondary school students*. NIDA, Rockville, MD.

Jose, B., Friedman, S.R., Neaigus, A. *et al.* 1996: Collective organisation of injecting drug users and the struggle against AIDS. In: Rhodes, T., Hartnoll, R. (eds). *AIDS, drugs and prevention*. Routledge, London.

Junod, P., Rochette, P., Cots, P. 1997: Continuous medical education in a multidisciplinary team. Presentation number 65. Third International Conference on Home and Community Care for Persons Living with HIV/AIDS, Amsterdam.

MacKenzie, P.A. 1997: Primary care and youth services working together to provide young focused prevention. The Shropshire Health for Youth project presentation. Presentation number 278. Third International Conference on Home and Community Care for Persons Living with HIV/AIDS, Amsterdam.

MacIver, N. 1992: Developing a service for prostitutes in Glasgow. In: Bury, J., Morrison, V., McLachlan, S. (eds). *Working with women and AIDS*. Tavistock-Routledge, London.

Metzger, P., Vaddhanaphuti, C., Duangdeelawerate, A., Soontorn-prakornkit, R., Wongsa, B. 1997: *The potential for integration of community based care for people with AIDS into the primary health care activities of suburban health centres and slum communities. Amphur Muang, Chiang Mai, Thailand.* Presentation number 217. Third International Conference on Home and Community Care for Persons Living with HIV/AIDS, Amsterdam.

Mwondela, D.P. 1997: *Results from newly established home care activity.* Presentation page 223. Third International Conference on Home and Community Care for Persons Living with HIV/AIDS, Amsterdam.

Omar Saho, S. 1997: *Sex, prevention, STDs and AIDS preventive work among refugees, asylum seekers, migrants and ethnic minorities to affective state in HIV-seropositive IDUs.* Presentation number 35. Third International Conference on Home and Community Care for Persons Living with HIV/AIDS, Amsterdam.

Ovretveit, J. 1993: *Co-ordinating community care, multidisciplinary teams and care management.* Open University Press, Buckingham.

Pascual, J. 1997: *Directly observed treatment (DOT) at home for tuberculosis patients with 190 AIDS in Catalonia (Spain).* Presentation 017. Third International Conference on Home and Community Care for Persons Living with HIV/AIDS, Amsterdam.

Peck, D.F., Plant, M.A. 1987: Unemployment and illegal drug use. In: Heller, T., Gott, M., Jeffrey, C. (eds). *Drug use and misuse, a reader.* J. Wiley, Chichester.

Pictrantoni, L., Malaguti, E. 1997: *Psychosocial needs and new hopes in a community house for homeless people with AIDS.* Presentation number 237. Third International Conference on Home and Community Care for Persons Living with HIV/AIDS, Amsterdam.

Prussick, A., Moth, T. 1997: *The HIV/AIDS graffiti project.* Presentation page 239. Third International Conference on Home and Community Care for Persons Living with HIV/AIDS, Amsterdam.

Stowe, A., Ross, M.W., Wodak, A., Thomas, G.V., Larson, S.A. 1993: Significant relationships and social supports of injecting drug users and their implications for HIV/AIDS services. *AIDS Care* **5**, 23–33.

Strang, J., Gossop, M. 1994: The British system: visionary anticipation or masterly inactivity? In: Strang, J., Gossop, M. (eds). *Heroin addiction and drug policy. The British system*. Oxford University Press, pp. 342–51.

Thomas, R.M. 1992: HIV and the sex industry. In: Bury, J., Morrison, V., McLachlan, S. (eds). *Working with women and AIDS*. Tavistock-Routledge, London.

Tibamanya, O.H., Nuwagaba, D. *Fighting HIV/AIDS through music, dance and drama*. Presentation page 251. Third International Conference on Home and Community Care for Persons Living with HIV/AIDS, Amsterdam.

Watters, J.D., Downing, M., Case., P., Lorvick, J., Cheng, Y.T., Fergusson, B. 1990: AIDS prevention for intravenous drug users in the community. Street health education and risk behaviour. *American Journal of Community Psychology* **18**, 587–96.

Woerkom, J.R.M., van Tiemeijer, J. 1997: *AIDS care for drug users, from the test onwards*. Presentation page 293. Third International Conference on Home and Community Care for Persons Living with HIV/AIDS, Amsterdam.

Young, J.C. 1997: *Making space for PLWHIV/AIDS, issues related to setting up a drop-in*. Presentation page 261. Third International Conference on Home and Community Care for Persons living with HIV/AIDS, Amsterdam.

Index

Page numbers in **bold** type refer to figures; *italic* type refers to tables